MSU Program In Public Health
517.353.4883

The Practice of International Health

The Practice of International Health

A Case-Based Orientation

Edited by

Daniel Perlman, Ph.D.

Associate Director
Maternal Mortality Reduction Initiative
Bixby Program in Population and Maternal Health
School of Public Health
University of California, Berkeley

Ananya Roy, Ph.D.

Associate Professor
Department of City and Regional Planning
University of California, Berkeley

OXFORD
UNIVERSITY PRESS

2009

OXFORD
UNIVERSITY PRESS

Oxford University Press, Inc., publishes works that further
Oxford University's objective of excellence
in research, scholarship, and education.

Oxford   New York
Auckland   Cape Town   Dar es Salaam   Hong Kong   Karachi
Kuala Lumpur   Madrid   Melbourne   Mexico City   Nairobi
New Delhi   Shanghai   Taipei   Toronto

With offices in
Argentina   Austria   Brazil   Chile   Czech Republic   France   Greece
Guatemala   Hungary   Italy   Japan   Poland   Portugal   Singapore
South Korea   Switzerland   Thailand   Turkey   Ukraine   Vietnam

Published by Oxford University Press, Inc.
198 Madison Avenue, New York, New York 10016
www.oup.com

Oxford is a registered trademark of Oxford University Press

Library of Congress Cataloging-in-Publication Data
The practice of international health : a case-based orientation / edited
by Daniel Perlman, Ananya Roy.
p. ; cm.
ISBN 978-0-19-531027-6
1. World health—Case studies.
2. Public health—Case studies.
I. Perlman, Daniel, 1950–
II. Roy, Ananya.
[DNLM: 1. World health—Personal Narratives. 2. International
Cooperation—Personal Narratives. 3. Public Health Practice—Personal
Narratives. WA 530.1 P895 2008]
RA441.P73 2008
362.1—dc22
2007037556

Printed in the United States of America
on acid-free paper

CONTENTS

FOREWORD

It has been observed that public health is less a discipline than a collection of problems. While global health, as now emerging, may constitute an improvement over what was once widely termed "international health," it nonetheless remains a worldwide collection of problems. Although universities across the world now tout programs in global health, there is to date no agreed-upon definition of the boundaries of topics meaningfully examined under this rubric, and still less accord regarding the metrics and methodologies best suited to explore the problems and analytical challenges that this emerging field poses. Very few have mentioned, much less explored, the ethical challenges that will face affluent research universities seeking a toehold in the poorest reaches of the world, most of them former colonies.

Contributors to *The Practice of International Health* acknowledge both the importance of understanding the problems routinely classified under this rubric as well as the limitations of international health as a framework. What Daniel Perlman and Ananya Roy term "place-based research" answers what was, for them and for many of us, a pedagogic imperative: as teachers of public health, Perlman and Roy found that the materials used in the classroom were too theoretical and dry—too "experience-distant"—to prove compelling to students who had experienced neither the developments described nor the far-away places being discussed. This volume is the fruit of a five-year-long collaboration between the editors and a group of case writers with deep expertise in the field. Chapter authors respond to these challenges in the form of case studies anchored in a particular time and place but which remain very much alive to history and social context in general. The book stands as an antidote to a pedagogic challenge encountered in almost every school of public health in the world.

The twelve chapters are grounded in nine geographically distinct settings (not counting the culturally and historically specific considerations of global meetings such as "Beijing + 5" or multi-site efforts such as polio eradication) and collectively offer a history of international health that situates place-based studies in broad context, while conveying the vividness of experiences told through first-person accounts. Even the more technical subjects never lose the sense that the questions and problems raised by these situations remain profoundly relevant to current debates. Ciro de Quadros' account of his involvement in both smallpox and polio eradication efforts, for example, directly addresses the question of whether "vertical" disease-control programs are more effective than "horizontal" or integrated primary health-care programs; yet his experiences simultaneously and importantly speak to the current and often acrimonious "either-or" debates about the AIDS prevention-and-care programs that have been funded for the first time over the past five years in poor countries.

The editors are to be congratulated for their efforts to embed these case studies in a scholarly, but eminently readable, "connective tissue." The metaphor is mixed, but how else to describe their foreshadowing of accounts such as Ciro de Quadros' in a broad and critical history of development ideologies? By comparing the differing fates of contemporaneous efforts to eradicate smallpox and malaria, Perlman and Roy cast light on various models of development that have emerged since the 1944 Bretton Woods meetings and culminated in the rise, apparent by the early 1990s, of the World Bank as the preeminent and most well-funded international health agency. How a bank might become a health agency is a question worth asking if we hope to understand international public health today—particularly since some would argue that ideologies regarding cost-effectiveness continue to determine which programs and efforts are likely to be funded and which are not, while others would interrogate the peculiar "conditionalities" attached to banks' largesse.

The narratives in this book range from memoir to ethnography to report. They weave together different voices that engage the reader's imagination. The cases are diverse, and include Julie Cliff's beautifully written exploration of *konzo*, an epidemic of spastic paralysis in Mozambique caused, as she and her co-workers in Mozambique discovered, by cyanide poisoning from inadequately prepared cassava; Jane Galvão's elegiac tribute to a friend and colleague well known in Brazil for his efforts to address an AIDS epidemic that only three decades ago threatened to take the lives of more than three million in that country but did not; Sandy Lane's compelling effort to bring lessons from international health back to the urban United States; Gopi Gopalakrishnan's description of how Janani, a non-profit Indian society, ingeniously used what were termed "free-market" mechanisms to improve access to family planning and abortion in Bihar, India; and Alejandro Ceren and Meredith Fort's account of the process by which *Instancia Nacional de Salud*, a coalition of community-based organizations, responded to the Guatemalan government's top-down health care reform by creating an alternative program that integrated Mayan medicine into a comprehensive primary health-care structure.

Historically important projects such as Gonoshasthaya Kendra and other poverty-alleviation efforts permeate the case-studies, as do accounts that address the geopolitics of gender inequality. Indeed, the essays in this volume by Assefaw Tekeste Ghebrekidan, who writes from the Eritrean Sahel, and Suneeta Krishnan, who focuses on rural southern India, are eloquent additions that share lessons not only about the specifics of important projects but also about humility, partnership, and the sometimes difficult clashes between health-care workers' personal beliefs and their patients' cultural practices (very often concerning women's rights and women's health).

Many of the topics addressed in this book reflect four recurring themes that Perlman and Roy signal as "key contributions" that are more like recurrent themes in the musical sense (as being written into the score). These are: moving beyond the medicalization of health; considering the geopolitics of health; adopting a case-based approach; and taking a hard look at the ethics of practice. It is, however, equally important to recognize the existing gaps in public health literature that these cases fill. One of my favorite chapters, by Benjamin Mbakwem and Daniel Smith, is an intentionally humble account of corruption in Nigeria. Their dialogue constitutes a veritable sociology of International Health, Inc. (not their term) and starkly juxtaposes the nearly invisible corruption of the entire endeavor—the lavish lives and salaries of the expatriate experts, the consulting fees, the air-conditioned vehicles, the vast disparities in salaries—with the visible corruption of locals (viz., a Nigerian woman working for USAID who gets her son a job because his last name is different). The latter sort of corruption is the subject of endless discussion among the expatriates, they note, while the former sort is largely ignored. Quite similarly, Aruna Uprety's heartfelt narrative recounts the specific strategies and tactics that she and her colleagues employed during their eighteen-year struggle for the right to safe abortion in Nepal. None of these tactics and none of this story, which reduced mortality among young women dramatically, can be found in standard medical or public health textbooks. Mbakwem and Smith aver that they are not "heroes of public health," yet the frankness of both their account and Uprety's narrative leads me to believe that is exactly what they are.

I could go on but, as noted, Perlman and Roy supply these chapters with the intellectual scaffolding they demand.

The variety of styles and topics represented in these case studies paint a picture of international health as the complex and confusing collection of problems that it is. Instead of trying to tidy a collection of problems into a discipline, this volume acknowledges the messy social realities, the discord, and the discrepant claims of causality that have always marked international health—a cacophony of voices from health workers, policy makers, drug manufacturers, afflicted communities, bank presidents, researchers, and—rarely—poor and afflicted communities. Indeed, the chapters, and the introduction and section headings, are in and of themselves instructive and revelatory. They are written in a lively and engaging style, alive with the voices not only of victims but also of practitioners and protagonists.

Together, these chapters limn the outlines of what should come to constitute a new field.

What might this field look like, when and if the resources necessary to build it are ever made available? Research would move beyond case studies to rigorously multidisciplinary *biosocial* investigations of complex phenomena. Of the chapters in this book, Julie Cliff's is the one closest to such an analysis, and her topic, a mysterious epidemic of spastic paralysis in war-ravaged Mozambique, demands nothing less. But we shouldn't save our broader, "resocializing" overviews for first-person reflections only; we should instead link them rigorously to the clinical, epidemiological, and laboratory work required to help unravel many of international health's knottiest problems. I refer not to mysterious epidemics but rather to the pathologies now causing millions of deaths, registered mostly among children and young adults, each year.

Allow me to give a couple of examples from our work. In about half of the places in which we work malaria is the leading diagnosis. Biosocial research on malaria's resurgence or retreat would necessarily draw not only on molecular-level inquiry, but also on the exploration of population movements, the use and banning of certain insecticides and international trade regimes, the availability not only of bed nets but also of diagnostics and medications, and the damming of rivers. That much is agreed upon. But as someone working in malarious areas, in both Africa and in Latin America, I know there are more slippery problems and discrepant claims. It would be impossible to count the number of times I've heard my peers (as opposed to my patients) in public health and medicine assert that bed nets should be sold rather than distributed as public goods for public health. "People don't value things unless they pay for them," we're told authoritatively. But this is an ideological assertion, not a fact: how did it come to have so much traction in what are now termed "resource-poor settings"?[1]

Exploring malaria in biosocial terms would require the expertise of epidemiologists, anthropologists, specialists in policy and policy adoption, laboratory-based researchers, etymologists, clinicians, and ecologists who understand history and the political economy. It requires what has been termed a sociology of knowledge: how and when did x, y, or z claim (or paradigm) come to hold such sway?

And all this is before we would even begin to consider the ethical challenges posed by transnational research that links rich-world universities and standard-setting agencies to poor villagers facing recurrent bouts of malaria without even the most meager resources at hand unless they become (willingly or no) the subjects of inquiry themselves.

Elsewhere, in research and writing, I've sought to adopt a biosocial approach to AIDS, tuberculosis, and emerging infectious diseases. I've argued that without such approaches, we will understand neither the burden of disease nor how best to respond to it.[2] Drug-resistant disease—whether due to these pathogens or others—is the obvious case in point. Just a few decades ago, it was unheard of, since resistance to antibiotics occurs only after pathogens are challenged with these agents and must adapt or fade. Such challenges have become widespread only in the past few decades, as policies and practices have brought new drugs, from sulfa to chloroquine to antiretrovirals, into public health programs in settings of poverty. In other words, policy decisions, health-seeking behavior, and many other forms of human behavior have molecular-level consequences.

Beyond research and writing, a biosocial view stems from and informs practice. We came to understand this while working in rural Haiti in the early 1980s. We knew then that tuberculosis was the leading infectious cause of adult death there. And while we did not know for sure that AIDS would soon displace tuberculosis as the leading killer while at the same time driving up rates of TB, we had a good idea that this would come to pass. What was different about the two diseases was the simple fact that one of them was curable during that time and had long been so. Yet we were failing, in 1987, to cure more than half of the case of TB we diagnosed. Taking a biosocial view led us to explore why TB remained, in the catchment area we served with the best of intentions, so lethal.

At least three discoveries ensued. We discovered, to no local surprise, that the biggest co-morbid disease was not HIV infection but hunger. The only known treatment for hunger was food, so we added food to the formulary, prescribing it as part of the TB cure. We discovered a host of hidden costs to our ostensibly free TB program: transportation costs (physical, for walkers, and economic); childcare costs (the great majority of our patients had children and needed a plan before coming to clinic); the cost of spending an entire day (and sometimes more) waiting for the disbursement of a therapy that did not vary from month to month; and payments to local "injectionists," since intramuscular injections of streptomycin were then part of the therapy.

We sought to address each of these readily surmountable barriers through incentives and disbursements and protocols.[3] Finally, we learned that clinic-based staff could not supervise the progress of either programs or patients in rural Haiti: we needed to train community health workers (who we called "*accompagnateurs*") to do so. When we heard calls, again from our well-paid peers but never from the poor, for community health *volunteers* "since only voluntarism was sustainable in such a poor country," we recognized such calls as ideology, not fact. We knew, through experience, that *accompagnateurs* could address many of the problems facing their own communities and that they might become the protagonists of the struggle to promote primary health care for all.

The experience of setting up a community-based TB program in rural Haiti—an ostensibly "vertical" program that strengthened "horizontal" primary health care, to return to the discussion raised by Ciro de Quadras—stood us in good stead when we later contemplated the other chronic diseases facing the world's poor: not only AIDS and TB (or recurrent malaria, which ends up causing chronic anemia, as do helminths and back-to-back pregnancies) but also complications of coronary artery disease, rheumatic heart disease, diabetes, and major mental illness.[4] For each of these pathologies, we have, finally, effective preventions and therapies. All are "deliverables." You would think that systems developed to address chronic pathologies in settings of great poverty and turmoil should be very much in vogue with efforts to address such pathologies in Africa and elsewhere. That these systems are not yet universally adopted—and that "social marketing" appeals for more "cost-effective" interventions and "cost recovery" through users' fees imposed on the sick and poor, and warnings of "unsustainability" have far more clout THAN WHAT? among decision makers—are two of the key topics that need to be addressed by biosocial research.[5]

Understanding that policy might lag, and that the clock was ticking for the vulnerable, we proceeded to set up programs to address health disparities in ten countries; all are going well. But we find ourselves swimming against a constant undertow of censorious opinion. Again, these opinions never come from our patients, their families, or their communities, from whom a very different set of opinions emerges. They come from our peers—experts in development, international public health, and health policy. They come from those likely to read or author books and articles on these topics.

That's why this book is both instructive and heartening. *The Practice of International Health* offers an inspiring example of what may be accomplished when scholars with field experience break free of rigid disciplinary boundaries in order to examine what any observer would agree are the key problems in international health. This case-based approach is precisely the one that will allow us to build a new field focused on broad understandings of these problems and on the solutions that might follow.

This book is ultimately, by conscious design, a call to action. As noted, "the ethics of practice" serve as a recurring theme. Each of the case studies reveals how vexed were the situations encountered and how personal and pragmatic engagement were critical to identifying what might constitute ethical practice in these far-flung settings. The authors and editors alike remind us that simply studying those who face appalling disparities of risk is not enough, and never will be enough. The need for and vibrant potential of practice that resonates in every page of this book signals its profound relevance to students and teachers of public health, and to, one hopes, policy makers and funders as well.

Paul Farmer, M.D., Ph.D.
Presley Professor of Social Medicine
Harvard Medical School

PREFACE

This book started as a concern with the pedagogy of international health. How is the practice of public health in Asia, Africa, and Latin America taught in the research universities and colleges of Europe and North America? How can the realities and sheer inequities and injustices of a global system of health be conveyed to a more privileged audience while avoiding the apocalyptic narrative of crisis, emerging epidemics and dying children? For while there are indeed children dying by the minute in many parts of the world, including here in the Americas, how may we also convey the bold and brave work of so many nurses, doctors, epidemiologists, activists, and health workers who make up the practice of health? How do we tell and teach the stories of those who have not received the global awards, the Gates Foundation grants, of those that deal with diseases that have no simple branded interventions such as an insecticide-treated mosquito net? And what do we learn from the failures and betrayals embodied in these stories of practice – as much as we may learn from their successes and achievements?

This book is the outcome of a five-year collaboration between the editors and an informal network of NGOs, foundations, development institutions, and social movements in Asia, Africa, and Latin America. It is not comprehensive in its coverage of health issues and practices. No book can perhaps be comprehensive. Instead, our selection of partners and stories is strategic. In picking organizations and programs to showcase, we searched, not for "best practices" but rather for organizations that are guided by an ethical compass. This ethical compass was not a particular position on a particular issue, not a litmus test of any kind, but rather the fundamental question of whether or not an organization or program was political.

What do we mean by the political? We do not necessarily mean electoral politics or political machines. In somewhat simple fashion, we mean the political to be the allocation of resources and power. The political is about the decisions that shape who gets what and is also about who gets to make decisions about who gets what. In this sense, the practice of international health is political rather than technical, political rather than bureaucratic, political rather than academic. There are many ways of being political, and indeed some of the organizations and programs highlighted in this book would not explicitly present themselves as political. There are of course those that have thrown themselves into the messiness of political action, those that cannot set themselves apart from the people they seek to diagnose and cure. And then there are those that work from the top, seeking to redesign structures of health-care delivery. This too is political. And there are those that work through mainstream institutions, including the market. And this too is political, for it ultimately shapes the allocation of resources and power.

This focus on the political is missing in most classroom texts on global health. The choice between interventions is presented as a question of efficacy that can be measured and scientifically evaluated. But the world is not that simple. Choices are often based on ideology, values, and national and organizational interests. How then is a student to develop his or her own ethical compass with which to navigate through potential alternatives? How are they to place themselves in relation to the fiercely contested political debates underlying technical and programmatic alternatives? We hope that the this book will inspire our readers to follow the example of our authors and consciously plot the coordinates of their practice and reflect on the complex ethics of their work.

In the shadows of many of these organizations are inspiring individuals, some charismatic, others modest. This book is also an account, and often a reflexive self-account, of these individuals. Their narratives reflect the degree to which the practice of public health involves the cross-border flow of ideas, resources, and people. Too often, however, the direction of that flow runs from north to south, from developed core to underdeveloped margins. The case studies that follow show just how much there is to be learned from the innovations, solutions, and experiments that Asian, African, and Latin American practitioners have pioneered. In doing so, they give voice to the real experiences of public health practitioners and the day-to-day dilemmas and challenges they encounter.

We came to this book with different interests and experiences with the hope that such diversity will enrich the pedagogy that is at stake here. The knitting together of different voices would not have been possible without the dedication and support of the many colleagues who helped at every stage of the development of this text. We are grateful to Michael Watts, and the Ford Foundation "Crossing Borders" grant program that he administered, for sponsorship of the case writers' workshop that first allowed us to bring the authors together. Sarah Shannon and Todd Jailer of the Hesperian Foundation introduced us to several of the case writers, who had translated *Where There Is No Doctor*—a village health-care handbook written by David Werner and published by Hesperian—into their local languages. The warmth and simplicity of David Werner's prose and illustrations, which grew from the his desire to make the handbook available to as wide an audience as possible, inspired our attempt to give the present book a narrative flavor that will make it accessible health workers, nurses, outreach workers, physicians, volunteers, and government health officers. If we have succeeded, and the case studies are lucid and storylike, it is due to the extraordinary efforts of Nina LaCour, Sarah Leavitt, Ana Maria Ventura, Katherine Lee, Kate Robertus, Elena Conis, and Tanya Pluth, who worked closely with the authors as they applied the tools of fiction (plot, characterization, and dialogue) to their narratives. We are indebted to Meredith Fort for her help in researching and conceptualizing the linking chapters. We also wish to thank Malcolm Potts, Julia Walsh, Nami Jhaveri, Sandra Lane, Kira Foster, Marena Zavaleta, Kevin Williams, Claire Norris, Nap Hosang, Negar Ashtari, Jane Maxwell and numerous others for their encouragement and support during the writing of this book.

Daniel Perlman and Ananya Roy
Berkeley
July 2008

CONTRIBUTORS

Sarah (S. L.) Bachman has written for newspapers, magazines and academic publications in the United States, Japan and Bangladesh. She received her undergraduate degree from Yale College, and a master's degree in journalism from the Columbia University Graduate School of Journalism. Her writing about health care, child labor, and economic development has been inspired by Gonoshasthaya Kendra since she first arrived at GK's front gate on the Dhaka-Aricha road in 1977.

Alejandro Cerón is a general practice physician trained at San Carlos University in Guatemala where he graduated from the School of Medicine in 2000 and the School of Public Health in 2006. Starting in 2001 he worked as a physician in the government's program to extend service coverage to rural areas called SIAS-Extensión de Cobertura. Starting in 2002 he began working with the Instancia Nacional de Salud to coordinate a project on monitoring the right to health in Guatemala, and from 2003–2006 he was the Coordinator for the implementation of the Instancia's Inclusive Primary Health Care proposal in the Boca Costa of Sololá with the Clínica Maxeña.

Currently he is a doctoral student in Sociocultural Anthropology at the University of Washington. He conducts research on the right to health and access to medicines in Central America and keeps in close touch with the Instancia's proposal implementation team.

Zafrullah Chowdhury was born and brought up in then East Bengal, India. After graduating with a medical degree from the University of Dhaka in 1964, he studied in the United Kingdom to become a Fellow in the Royal College of Surgeons. In 1971, Zafrullah joined in the war of liberation for Bangladesh, and with Dr. M. A. Mobin and other colleagues, set up a 480-bed field hospital for freedom fighters and refugees. This experience transformed Zafrullah Chowdhury from a vascular surgeon operating in sophisticated operating rooms in the finest western hospitals to a village-based general-surgeon-cum-obstetrician and public health advocate. After the war ended in 1972, Zafrullah and colleagues established Gonoshasthaya Kendra (GK, The People's Health Center), which translated the wartime field hospital experiences into the development of a rural health care delivery system and associated income-generating enterprises, such as a pharmaceutical factory and university.

Zafrullah was awarded the Swedish Youth Peace Prize in 1974, the Ramon Magsaysay Award in 1985, The Right Livelihood Award in 1992, and Bangladesh's highest honor, the Independence Day Award, in 1997. In 2002, he was declared a Public Health Hero by the School of Public Health of the University of California, Berkeley. His books include *The Politics of Essential Health: The Makings of a Successful Health Strategy: Lessons from Bangladesh* (Zed Books, 1995), and, with co-author Rafiqul Huda Chaudhury, *Achieving the Millennium Development Goal on Maternal Mortality: Gonoshasthaya Kendra's Experience in Rural Bangladesh* (Gonoprokashani, 2007).

Julie Cliff is an Australian physician and public health specialist who has worked in Mozambique since 1976. She is currently based as a teacher and researcher in the Faculty of Medicine, Eduardo Mondlane University, having previously worked in Maputo Central Hospital as an infectious diseases physician and in the Ministry of Health as an epidemiologist.

She has worked on cassava-related diseases since 1981, when she investigated a large epidemic of konzo, a paralysis due to eating cassava. Her other research has been in infectious diseases, mostly in applied field research and policy. She is a Fellow of the Royal College of Physicians in London, holds an Honorary Doctorate from Monash University, Australia, and is an Officer of the Order of Australia. Monash University and Health Alliance International have supported her work in recent years.

Meredith Fort is a health policy advocate and public health practitioner. Since 1997 she has supported community-based health programs in Guatemala. Starting in 2001 she carried out health policy research with the Instancia Nacional de Salud and from 2003–2006 she worked with the Evaluation and Supervision component of the implementation of the Instancia's Inclusive Primary Health Care proposal. She continues to support the efforts of the implementation team.

Currently she is a doctoral student in the Health Services Department of the University of Washington School of Public Health and Community Medicine and works with the Seattle-based Health Alliance International where she conducts research on key social and health policy issues to support effective health service delivery in low-income countries.

Jane Galvão is currently the Senior Program Officer for HIV/AIDS/STI at the International Parenthood Federation (IPPF) in New York and works with IPPF member associations in the Latin America and the Caribbean Region. She holds a Ph.D. in Collective Health and an M.A. in Social Anthropology, and has been actively involved in HIV/AIDS programs in her native Brazil for a number of years. In Brazil, she worked with non-governmental organizations dedicated to AIDS. She was the Executive Director of the Brazilian Interdisciplinary AIDS Association (ABIA) from 1993 to 1999 and served with the National AIDS Program, at the Brazilian Ministry of Health, 1999 to 2001. In 2001 she undertook a postdoctoral fellowship in the Fogarty International AIDS Training Program at the School of Public Health, University of California, Berkeley, and was a researcher and postdoctoral fellow at the Institute for Global Health, at the University of California, San Francisco, from 2002 to 2004. Jane has authored and coauthored numerous publications and articles on AIDS, health, and human rights, both in Brazil and internationally.

Assefaw Tekeste Ghebrekidan was born in Eritrea and earned his medical degree at Haile Selassie I University in Addis Ababa, Ethiopia. He returned to Eritrea to practice medicine at Massawa General Hospital and later served as a physician in the Eritrean Popular Liberation Front (EPLF), which led the country's thirty-year war for independence from Ethiopia.

From 1982 to 1991, Assefaw served as Head of Medical Services for the EPLF and Head of Civilian Health Services for Eritrea. He was a key architect in rebuilding the national health care system before and after the country's liberation in 1991. In addition to providing emergency services, primary care, and preventive health services based on community need, Eritrea's health system during the liberation war had become a model of operational efficiency and effectiveness for other developing countries.

In 1992, Assefaw became Secretary (Minister) for the Department of Social Affairs in the Provisional Government of Eritrea. In 1994, he returned to academia as the Dean of the Faculty of Health Sciences at the University of Asmara. Since 1999, he has been a Research Fellow in the School of Public Health at University of California, Berkeley. In January 2003, Assefaw earned a Doctor of Public Health (Dr PH) degree for his study of corruption and its effect on health in sub-Saharan Africa. In May 2005 he joined the Touro University in California as the Director of the MPH program in the College of Health Sciences.

Gopi Gopalakrishnan has over 20 years of experience in using private sector resources to deliver products and services to the poor. He moved to Bihar, the poorest and most rural Indian state and home to 110 million people, in 1995 to set up the Janani program. The program, which is arguably the largest initiative in the world that leverages private sector resources to target the poor, has come to be recognized as one of the most innovative systems for addressing the huge unmet need for family planning. In 2006, Gopi moved to Vietnam as the Country Director of DKT International.

Nuriye Nalan Sahin Hodoglugil was born and raised in Turkey. She graduated from Hacettepe University Faculty of Medicine in 1992, received her master's degree in Cultural Anthropology in 1996 and her MPH in 1998. She had the privilege to be mentored by and work with some of the most dedicated women's health experts in Turkey, whose mission was to improve women's status through health. She developed an immense interest in reproductive health, because it seemed so defining for almost everything else in women's lives, and was one of the main platforms where gender-equity struggles were being fought. Nuriye trained reproductive health providers for the Turkish Ministry of Health, and taught courses in women's health as a professor at Hacettepe University in Ankara. She is currently studying Public Health at the University of California, Berkeley and conducting research on HIV prevention among young women in Zimbabwe for the University of California, San Francisco. She is also the mother of two wonderful children.

Suneeta Krishnan, a social epidemiologist, received her PhD from the University of California, Berkeley in 2000. Her research focuses on the development of sustainable and replicable interventions to promote young people's reproductive and sexual health using strategies that address and respond to structural inequalities, such as economic empowerment, health education, and increased access to and utilization of contraceptive and barrier method technologies. Suneeta is a researcher at Research Triangle Institute, San Francisco and has an adjunct appointment at the University of California, Berkeley. She is also Visiting Faculty at the Indian Institute of Management, Bangalore's Center for Public Policy (IIMB-CPP). She is a recipient of the Presidential Early Career Award for Scientists and Engineers (2004), the highest honor the US government bestows on researchers just beginning their independent careers. In addition, she received the Henrik Blum Award for Distinguished Social Action from the University of California, Berkeley for her work with Swasthya—A Community Health Partnership.

Nina LaCour worked as the associate editor of this book. She is a writer and high school English teacher. A Bay Area native, Nina has taught and/or tutored at 826 Valencia, Berkeley City College, Alameda County Juvenile Hall, and Mills College, where she earned her MFA in 2006. Her first novel is forthcoming from Dutton Books in 2009.

Sandra D. Lane is Chair of Health and Wellness and Professor of Social Work and Anthropology at Syracuse University, as well as Research Professor in the Department of Obstetrics and Gynecology at SUNY Upstate Medical University. She is a medical anthropologist/epidemiologist, whose research addresses racial, ethnic and gender disparities in the Middle East and the urban United States. Her book, *Why are our babies dying? Pregnancy, birth and death in America*, was published by Paradigm Publishers in 2008. From 1997–2002 she was Project Director of Syracuse Healthy Start, an infant mortality prevention project with the Onondaga County Health Department. She was also the Reproductive Health Program Officer in the Ford Foundation's Cairo (1988–1992), Egypt field office with responsibility for Egypt, Sudan, Jordan, Yemen, Lebanon, and the West Bank and Gaza.

Benjamin C. Mbakwem is the founder and program director of Community and Youth Development Initiatives, a Nigerian non-governmental organization dedicated to combating the HIV/AIDS epidemic among Nigerian youths. Previously, he worked for the U.S. non-governmental organization, Africare. He is the recipient of an Ashoka Foundation fellowship for social entrepreneurs and an Emory University Community Partnership Leadership fellowship. He serves as a regular advisor to the Imo State government's programs on HIV/AIDS, and frequently works as a trainer for UNICEF and other agencies' HIV/AIDS prevention programs in Nigeria.

Daniel Perlman is a medical anthropologist with three decades of experience working with community health-care programs in Asia, Africa, and Latin America. His case-based courses at the University of California, Berkeley, have explored the social dimensions of international health, public health practice in the developing world, and the ethics of international health research. He presently lives six months a year in northern Nigeria where he co-directs the Population and Reproductive Health Partnership, an NIH funded collaboration between the University of California, Berkeley School of Public Health and the Ahmadu Bello University Teaching Hospital. Daniel has served as consultant for governmental and non-governmental organizations, including the Center for Victims of Torture, Centers for Disease Control and Prevention (CDC), Family Health International, and Centro de Atención Psicosocial. He is completing an ethnography of a rural rehabilitation center organized and run by disabled villagers in the foothills of the Sierra Madre in western Mexico.

Ciro A. de Quadros is Executive Vice-President of the Sabin Vaccine Institute (SVI). Before joining the SVI, he was Director of the Division of Vaccines and Immunization of the Pan American Health Organization in Washington, DC. He completed his medical studies in Brazil in 1966 and received a Master of Public Health degree from the National School of Public Health in Rio de Janeiro in 1968. He was involved with the pioneering experiences for the development of the strategies of surveillance and containment for Smallpox eradication and in February 1970 joined the World Health Organization (WHO) as Chief Epidemiologist for the Smallpox Eradication Program in Ethiopia. He transferred to the Pan American Health Organization (PAHO) in February 1997 to serve as the Senior Advisor on Immunizations. He directed the successful efforts of polio and measles eradication from the Western Hemisphere. Ciro has received several international awards, including the 1993 Prince Mahidol Award of Thailand and the 2000 Albert B. Sabin Gold Medal. In 1999 he received the Order of Rio Branco, the highest civil award given by the Government of Brazil.

Ananya Roy is Associate Dean of International and Area Studies and Associate Professor of City and Regional Planning at the University of California, Berkeley. She specializes in the study of international development. Ananya is the author of *City Requiem, Calcutta: Gender and the Politics of Poverty* (University of Minnesota Press, 2003) and co-editor of *Urban Informality: Transnational Perspectives from the Middle East, Latin America, and South Asia* (Lexington Books, 2004). In 2006, Ananya was awarded UC Berkeley's Distinguished Teaching Award, the highest teaching honor the campus bestows on its faculty. She is currently the Curriculum Director of the newly established Blum Center for Developing Economies, which seeks to train the next generation of University of California, Berkeley students to engage in rigorous and reflexive ways with global poverty and inequality.

Daniel Jordan Smith is associate professor of anthropology at Brown University. He has worked in Nigeria since the late 1980s, first as a public health worker with a nongovernmental organization and later as an anthropologist, conducting research on HIV/AIDS, rural-urban migration and family organization. He has published widely on Nigeria in journals such as AIDS, American Journal of Public Health, Africa, American Anthropologist, American Ethnologist, Cultural Anthropology, Culture, Health & Sexuality, Medical Anthropology, Population and Development Review, and World Development. His recent book, *A Culture of Corruption: Everyday Deception and Popular Discontent in Nigeria*, is published by Princeton University Press.

Paromita Ukil apprenticed as a journalist with The Telegraph newspaper of Kolkata soon after completing her BA in English. Paromita then moved to rural north India, worked with village artisans and taught young children and out-of-school adolescents. The years spent in villages gave a close-up experience of poverty and its implications. She now combines her skill and experience to document healthcare in rural India.

Aruna Uprety is medical doctor with a post-graduate degree in Social Studies. She has held numerous positions in the health care field working with programs that address reproductive health, nutrition, HIV/AIDS, safe motherhood, communicable diseases, and primary health care. In addition to Nepal, Aruna has worked in Afghanistan, Iran, India, and Sri Lanka, and China in a multitude of positions, including medical coordinator, program officer for monitoring and evaluation, technical adviser, and project manager. She has advocated for the legalization of abortion in Nepal since 1986. Aruna has written articles on health issues for popular health journals and has conducted radio health programs for the rural community.

The Practice of International Health

INTRODUCTION

Daniel Perlman and Ananya Roy

This book represents an unusual collaboration between two different approaches to public health: that of a profession based on scientific knowledge and techniques and a contrasting view of public health as a messy political practice entangled in the complex aspirations of communities and societies. We hope to show how the practice of public health inevitably engages with public issues such as social struggle, political intrigue, and ethical calculations. We intend to foster a conversation across the often separated domains of professional practice and social science theory and to explore how understandings of concepts such as "gender inequality" or "development paradigms" or "social markets" allow for a deeper understanding of health practice.

This book culminates a 5-year collaboration between the editors—academics at a large North American university—and an international network of case writers—physicians, epidemiologists, activists, and public health professionals. The practitioners provide the narratives and analyses, but they also engage the theories, institutions, mandates, and models of North American and European scholarship. This collaboration reflects the degree to which the practice of public health involves the cross-border flow of ideas, resources, and people. Too often, however, the direction of that flow runs from north to south, from developed core to underdeveloped margins. The case studies that follow show just how much there is to be learned from the innovations, solutions, and experiments that Asian, African, and Latin American practitioners have pioneered. In doing so, they give voice to the real experiences of public health practitioners and the day-to-day dilemmas and challenges they encounter.

Such unusual collaborations make possible an alternative approach to the international study and practice of public health, an approach that reveals a less certain and less coherent—but perhaps more revolutionary—discipline and profession. In particular, the case studies in this book make four important contributions, as outlined in the paragraphs below.

BEYOND THE MEDICALIZATION OF HEALTH

International health research has been primarily geared toward the calculus of disease and cure. This "medicalization of health" has meant that the material basis of key issues—be it clean water, contraception, or the AIDS epidemic—is often unaddressed. Questions of social inequality or political power have not had as much coverage as technical factors in this discipline. The teaching of international health has been concerned with diseases but not places, with scientific solutions but not historical moments, and with pioneering heroes but not institutional contexts. And yet there are exceptions that provide insight into how diseases and cures are inextricably linked to the cartographies of social, economic, and political power. Such figures as Rudolf Virchow, Joshua Horn, and more recently Paul Farmer have extended social medicine and the political economy of health into public health, showing how diagnosis is not simply epidemiological but rather geopolitical, not simply concerned with pathology but rather with what Farmer calls "pathologies of power." Each case study in this book is as much a social inquiry as a technical inquiry; each is as concerned with communities, families, markets, states, discourses, and ideologies as it is with disease, diagnosis, prevention, and cure.

THE GEOPOLITICS OF HEALTH

International public health practice is founded on the belief that scientific knowledge can have universal applicability and that diseases can be prevented and cured if such knowledge is widely disseminated. The long history of difficulties associated with the implementation of medical findings in diverse settings suggests that this is not always the case.

To address this issue, this book emphasizes place-based research. Its case studies are explicitly grounded in the material realities of specific sites. In locating health theories and practices, we question assumptions of universality, showing how the same health dilemma—for example, access to antiretroviral drugs for the treatment of HIV/AIDS—plays out in different places in fundamentally different ways. Why is there good access to such medications in Brazil and poor access to the same drugs in sub-Saharan Africa? Why are certain scientific practices stymied at the local level—for example, through local customs and norms that insist on female circumcision? Such geographical investigations not only reveal the grounded complexities of particular places but also indicate the multisited development processes through which the agenda of international health is made. So we ask, for example: How was the fate of women's health in Turkey linked to the global gender agenda that was formulated in United Nations conferences? How did local doctors in Nepal advance access to safe abortion by leveraging this global agenda?

Geography also encompasses history. Place-based complexities and transnational transactions take on very different forms at different historical moments. We link the conventional timeline of international health (diseases, discoveries, and policy debates) to another timeline: that of economic change in a world system managed by powerful institutional ideologies in the wealthy, technologically developed nations. We conceptualize international health as existing within the larger endeavor of international development. If development has had its distinctive phases, so has international health—from the modernizing belief in top-down policies in the 1950s to a basic needs formula in the 1970s to current practices of economic liberalization.

A CASE-BASED APPROACH

In our teaching at the University of California, Berkeley, we have encountered many of the pedagogical challenges commonly faced in university-based training in international health. Our lectures were too theoretical and cut off from the practice of international health.[1,2] Few of our students had lived in Asia, Africa, or Latin America. Their questions and comments in class were often abstract or even fanciful. We turned to case-based teaching to address some of these pedagogical deficiencies and began writing draft case studies with an international group of colleagues. We found—as business schools have known for decades—that the case method of teaching helps ground class discussion in the "stubborn facts" of the case studies[3] and exposes students to the day-to-day issues they will likely encounter in their new profession.[4,5]

Our collaboration with the case writers—a network of highly committed and talented practitioners from around the world—culminated in a workshop held on the UC Berkeley campus in 2004.[6] Through discussion and debate, we hammered out the text's conceptual framework, which emphasizes historical and social context, place-based research, and local authorship. In contrast to conventional case-study materials, which present a polyphony of voices, we agreed that each case should present a single viewpoint, deciding to let the reader think critically about the strengths and limitations of that perspective. To facilitate this process, each of the book's three parts begins with an overview of the section themes and relates the cases to one another. These introductions place the practice described in the cases in the context of major policy initiatives, such as the Alma-Ata Declaration, adopted at the International Conference on Primary Health Care of 1978; the World Bank's 1993 development report titled *Investing in Health*; the Program of

Action that came out of the United Nations Conference on Population and Development, held in Cairo in 1994; and the United Nations Millennium Development Goals.

To make the book accessible to a wide variety of readers, we have encouraged the authors to write in a lucid, story-like style. The result gives the cases a vivid narrative flavor that should prove helpful to readers who have not lived in the countries being discussed.

THE ETHICS OF PRACTICE

The stark inequalities that mark the world of international health present an ethical crisis of grave urgency. What action is needed in a global system where, in so many countries, per capita expenditures on health are less than the cost of delivering a new vaccine or an insecticide-treated mosquito net? What action is needed as thousands die every day of treatable diseases, making a mockery of human dignity? Is the "medicalization of health," with its technological solutions, equipped to take on such seeming irrationalities? Can it explain how and why the world watches as people die?

This book is a call to action. But the ethics of its call to action is significantly different from the missionary zeal that has accompanied old and new efforts of international development and international health. The book is a series of inspirational and cautionary tales drawn from public health practice. Each case presents difficult ethical choices, in which practitioners and activists reflect upon the ambiguities and dilemmas that they inevitably confront. We intend to provide not a blueprint for best practices but rather a map of historical and geographical coordinates of reflexive practice. To this end, we hope that readers will engage in active rather than passive reading, that–like our authors–they too will plot the coordinates of their practice, reflect on the complex ethics of their work, become aware of their geopolitical location, and in doing so tackle the challenges and imagine the possibilities embedded in their place on the map.

PART I

Health and Development

Daniel Perlman and Ananya Roy

The relationship between health and development seems at first glance obvious: an improvement in health indicates successful development; conversely, the development of economies is one of the most important ways in which standards of living, and thereby standards of health, can be improved. However, at second glance, the relationship between health and development is more complex. It involves at least four persistent dilemmas: What are the relationships among underdevelopment, development, and ill health and how have these definitions influenced health policy? How does the distribution of development's benefits and deficits impact the distribution of access to good health? Which groups own development and how do their interests shape health policies and practices affecting underserved populations? What institutional form does development take and how does this influence the outcomes of public health? Opinions on these issues among scientists, economists, medical personnel, and both public health and development specialists have varied dramatically over the last 60 years.

FRAMING THE PROBLEM

Since the late 1940s, the term *development* has been contested. The changing meaning of the term reflected not only political shifts but also the enormous changes in technology during the twentieth century. In the 1940s, as the large international institutions of development—the World Bank, the International Monetary Fund, and the United Nations' World Health Organization (WHO—were set up, development theorists and practitioners equated "development" with "modernization." They imagined modernization as a ladder of economic growth, with poor countries occupying the bottom rungs of the ladder but able to climb their way up through an expansion of their economies. Modernization theorists pinpointed urban industrial centers as the centers of economic growth, which they theorized would eventually spread throughout rural hinterlands and create a national "equilibrium." With economic growth would come social change, creating "modern" citizens free of the backward traditions of the rural countryside. This modernization of economy, infrastructure, and citizenship would result in better health and better access to health services as a natural consequence. Modernization persisted as the dominant development discourse and practice in the 1950s and 1960s. Its primary indicator was a simple statistic, Gross National Product (GNP) per capita, capturing improvements in the average standard of living. Such faith in economic growth, in industrialization, and more broadly in science and technology was especially evident in the sphere of public health.

Under the banner of "health and development," international agencies initiated the wide scale transfer of western preventive and clinical practices to the global south. The mid-twentieth century can be described as a "golden age" of medicine, in which discoveries about infection control, epidemiology, vaccines, and pest control transformed medical practice. Public health officials attributed high morbidity and mortality rates to individual pathology caused by specific microorganisms and believed that health could be restored by the destruction or control of these organisms.[7] With the emergence of new vaccines, penicillin, DDT, and other scientific technologies, one widely used medical textbook published in 1953 foresaw the "virtual elimination of infectious disease as a significant factor in social life."[8]

No international health agency better reflected the period's faith in the power of science to alleviate human suffering than the Rockefeller Foundation's International Health Board (IHB). The IHB gained recognition by attacking diseases—yellow fever, hookworm, and malaria—one by one in poor countries.[9] Perhaps the most celebrated of the Rockefeller initiatives were Fred Soper's antimalarial eradication campaigns against the *Anopheles gambiae* mosquito. After using pesticides to eliminate this mosquito from Brazil and then Egypt during the 1930s and 1940s, Soper became convinced that malaria could be eradicated from the planet. In 1953, the Brazilian malariologist Marcolino Candau—who had worked for Soper during the *A. gambiae* eradication campaign of the 1930s—became the director general of the World Health Organization and launched the Global Malaria Eradication Program as his first major initiative. The Intensified Smallpox Eradication Program followed in 1967. Within years, "smallpox was pushed back to the horn of Africa and then to a single natural case" in Somalia in 1977.[10] The global eradication of smallpox was certified 2 years later. There were a number of characteristics of the disease and vaccine that facilitated the eradication of smallpox. Transmission was person to person (with no animal reservoir), there were no carriers without symptoms, the disease was easy to diagnose, the vaccine did not require a cold chain, and only one inoculation was required. Still, the director of the program has reflected that "eradication was achieved by only the narrowest of margins."[11]

THE DISTRIBUTION OF DEVELOPMENT

The early results of the Global Malaria Eradication Program were remarkable. The campaign saved millions of lives. But the eradication of malaria was a much more complicated project than that of smallpox, and consolidation of these achievements proved difficult. Many countries in Asia, Latin America, and Africa lacked a basic health infrastructure, which hindered effective surveillance and treatment. Pockets of malaria remained and then spread. Logistical, managerial, and technical problems plagued the program.[12] But it was the mosquito's adaptive genius—it became resistant to DDT—that ultimately led to the downfall of the global campaign.

The failure of the Global Malaria Eradication Program came at a time when more and more specialists began to question the emphasis on "growth at all costs" that had prevailed since the Second World War. By the 1970s, after decades of modernization and economic development, much of the Third World was still in "a state of advanced crises characterized by static or worsening life conditions."[13] Over 800 million people were living in extreme poverty. The vast majority of the population of Asia, Africa, and Latin America lacked access to modern health services. Far fewer had clean drinking water and sanitation services. The preventable deaths that resulted were "the equivalent of 20 nuclear bombs exploding every year in the world of underdevelopment without making a sound."[14] Clearly the focus on raising GNP and spreading medical technology, although it did lead to some successes, did not achieve the goals promised by its promulgators.

This was the context in which a new development paradigm, basic needs, challenged the postwar emphasis on modernization. In the 1970s, under the leadership of Robert McNamara, the World Bank became increasingly interested in the distributional impacts of development: Was development reaching the poor? Was it meeting basic needs? In the basic needs framework, development was redefined as something much more than economic growth. It was now envisioned as human development, as a set of investments in human capital. Not surprisingly, health was a significant component of the human capital approach to development. The Human Development Index emerged as an alternative indicator of development and was concerned with trends such as literacy rates and infant mortality rates.

Deep inequities in health status and access to health services represented more than just limitations of the health system: they pointed "to the inability of societies to cope with the underlying causes of ill health and its unfair distribution."[15] Emphasis shifted from "vertical" programs in which technological know-how is distributed from centers of power to "horizontal" community-based initiatives. The then director general of the World Health Organization, Halfdan Mahler, was a passionate advocate of human rights in health-care access. Under the slogan "Health for All by the Year 2000," the International Conference on Primary Health Care[16] held in Alma-Ata, Kazakhstan, in 1978, called for universal access to comprehensive care (preventative, primary, secondary, and tertiary) within an integrated health service that facilitated referrals throughout the health-care system. The conference declaration also advocated equitable socioeconomic development, community participation in health-care decision making, and such policy initiatives as the decentralization of health services and coordination among various sectors of the health-care system, with an emphasis on food supply, basic sanitation, access to clean water, and health education.

The People's Republic of China served as an important source of inspiration to architects of the concept of "primary health care" as defined at Alma-Ata. Western health delegations returned from China impressed that dramatic health improvements need not depend on highly trained and highly paid professionals. China had an estimated 40,000 physicians trained in western medicine for a population of 540 million in the years following the Chinese Revolution. Infectious diseases, the source of much of China's morbidity and mortality at the time, are easily treatable or prevented. A million peasants were given basic training in prevention, diagnosis, and care. The "barefoot doctors" worked next to their comrades in the fields and referred problems beyond their expertise to the commune health centers. Inspiration for primary health care also came from small community-based health-care programs in Asia, Africa, and Latin America. Gonoshasthaya Kendra was one case study presented at the conference and used as a model for primary health care. The high level of training of the Gonoshasthaya Kendra paramedics and the high number of referrals and counterreferrals between the paramedics and the primary, secondary, and tertiary care facilities was especially notable. Although such a referral capability was much talked about in the literature, Gonoshasthaya Kendra was one of the few health programs in which the referral system actually worked.

Basic needs approaches such as primary health care questioned whether development initiatives actually reached the poor whom they targeted. An even more radical critique came from dependency theory, a Marxist framework developed by Latin American social scientists in the 1950s. Dependency theorists argued that the problem was not underdevelopment but development itself; indeed, they posited that the poverty of the underdeveloped world was created and sustained by the exploitative policies of the developed world. In sharp contrast to the "equilibrium" imagined by modernization proponents, dependency theorists conceptualized the world as divided into "core" and "periphery," where core countries extract resources from the poor margins, keeping them impoverished. Such a critique is radical because it implies that "development" cannot end poverty and deprivation; rather, development itself produces deep and persistent inequalities. Julie Cliff's brilliant analysis of konzo makes tangible this "development of underdevelopment." The development of Mozambique, according to the strictures of the global economic system, has meant that its rural poor are left to rely on bitter cassava as a primary food source, a bitter harvest that poisons and paralyzes. Konzo's maimed bodies are a poignant reminder of the unjust distribution of development.

Such critiques as dependency theory and social medicine[17] understand pervasive ill health in poor countries not as a product of cultural backwardness or of the use of the wrong type of technology, as modernization theorists posit, but rather the outcome of "a pattern of world wide relations in which the few control quite a lot and the many control very little."[18] From this perspective, the global economy "operates according to specific rules, such as the accumulation of capital and exploitation of wage laborers, that give it a certain predictable logic," a logic that heavily influences both the kinds of health problems affecting a population and the organization of services developed to address them.[19] Paul Farmer calls these rules and logic "pathologies of power." Thus, critics of the Global Malaria Program questioned its focus on pesticides to eliminate malaria through eradication of the mosquito. They saw social and economic conditions like housing, nutrition, and agricultural production as important factors in determining which people became most susceptible to infection. These critics argued that the exclusive focus on the natural history of malaria would not uncover the true origins of the pattern of disease, which lay in the organization of society.

This debate remains at the heart of many public health controversies. Should the focus of international health be on disease eradication and control or on combating the social inequalities that underlie much of the world's ill health? The debate can be traced at least as far back as the work of Rudolf Virchow and Robert Koch, two renowned German physicians of the latter nineteenth century. Virchow is best known in North America as the father of modern cell biology and pathology. In Latin America he is remembered as the founder of social medicine. In 1847, during a typhus epidemic, Virchow became convinced that the then recent discovery of microscopic organisms alone could not explain pathologic processes. He came to believe that poverty and political disenfranchisement formed part of a complex web of causes that generated much of the disease, disability, and early death he witnessed. However, his interest in social issues of disease causation fell out of favor three decades later, when Robert Koch identified the causal agents of tuberculosis and cholera, then two of Europe's deadliest diseases. This revolutionary discovery greatly diminished the role attributed to social and environmental factors. "It was once customary to consider tuberculosis as the manifestation of social ills," Koch wrote with Virchow in mind, "but in the future, the fight against this terrible plague will no longer focus on an undetermined something, but on a tangible parasite."[20] As we shall see, although the identification of the tuberculosis bacillus and the use of streptomycin initially had a major impact on infection rates, today the combination of drug resistant bacilli and the spread of AIDS have made tuberculosis once again a major infectious cause of death throughout the world. Virchow's point of view once again finds champions in the twenty-first century, but for most of the twentieth century, Koch's more strictly medical model held sway.

In 1987, anthropologist Peter Brown reframed this debate in terms of what he called "microparasites" and "macroparasites." In a study of malaria in postwar Sardinia, Italy, he asked would an attack on "microparasites"—disease organisms such as viruses, bacteria, helminthes, and protozoa—or one on "macroparasites"—economically exploitative relationships between landowners and workers—more efficiently eliminate malaria?[21] Brown found that exploitation by the landlords was a greater drain on the energy of workers than the parasitism of the malaria bacillus, as they consumed roughly 3.5 times more of the energy produced by the farmers than malaria. In addition, a number of economic development initiatives such as forest clearing and expansion of irrigation systems actually increased the incidence of malaria because they provided more of the pools of partly shaded water that mosquitoes use to breed, thus increasing the population more than DDT reduced it.

Did Koch have a point when he argued that with the advancement of scientific technology there is no longer a need to focus on such hard-to-achieve objectives as reducing social inequality in order to reduce morbidity and mortality in the global south? Is it sufficient to conceptualize disease as individual pathology caused by microorganisms within the body, and health as the absence of disease processes, or their elimination through technological intervention?[22] Or is Brown more on target when he asks, tongue only partly in cheek, whether vertical disease control programs should be seen as adaptive strategies of the macroparasites to reduce competition from their microparasitic competitors?

WHO OWNS DEVELOPMENT?

We have already discussed theories of development as a process of economic expansion and growth; development as an improvement in the human conditions of life and work; development as a transformation of societies and cultures. But development is also a "project." It involves the allocation of millions of dollars of development assistance through powerful institutions. It constitutes an apparatus of knowledge that evaluates progress, measures success, and imposes conditions. It represents a system of governance in which national and regional visions of development are coordinated at a global scale. Since development is not only a process but also a project, we must ask the question, "Who owns development?" Whose interests predominate in the design and targeting of development projects?

The project of development was launched by the United States with the assistance of Western European countries and the British Commonwealth in 1944, at the cusp of the Second World War and the Cold War, in an era of fading colonialisms and rising American global power. Known as the Bretton Woods regime (after the site of the landmark meeting), this project involved the establishment of two key institutions: the International Monetary Fund and the World Bank, which were to implement modernization policies and catalyze economic growth. While the founding meetings envisioned these organizations as multilateral institutions with representation by all countries, rich or poor, many governments of the global south perceive both as primarily representing American economic and political interests. Given the history of the United States and the British Commonwealth as colonial nations, this perception is neither groundless nor surprising. The flow of official development assistance (ODA) in both loans and grants goes from the United States and Western Europe to former colonies and comes with political conditions that can be enforced by the economic and political dominance of the former colonizers. The political-economic orientation of such aid has been heavily influenced by political changes in the United States and Great Britain. For example, during the "conservative revolution" of the Reagan-Thatcher years, conditions of aid included reducing protective tariffs in order to open economies, cutting spending on social services, reducing funding to family health services that included abortion, privatizing both industry and health services – all ideological priorities of the political ideologies then dominant in the United States and Great Britain.

Such ownership has led critics to compare twentieth-century development with nineteenth-century colonialisms. The analogy is provocative and instructive. Colonialism was much more than military conquest and occupation. It was also political rule, economic expansion, and projects of improvement and philanthropy. This liberal moral order of colonialism had two key components: a sense of trusteeship whereby colonial administrators (including doctors) felt that they were carrying the "white man's burden" to advance the mission of civilization and a discourse and imagination that identified, mapped, counted, categorized the backward, the uncivilized, the poor, the unclean, the unhealthy. Colonial projects, and later development projects, reflect the ideologies of the United States and Western Europe. It was in the colonial era that western officials began to see health as a "public" project, one that involved the colonial state. It was in the colonial era that the concepts of "poverty," "hygiene" and "spatial order" were constructed and implemented. And it was in the colonial era that officials imagined that they could create in colonized areas a utopia populated by "improved" and "modernized" subjects who shared western values such as literacy, women's rights, democracy, hygiene, etc. The project of twentieth-century development continues these legacies of colonialism. Like colonial officials before them, development specialists also enjoy a geopolitical distance from the poor countries in which they work. To most of the citizens of the United States, Western Europe, and the British Commonwealth whose taxes support development projects, these poor countries are both geographically remote and politically vague. The agencies which supported the failed agricultural policies of the World Bank and the International Monetary Fund (IMF) in sub-Saharan Africa were not held responsible for the spread of the disease of konzo, which Julie Cliff describes with such passion in Part One, because most citizens of western nations were unaware of how the situation looked from the point of view of the targets of the policies. Cliff demonstrates how the outbreak of konzo was not only epidemiological but also geopolitical.

But there have also been efforts to transform the ownership of development. The term *Third World*, designating the main countries targeted by development aid, has both an economic and a political meaning. On the one hand, it refers to developing countries, the impoverished half of humanity, the object of development. On the other hand, it refers to countries in the global south that, at the height of the Cold War, embraced "nonalignment," refusing to pledge allegiance to either the capitalist West or the communist bloc. This double meaning indicates the complex political struggles through which development often proceeds. Part of the postcolonial struggle has involved attempts by the targets of development to shape policies to better reflect their interests rather than those of the former colonizers.

Gonoshasthaya Kendra, described in Part One, is an uplifting example of this postcolonial development—of human and social development in tandem with the search for sovereignty and self-determination. Bangladesh, one of the poorest countries in the world, is also home to some of the most innovative, impressive, and important poverty-alleviation organizations, such as Gonoshasthaya Kendra, Grameen Bank, and BRAC. Each of these organizations has created a formidable institutional structure that is centralized and yet highly decentralized, that cares about poverty and yet does not accept or dole out charity, that seeks to create social change such as women's empowerment and yet works effectively at the grassroots level in a conservative social milieu. The story of Bangladeshi institutions is an astounding history of charismatic middle-class pioneers: Zafrullah Chowdhury, Fazle Abed, Muhammad Yunus, seeking to build a new nation with a new vision of development.

The issue of sovereignty is applicable not only at the scale of geopolitics but also at the more intimate scale of the relationship between the state and its citizens. It is this relationship that puts the "public" in public health: the power and capacity of the state to determine and implement the public interest. In Part One, Assefaw Tekeste Ghebrekidan tells the story of how the postcolonial state sought to develop and modernize pastoralist nomads by settling them in camps, complete with health services. But for the nomads, such development was an erosion of their way of life, of the foundational notions of freedom and liberty. Tekeste's story is also a narrative about the encounter between a progressive imagination of women's rights (the Eritrean People's Liberation Front) and the more conservative customs and traditions of the "people" (in this case the nomadic tribes).

A progressive imagination of development sees it as the expansion of local people's choices. This is the Nobel Prize–winning work of welfare economist Amartya Sen: development as freedom. However, such a view of development requires allowing local people to make choices that may contradict or even offend the cultural politics of development agencies. For example, what if local people, like the Eritrean nomadic tribes described by Assefaw Tekeste, choose to continue to practice female genital surgeries, abhorrent to most westerners? The Eritrean Liberation Front was unable to override that choice because the practice was so important to the tribes that eradication attempts would imperil partnership with the tribes in efforts to provide them with basic medical and educational services. The implications of local ownership of the development process can include continuing political dominance of traditional leaders who promulgate gender, ethnic, or age-related discrimination repugnant to development agencies and officials. These issues of local versus international sovereignty remain both complex and unresolved.

PLANNERS VERSUS SEARCHERS

In a recent book that is generating much controversy, William Easterly[23] notes that the real tragedy of development is this: that despite the deployment of so much money and so much knowledge, little has been accomplished in terms of the reduction of poverty and the elimination of disease and suffering. He argues that the problem lies in "Big Western Plans" that seek to create a "Big Push," one that will for once and for all end underdevelopment. Easterly insists that such plans are neocolonial; they are imbued with colonial ideas of trusteeship, of a "white man's burden." And perhaps even more important, such plans are doomed to failure. As instances of utopian social engineering, they cannot address the complex and variable realities of poverty and disease on the ground. In the place of planners and their big plans, Easterly calls for searchers and their incremental ideas and practices, piecemeal efforts initiated at the grassroots, often by the poor themselves.

Easterly's distinction between top-down versus bottom-up efforts has long haunted the domain of public health. Ciro de Quadros, in Part One, notes that the success of smallpox or polio eradication rested on vertical, top-down programming and that such verticality was not at odds with community consultations and grass-roots initiatives. Indeed, de Quadros argues that vertical programming around "banner" diseases could strengthen primary health care infrastructures. Against de Quadros, Easterly would argue that many top-down programs, such as malaria eradication, did not achieve much success. The Global Malaria Eradication Program built its own infrastructure in many countries and rarely elicited indigenous understandings and expertise.

In contrast, the cornerstone of primary health care was to be community involvement in the design, implementation, and evaluation of the development activities affecting them. Though conceptions of community participation varied greatly, most governmental programs saw participation as a means to increase project efficiency and the sharing of costs.[24] Two country-by-country surveys in Latin America found that virtually every large government and internationally sponsored primary health care program had failed or collapsed.[25,26] Many of these programs stressed the importance of building on the shared values and cooperative activities that were said to form the core of rural village life; few of these communities, however, were homogeneous. Most were characterized by some form of social stratification based on wealth, ethnic origin, religion, or sex. In such settings, local elites dominated village health committees. Community participation became a vehicle for village leaders to solidify their power and pursue their own interests within the larger social hierarchy.[25] Gonoshasthaya Kendra and the Eritrean People's Liberation Front health services, however, saw participation as way of bringing about a more equitable distribution of power and resources through "a long-term process in which community confidence, solidarity, responsibility and autonomy are gradually built up."[27]

Within a few years the policy pendulum started back toward a more vertical, disease-based focus. The process began at the Rockefeller Foundation's Bellagio Study and Conference Center, Lake Como, Italy, in 1979. A meeting— attended by the leaders of major donor institutions, including the World Bank, USAID, and UNICEF—was held to discuss alternatives to Alma-Ata. The organizers believed the concept of primary health care was overly idealistic and difficult to quantitatively monitor and evaluate and sought to identify cost-effective technical interventions that had specific and quantifiable health targets.

The starting point for discussion at the conference was a paper titled "Selective Primary Health Care, an Interim Strategy for Disease Control in Developing Countries."[28] The authors advocated that emphasis be placed on the prevention and treatment of pediatric conditions and selected diseases through simple and low-cost technologies, such as immunization and oral rehydration for diarrheal dehydration in infants and children. "The goal set at Alma Ata is above reproach," they stated, "yet its very scope makes it unattainable." In "an age of diminishing resources," the authors suggested that the best way to improve health by the year 2000 was to select a limited number of high-impact interventions that target diseases on the basis of prevalence, morbidity, mortality, and feasibility of control (including efficacy and cost).

UNICEF, under the leadership of James Grant, soon operationalized the concept of Selective Primary Health Care under the acronym GOBI, for "Growth monitoring to fight malnutrition in children, Oral rehydration techniques to defeat diarrheal diseases, Breastfeeding to protect children, and Immunizations)."[29] GOBI was later expanded to include Family spacing, Female education and Food supplements (GOBI-FFF). Ciro de Quadros' vision for a polio free Americas fits perfectly into this approach.

Today, there seems to be a revival of de Quadros' vision in the various global initiatives to end poverty and disease (and it is this "Big Push" that Easterly critiques). From the Gates Foundation to the Clinton Global Initiative to the Millennium Project to the Make Poverty History Campaign to the Global Fund to Fight AIDS, Tuberculosis, and Malaria, there is now a flurry of global activities that tackle "banner" diseases. As in the case of de Quadros' polio eradication program of the 1970s, there is today an internationalization of public health. In other words, the diagnosis and cure for banner diseases no longer lies within national borders. It is a global responsibility. Unlike de Quadros' efforts, these new global campaigns are the domain of an emergent global civil society: nonprofits and nongovernmental organizations, rather than the domain of national governments or even international development institutions such as the WHO or UN or World Bank. In other words, there is an ongoing transformation of the meaning of the word *public* in public health. These "new" development actors claim to care about the distribution of development and about the ownership of development. The question for the new millennium is whether such promises will be fulfilled or whether the legacies of nineteenth century colonialisms and twentieth century development will endure.

1   Nomads and Nationalists in the Eritrean Sahel

Assefaw Tekeste Ghebrekidan

Shielded by high mountain ranges that make a dramatic descent into the western lowlands and Red Sea plains, the Sahel is one of Eritrea's most inaccessible regions. It is a land of two winters, with June to September rains in the highland plateau and November to February rains in the lowlands, which draw the 27 clans of the Tigre ethnic group like a magnet. They travel along arid paths from the highlands of the Sahel in groups of three or four families, taking different routes to ensure that all their livestock have sufficient grazing room. The women are wrapped in brightly colored dresses with only the sun-darkened skin around their eyes showing; the men, tall and thin, herd goats across the dusty ground; children trek alongside their parents, likewise tending to the herds. In June, they pack up and return to the Sahel for the rainy season there. The Tigre pastoralists make this trek every year, stopping only a few weeks at a time in any one place. Because their livestock is their primary asset and serves for everything from their daily livelihood to dowry payments, they follow the rainy season to wherever the grass is green. They have lived this life for generations. They would not live any other way.

In 1972, a new "clan" came to the Sahel: the Eritrean People's Liberation Front (EPLF). The EPLF chose this inaccessible region as a base for guerrilla operations against Ethiopia, which had illegally annexed Eritrea as a province. The war went on for over 30 years—the span of an entire generation—during which Ethiopia was backed by the United States and provided with modern weaponry from 1961 to 1975 and by the Soviet Union thereafter. In 1993, after a national referendum supervised by the United Nations produced an almost unanimous vote for its independence, Eritrea was proclaimed a sovereign state.

The guerrillas' mobility was compatible with the nomadic life of the pastoralists, but unlike the latter's, the guerillas' movements were not dictated by the need for grass; instead, they were governed by the strategic rules of warfare. Their lives depended on blending in with the pastoralists. Their ideology was one of social change, with emphases on literacy, self-reliance, and women's rights. They lived the nomadic life for less than one generation. It was a step toward living in a completely different way.

Thirty years of war were unthinkably ruinous and tragic for Eritrea. I was there, yet even I can scarcely conceive of the devastation wrought in terms of lives, suffering, and property damage. Although I will never forget the horrors I witnessed, serving as a medical cadre among the pastoralist communities is one of my most cherished memories. The beauty of the impromptu cooperation between a liberation front and a marginalized population utterly unaware of politics has forever changed me.

I was born at the northern flanks of the central highlands, where the lands of farmers merge with the trails of the nomadic pastoralists. At age 19, I went to Ethiopia to study medicine. The hospital where I was placed after graduating from medical school, in the port of Massawa, was not far from my home in the highlands, and I lived comfortably. As one of only 16 doctors in Eritrea at the time, I had my own home and a car, luxuries that most of the population could not afford. This ended for me, though, after my arrest by the Ethiopian government.

I had been a clandestine member of the EPLF since the age of 19. From the time I began working as a physician in Massawa, through my promotion to hospital director, until I was uprooted and sent back to Ethiopia, I had been meeting secretly with *Tegadelti* (liberation fighters), who would sneak into the city in the dark of night.

I would meet with *Tegadelti* in my home to talk about the marvels in the Field, and I would hand off medicine, microscopes, and other necessary provisions for the camouflaged hospital in the Filfil, a nearly inaccessible region in north central Eritrea, shielded by high mountain ranges and thick forest that descended dramatically into the coastal plains.

Not long after my arrest, I was contacted by the Front to plan my escape from Ethiopia. They arranged for me to fly back to Asmara, the capital city of Eritrea, via a circuitous series of local flights. I then met up with a man who guided me north, and we began our walk that very day toward the base of the Front. It was a long walk across rocky terrain, throughout the afternoon and into the evening, with a 4-hour rain that pelted my skin and soaked my clothes.

We finally stopped walking when we saw light from the house of semisedentary farmers. The woman inside gave me dry clothes and a plate of sorghum porridge, all the while quietly continuing her work. Finally she looked up at me and said simply, "Why are you here?" Her hands were tough, their papery skin dry against the stones she used to grind sorghum for the next day's meal: sorghum bread, more sorghum porridge. She eyed me from her place on the floor mats, where she'd been on her knees, grinding endlessly. "Look at you. Your skin is so soft. Why did you come to this misery?" Her eyes narrowed, her mouth turned down. I tried to explain to her about our position as a colonized people, that life without liberty is worthless. My explanation did not impress her. "Why don't you just go live somewhere else as a doctor? You can live comfortably," she said. In the morning I thanked her for her hospitality and continued my journey toward the Sahel and the spartan life of poverty that awaited me.

There were a number of new recruits heading north to join the Front, and we were lucky that our guides knew the route well. We had camels to carry all of our supplies—food, drink, everything. However, we were forced to walk at night, as it was imperative that we avoid the Ethiopian army and the merciless heat of the lowlands. Although our guides were knowledgeable, their task became difficult when winter clouds passed by overhead, rendering navigation by the stars nearly impossible. But the camels knew their direction, and their inner compass led us safely to our destination.

The first night of our journey was intolerable. Many of the recruits whispered to the guides that they needed water. I understood. My own thirst was desperate. Being in the lowlands made it worse, and our dehydration was fierce. We each had a cup that held barely more than three handfuls of water. "You will drink one of these at a time and only when needed most," the guide explained, holding his own cup up against the moonlit panorama of desert. "But no more." He kept to his word.

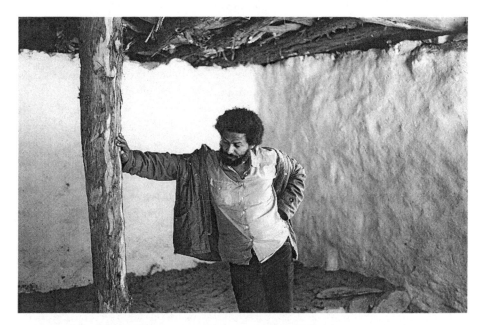

Assefaw Tekeste in an underground health center in 1985. (Photo: Peter Wolff.)

There it was, the guerilla base in the Sahel, and I found that a friend of mine was already there. I sat with him, grateful for a moment's rest after so many days of walking, and we talked. It surprised me when he very suddenly took off his trousers. I watched him, silent for the moment, as he began to pick tiny lice from the cloth, killing them in the heat of the afternoon.

"You know," I told him, "Having lice doesn't make you a revolutionary. There's no reason for this. Simple cleanliness is all it takes to avoid lice." My arms were draped across my knees, and my own clothes were free of contamination.

My friend laughed and squashed yet another louse between thumb and forefinger. "Take your time, maybe few months, Assefaw," he said. "You will do what I am doing and a newcomer will ask the same question to you. "

In less than 3 months my hair, clothes, and everything were covered with lice. With no running water and the opportunity to bathe arising only once every 6 or 7 months, it was impossible to keep the bugs from communing on my body, on my single shirt and only pair of trousers. It was simple to be an idealist back in the city. In practice, it was uncomfortable to say the least. This was the life I had chosen, one of blending in willingly with the poor, surrendering fleeting personal leisure for a permanent, gratifying communal life in a liberated country. And so I shared the poverty, and despite the inconveniences it posed, I felt alive to the fullest.

AN UNLIKELY ALLIANCE

Morning in the Sahel bled the bone-aching cold of night into the blistering heat of day. Days rolled into months. The underground hospital served as our base. The nature of our struggle forced us to work from the most difficult and barely accessible locations—the terrain was inhospitable but defensible. It did not take long before that stony land became our home. We lay low during the day, coming back to life at night, between dry valleys and mountains slippery with erosion.

The paths of the nomads were ample, winding throughout Eritrea in the highlands and down the mountain flanks into the lowlands. Some of the clans crossed to the Sudan, oblivious of the borders, while others stayed only within the country. There were spots where the tribes would stay for months, where there were ample grasses to sustain their livestock. The pastoralists' sense of cultural identity is deeply rooted in this way of life, an inextricable mix of age-old tradition and necessary adaptations to the exacting conditions of the environment. Neither the term *pastoralist* nor *nomad* fully describes the complexity and diversity of their economic and social adaptations. Inevitably, their paths crossed our own—a meeting that sparked the beginning of change for all of us.

Historically, the pastoralists have had little if any access to modern health services. When the Front arrived in the region, it provided primary health care, then secondary and finally tertiary care. Those pastoralists who crossed into the empty lowlands of Sudan, had no health-care options. In the beginning, few but major ailments were treated by the barefoot doctors of the Front. Despite the pastoralists' skepticism, their recovery was convincing. Eventually a mutual bond was established.

One afternoon, some men came to the hospital from a pastoralist village where a woman had been in labor for 3 days. It took me hours to walk there under the sun of the Sahel, and when I arrived the husband looked at me and said, "I was expecting a woman. You cannot go inside the tent." I tried to explain that I could help her, that there was a strong possibility that she could die. An elder came and apologized for my having walked so far, and I was sent back to the hospital. But that night they came back, and again I made the trek, this time cold beneath the moon. Inside the tent, the woman held onto a rope that dangled from the ceiling, her legs bent into a squat. Her eyes were focused on the rope and her teeth clenched against screams; women in Sahel never utter a sound while giving birth. I could tell immediately that she was anemic. Her skin, her hands, her tongue, everything was so pale. There were five women gathered around, including a traditional birth attendant who was rubbing some butter onto the woman's belly.

I needed more space to do a vacuum extraction, so I told them, "She needs to be in the supine position. That's the only way this will work." The women refused. It was not the way they did things in the Sahel. Her husband told them to let me do my job, so we stretched her out into the supine position and I could see then that her hips were too small—the baby's head was stuck. I put on my gloves, washed her, and placed the cup over the fetus' tiny skull. The mother was very strong despite being anemic and in so much pain; she listened carefully, pushing when told. Her courage and tolerance to pain were remarkable. That facilitated the vacuum extraction, and the baby was born blue, not breathing, and nearly lifeless.

I placed my mouth over his tiny face coated in birthing fluid and breathed. I pressed on his tiny chest, his 7-pound body so slight under my hands, and after 3 or 4 minutes he was resuscitated. He lived, they never forgot about it, and that was how the trust between us was built.

Before the war, several of my colleagues had not known the Eritrean nomad community. Growing up in the cities, they assumed that all people were settled. Although I had known of the pastoralists before the war, I didn't know much about them. Like my colleagues, I thought that they simply didn't know a better way of life. With disdain, we sought to change them. We thought that settlement (the only way of life we knew) would be for their own good—they would have access to health care, education, and all the things we felt would solve their problems, make their lives better.

They intensely challenged our attempt to impose change. "We love our way of life. Don't interfere," the elders told us. "We didn't come to you. You came to us." And it was true. We had moved into their lands, we had been fed and protected, our wounded had been helped by them, and above all they had taught us how to live in that desolate terrain. We knew our position was that of learners.

Slowly, their world became intertwined with ours. Their camels carried most of our food and artillery. They were a natural target for the Ethiopian bombs that rained down on their livestock and their tents. Often, our fighters were carried into medical facilities by the nomads, open wounds dripping blood onto their clothing. Survival in the face of a common enemy linked us together. The nomads paid for liberation as much as we did, if not more.

One such case involved a child who had wandered with a baby goat a short distance from his family. He stepped on a land mine, and his delicate rib cage became a cave of bone fragments and muscle tissue. Blood spread slowly up his shoulder and across his abdomen. Miraculously, he survived.

The boy's parents carried him to the hospital. His younger sister was slung across the mother's chest and, as the boy lay unconscious, her screams were more deafening than anyone's. It was a delicate procedure—we had to treat this wound very carefully, tweezing the smallest bits of dead tissue and shrapnel from his flesh, which were placed into a shallow metal pan at the side of the operating table. It was then that I wondered about this war. How many Ethiopian children have starved in their poverty-stricken country to pay for the bomb that had injured this innocent child? The war of liberation was the only means of bringing an end to such atrocities. Fortunately, the shrapnel did not penetrate deeply enough to be fatal, and although it was a painful recovery, eventually the boy grew strong once again, with a thick scar braided over his chest and the loss one leg.

The Front, although initially few in number, had a medical service almost from the very beginning. We started by training medics who traveled with the military units and eventually developed a mobile service tailored to their needs. By 1982, we had over 20 mobile health teams, each consisting of a nurse, about five health workers, and—when available—an assistant midwife and several armed guards.

Although pastoralists in Eritrea make up one-third of the total population of 4 million, they are historically a forgotten people living on the margins of a colony. The center of power forgets them, and they forget the center. The presence of the EPLF in the Sahel represented, in many ways, a reversal of the status quo: for the first time there was a political center—that of the independence movement—located in the pastoralist region. Political power was concentrated at the margins. For both the pastoralists and for us, this shift was revolutionary. It meant that after liberation, the national government had to recognize the pastoralists for the first time. It meant that our ethnic groups—the Tigre pastoralists and the EPLF—had truly joined forces.

MEDICINE ON THE MOVE

In the beginning, there were no liberated areas. There were only guerillas moving across Eritrea's tough terrain, constantly changing location to avoid being targeted by the Ethiopian army. However, small areas were soon liberated and we were free to set up bases—hospitals and stationary health clinics—to which fighters and ci-vilians alike could come for free health care. Although those fighting for independ-ence no longer needed mobile health teams, we kept them intact and sent them out among the nomads to provide care for them during their long treks in search of greens for their livestock.

Having worked with the pastoralists for some time, we had become increas-ingly familiar with the health problems they faced. Endemic *falciparum* and *vivax* malaria sapped their strength by depleting their blood and overtaxing the supply of iron to their bodies. We also noticed that many of the nomads suffered from un-dernourishment. Their basic diet consisted of sorghum porridge with milk. Fruits were unknown to them, and the meager vegetables available were given to the livestock. Despite this, micronutrient deficiencies such as scurvy, goiter, and berib-eri were rare; however, during periods of drought, when livestock died and the milk supply decreased, undernourishment among the children rose quickly. Com-munity health was intimately linked to the health of the livestock—if the animals suffered, the people suffered.

They became afflicted by a variety of illnesses that could have easily been pre-vented if even the simplest of measures had been implemented appropriately. The extremes of temperature in this desert land coupled with undernutrition increased the people's vulnerability to respiratory tract infections, particularly pulmonary tu-berculosis and pneumonia, the primary causes of death among children. Schisto-somiasis, which had previously not been prevalent, was spreading quickly with the altered movement of the people during the war, and cases were arising in areas that had not been previously affected. Other vector-borne diseases, such as leish-maniasis, were common, and epidemics of meningococcal meningitis and cholera occasionally affected the western Eritrean lowlands.

The nomadic way of life also has many healthy aspects to it. Communicable diseases due to overcrowding—such as dysentery, typhoid, typhus, trachoma, and intestinal parasites—were rare. The people lived spread thin, denying the bugs pas-sage from one person to the other.

Despite these complex issues surrounding health provision for the pastoralists, they led a very simple life. It took some time for me to understand the appeal of this wandering from place to place, although a friend I made was very influential in helping to make this knowledge sink in. Each year, this friend from Biet-Abrehe passed by in search of the rainy season, his family in tow. One day he arrived on his way back from Sudan, a bottle of milk for me in hand. I thanked him for the gift, and we sat in a patch of shade with the underground hospital beneath us.

"You know," I said to him, "each year you pass by from highland to lowland. Your family is always walking along with you. Why don't you at least leave your wife and children here? We have the school, the hospital. They could get an educa-tion, medical treatment if they get sick. . . ."

He smiled at me and remained quiet for a moment. When he spoke, his voice was rough, like his callused hands. "You know, every time I go to the lowland end, you are here. I come back, and you are still here. What a boring life," he laughed, pointing to the underground bunker where I lived.

"Here's the thing. . . ." He lifted his left hand, gestured at the goats grazing on the hillside. "The goats are also a family. That goat, well, she has kids. I can take care of the adults, but the small goats, my wife has to take care of, and my children. So, we cannot split up. It's a family of goats as we are a family of people." It was wisdom gained by life experience.

What he told me made sense: they hadn't chosen the nomadic life for themselves, it had been dictated to them by nature. They could not be farmers in that arid land because there was not enough rain to support agriculture. While sedentary people often viewed them with contempt, no one can deny the productivity of the pastoralists: livestock became the main or only export commodity after Eritrean independence. And how can anyone scorn the pastoralists' lifestyle?

However, while I learned to respect the pastoralist way of life, I still could not come to terms with certain social and cultural practices that have a bearing on their health, particularly the health of women. Nomadic society, rooted in a patriarchal order that greatly circumscribes women's rights and power in the community, dictates that lineage and inheritance, thereby the transfer of rights and resources, travel along the male line. I would see the women in their seasonal villages grinding cereals between two stones to mill the seeds for porridge or bread, a task that often kept them busy until 3 or 4 o'clock in the morning. The nomadic women were also expected to bear children, take care of home and offspring, and prepare the food, including the laborious task of milling sorghum, tending and milking animals, fetching water and firewood, constructing and dismantling makeshift huts, and more.

As with many ethnic groups, the women were served food last. This uneven distribution of food within the family, combined with poverty, has damaging effects on the nutritional status of women in general and of pregnant and lactating mothers in particular. These conditions, coupled with strenuous work, make nomadic women disproportionately vulnerable to illness. Maternal and infant mortality rates in the region are extremely high (an estimated maternal mortality rate of 1,000 per 100,000 live births), which is aggravated by the severely limited accessibility of maternal and child health care, immunization, family planning, and general health education.

The patriarchal social structure and the low average education level of women further complicate their access to what few health services may be available. However, the revolution did make some differences in the emancipation of women. The female nomads who came to join the Front carried guns and donned clothes like ours. It was only a short time until a law was passed that at least 30% of each village council must be made up of women.

One of these councilwomen was Fatima, but everybody called her Mussolini. This Mussolini was only in her early thirties and not much taller than a medium-sized young girl, but she struck fear in many of the people she encountered. She was a divorcee—owing to her nonconformist will of steel—and so her lack of husband to complain about her status as a councilwoman, coupled with fair judgment, made her an excellent candidate for village office.

It was late at night when a dark shape scurried toward us under a desert moon. I could see that he was a pastoralist from the clothes he wore. He carried nothing but concern in the deep lines of a weathered face. He was from Brij, Fatima's village, and begged us to come quickly to treat his wife. I went.

We arrived at the man's tent an hour later. The woman had pneumonia and was critically ill with other complications. Her daughter mopped sweat from her mother's forehead with a bright yellow cloth. The woman shivered despite a thin blanket tucked around her bony shoulders and the perspiration that poured from her skin. I squatted on the floor of the hut and examined her. She was febrile and severely dehydrated. She was very ill, so I took the woman's husband outside with me.

"We must take your wife to the clinic," I told him. "She's dehydrated. She needs an intravenous infusion and maybe blood."

"I can't take her to the clinic," he said. He shook his head and shrugged. "I don't have anybody to help me and I can't take her alone."

"What do you mean you can't take her? She's your wife," I said. "If she doesn't go to the hospital, she'll die." He was a young man, in his late twenties at most, and he simply refused. I left the hut and walked over to Fatima and explained the situation to her.

"You go back to the clinic," she told me. "Don't worry. He'll meet you there."

I left, sure that I would never see the man or his wife again.

A short time later, to my surprise, the man did arrive, carrying his wife on his back. The effective outcome of sharing power with women struck me.

LEARNING TO LISTEN

I watched one of the pastoralists' healers late one night. Fire blazed while he chanted and cast herbs into the flames—a practice that seemed irrational and bizarre. I asked him about it later, with the pale moon illuminating his black freckles.

"I cannot tell you the secrets of my ways," he told me. He shook his head in refusal, crossed his arms.

"But if this truly works for healing sickness, isn't it better to tell others about it so more people can benefit from the practice?"

"No," he said. He continued to shake his head as he spoke. "Revealing secrets affects the potency of the therapy, and for this reason, I cannot tell you or anyone else."

Traditional healers were the prime health-care providers to the pastoralist communities. The fact that they charged excessive prices for their services, contrary to the practices of the Front, was in no way compensated by the occasional destitute family they helped for free or the fact that they did not charge for patients they failed to cure. Our stand against the healers was aggressive—we believed in doing away with some of the old habits and paving the way for improved modern health services. Typical of the arrogance of modern medicine, we prohibited their activities, sending fighters to arrest them in the most extreme cases. Consequently most of the healers fled their communities or went into hiding.

However, there were also traditional birth attendants, women who assisted in labor. They very rarely asked for payment up front and did not necessarily charge patients who could not afford to pay, and we began to wonder if the ban on traditional healing had not been a mistake. We were obliged to revisit the policy and reverse it. There was an attempt to reconcile our differences and integrate the beneficial aspects of traditional health practice with modern health services.

I went to one of the villages and began asking around about the traditional healers, where they had gone and how I might find them, saying that we had been wrong. Most of the nomads said, "No, we don't know where they are." Finally one man leaned close to me and said, "Well, there are three of them. But they don't operate openly because they are scared of you. Before, we had seven. But now there are just the three."

"Where did the other four go?" I asked. I was skeptical.

"Well, two of them fled to Sudan, and the other two you arrested. And the three that are still here, well, nobody's supposed to know that."

That night, I went in search of the traditional healers, entering each of their huts with the best of intentions. They all denied that they were practicing, though, and it was then that I knew: in our haste to ban traditional healing practices, we had lost their trust forever. We were never able to close the gap we had created.

I did know one traditional healer, though. His name was Sheik Abdul, a very rich man who was intelligent and cultured. He came to the hospital for his diabetes, a disease he knew he needed our help to control. He had been coming for some time, but when I saw him one morning I asked him to follow me. I began to examine him outside the outpatient department, where other pastoralists would see him.

He laughed and said, "You want to do this here? So everyone can see that I come to you?"

I smiled back at him and nodded.

"Okay, then," he answered, and allowed me to finish the exam.

When I was finished, I sat down next to him and said, "You know, I've been to your home; I've seen you giving treatments. And you have over 100 patients a day because they trust you. Here, we only see 30 or so people a day. And that's okay. But you know that there are some diseases you cannot treat, right?"

"Yes, sure. Tuberculosis, fever. . . . You can treat these things better than I can."

"So, when you have patients with these illnesses, do me a favor. Refer them to us."

He agreed, but only if I would refer psychiatric patients to him. In the end, many of the patients he referred received treatment from both of us, inevitably believing in the end that it was the traditional healing that cured them.

This daily interaction brought us together, resulting in a mutual respect and trust that enabled us to accomplish a great deal, especially in making it easier for them to understand modern health treatments, such as the one for tuberculosis (TB).

TB, a bacterial disease that is often spread through coughing or sneezing, was very common among the pastoralists and their livestock. Generally TB infects the lungs, although it can also affect the peritoneum, bones, kidneys, or any other organ. Most of our patients would come to see us after 2 or 3 months or more of a productive, grating cough, sometimes producing mucus tinged with blood. At that time, the treatment for tuberculosis took 18 months to complete. Patients were advised to come every 3 months for a checkup and to refill their prescriptions. After 5 years, we carried out an evaluation of the program, and to everyone's surprise, 97% of the pastoralists had completed their TB treatment—a remarkable demonstration of adherence in a nomadic community.

Sometimes, though, we seemed to have elicited too much faith. In one particular community, we had assured the people that if they attended the prenatal health clinic at the health stations and made use of the trained traditional birth attendants (TBAs), no more women would die in labor. But once a woman did die.

The family went to the clinic nearest their encampment and demanded to know what had happened. "We did everything we were supposed to do," they said. "She took her tablets, she attended your clinics, we had a trained birth attendant by her side. You told us she wouldn't die. Tell us what happened."

The birth attendant who assisted her, a very young girl, probably less than 20 years old, was asked about the night of the birth.

"We did everything we should have," she said, but she looked down at the floor, her voice hushed and unsure, fingers fidgeting.

Eventually, she took a deep breath, and looked back at me. The woman, she said, was her aunt. Her labor was delayed, and although she had been advised to deliver at the health center, she wanted to give birth at home. The traditional birth attendant did her a favor. In the middle of the birth, her aunt had collapsed and her breath had suddenly halted. The birth attendant began to cry, repeating that she had only wanted to do what her aunt wanted her to do—she thought she was respecting her request. Thus we had an answer for the young woman's tragic death.

The village, however, was not satisfied. They decided that the birth attendant should no longer serve there. The woman's husband was still angry: "This is only partially her fault," he said of the birth attendant. "If the medics stated that my wife should deliver in the clinic, they should have been paying closer attention. They should have been following her pregnancy to make sure she went in when it was time. We've done our part. It's time for you to do yours."

This attack, while humbling for our medical staff, was the point at which I realized the people knew their rights—and they considered it a right to understand that which they did not. It was a nascence of awareness, a healthy sign of social change, not to mention the sobering effect on the souls of us clinicians.

IRRECONCILABLE DIFFERENCES

The woman on the delivery table looked at me very seriously and without blinking said, "If you don't do it here, they'll do it back in the village."

I sighed and looked at the traditional birth attendant who had accompanied the young woman. Mere minutes after the birth of a healthy baby boy, the woman asked us to stitch closed her old infibulation wound. Infibulation was the practice of suturing the labia majora together—a traditional surgical procedure that allowed for an opening only small enough for urine and menstrual blood to pass through. Once married, the opening was enlarged just enough for the penis to fit through. However, this scar tissue would once again need to be cut in order to deliver babies; otherwise the possibility was very high that the inflexible scar tissue would simply rip apart and cause a large vulval tear, requiring surgical repair.

We campaigned vigorously against infibulating females, since it was one of our most critical reproductive health goals.

"It's clean here," the TBA said. "If I take her back to the village, they'll use thorns to suture it; your hands are blessed."

I looked between the two women, weighing the issue—under anesthesia, the procedure wouldn't be so painful, and in the clinic the wound had less chance of becoming infected. At the same time, though, I did not want to send the message to the other members of the community that circumcision and infibulation were right, or circumcision alone, the procedure in which they remove the clitoris of young girls. Either way, it would be wrong, and unfortunately this was the dilemma we faced.

Outside the delivery room, the argument persisted. Every 2 months, medical cadres met to discuss the progress of the campaign against infibulation and female genital surgery in various regions. The effectiveness of the campaign against circumcision and infibulation was assessed in the meetings of village councils. Although our results were unimpressive, there were some signs of change.

In Hager, it seemed that a health worker was not doing enough to dissuade the nomads from the practice of infibulation. Some of the Front members at the meeting pointed out that incidents of female circumcision were declining in most of the villages, but in the area which this man oversaw, it remained steady.

Upon the man's arrival back in his village, he announced to the pastoralists that there would be no more female circumcision. "It is against the law," he told them forcefully, "and anyone who is caught performing or condoning this ritual will be arrested." Clearly, this man wanted to be able to bring results at the next meeting, to show that he had made positive changes in the community.

However, his forcefulness was met with defiance, most surprisingly from the women. "It's none of your business," they stated, shaking their heads at the man. He persisted, though, and kept pressing the issue on the people, until one afternoon the women came out of their huts, raising not only their voices in defiance but also their skirts—hems lifted to their knees in an act of rebellion as they cried, "You can't tell us what to do with our bodies!"

Higher authorities eventually had to intervene, and it was decided that the women could do whatever they wanted with their bodies; it was our place to give advice, but we could not impose our will. This traditional practice was something I strongly disagreed with, but the women's resistance was a healthy sign of the power of the community.

Although 33% of the EPLF cadres and 52% of the medical cadres were women, we made limited progress on the topic of circumcision and infibulation. The pastoralist women claimed that the surgeries, which were mandatory for all girls, had no negative effects on their health, even though we knew that the procedure often caused complications such as excessive bleeding, urinary retention, infection, cyst formation, keloids, fistula, and deformation of the pelvis.

The women, for the most part, argued adamantly that it was simply not possible to choose to not be circumcised—it was tradition, cleanliness, religion, morality, health, and beauty for them. One woman once told me that it is done because they love their daughters and want to protect them from ostracism in the community. Besides she said, "If you had to keep your mouth open, bugs and spiders would get in there. The same is true of our genitalia." Although some local religious leaders have indicated that there is no verse in the Koran supporting the practice and a few even regard infibulation as anti-Islamic, the practice continues.

In private, we occasionally found women who complained about the practice. The relatively rare women who had been circumcised in later life were far less in favor of the practice. A few even admitted that they did not want their daughters circumcised. The anti-FGS (female genital surgery) trend was fairly restricted to younger women, including TBAs, who generally avoided performing FGS, but older TBA and non-TBA women in the clan remained true to the custom, performing the surgery without hesitation. Even after so many years of living and working with the pastoralists, our stand against subjecting girls to genital surgery never made much of an impact.

BIRTH ATTENDANTS AND BAREFOOT DOCTORS

The high demand for health professionals grew with the nomadic communities' awareness of their own rights. Over the years, we trained over 200 TBAs and 350 village health workers to serve the different nomadic communities with whom they lived. Because of our proximity, we were able to offer training as well as monitor their activities over extended periods of time. When it came to childbirth, the TBAs performed wonders and saved countless lives. They referred those in need of surgical intervention to the nearest hospital, although it was often inaccessible.

Training the women was very difficult owing to their high illiteracy rate. Hot afternoons dragged on, and the sweat dripped from the overworked body of the TBA trainer as she tried to explain to overworked brains concepts that would make so much more sense if only they could be written down. We used a system of symbols based on those used by the World Health Organization (WHO) and labored day after day with these symbols until a girl asked, "Instead of teaching us all these symbols, signs, and designs, why not just teach us how to read? After all, the alphabet is made up of symbols, isn't it?" So we did.

The TBAs played important roles in these communities, especially because they were often the only accessible and affordable source of health care for women in that society. They would often impart information on the prevailing side effects of female circumcision. Given the high birthrate among pastoralists, TBAs were encouraged to provide family planning education, although it was not always met with support.

Overall, the medical services offered by the Front were an enormous success. The mobile health teams and TBAs were received very positively. In time, the Front grew larger and stronger. As the forces of the EPLF gained the upper hand and commanded control of a wider territory, we were able to build stationary hospitals and clinics all over the Sahel. The nomadic population of Eritrea finally had health services and the fighters had a home and a family in the Sahel.

NOMADS AND NATION BUILDING

In 1991, when we won the war, everything changed.

Many Front members left the rural landscape that had been our home for so many years, a flood of people going back to the cities. Several committees representing the population in the Sahel made their way to Asmara to appeal to the leaders of the Front, who were now the government of Eritrea. Their questions were simple: "Why are the schools closed? Why aren't the health clinics helping us anymore? Where are the doctors?" They missed the spirited camaraderie they had had with the health workers and teachers. But the dynamics of relationship had changed. Now they were subjects living at the periphery, again forgotten by the center. One pastoralist, reminiscing about the level of commitment to the community evinced by the health cadres during the war and the current lack thereof, recounted a recent incident:

> One night in our village, a pregnant woman was bitten by a snake and we wanted to take her to Wade health station. However, because the health unit was far away and the patient was restless, we resolved not to take her. We sent a messenger to the health worker but he was unwilling to come. After some time, the woman passed away in front of our eyes. If the health worker had been one of us, he would have been available at any time and in any place.

There were few listening to the legitimate requests of the pastoralists. The government decided to settle all the nomadic communities permanently. We tried to persuade state officials that movement was the crux of the pastoralist lifestyle and that the settlement of nomadic communities in other countries, such as Libya and Somalia, had failed. But the political game had changed. The desires of the pastoralists were overruled by state proclamation. Having a say in their lives was considered an offense the new nation could not tolerate.

Many of Eritrea's pastoralists admit that nomadic life has become increasingly difficult and risk-prone. The impact of 30 years of war, responsible for many deaths and injuries and a landscape littered by land mines, has taken its toll. The nomads' ability to protect themselves against the risks of drought and advancing desertification has greatly diminished. Political instability in the Horn of Africa has forced many to flee their homes and traditional routes and to settle in neighboring countries. The Afar, relatively poor compared with the Tigre and the worst affected by drought, are resorting to salt mining, wage labor, and trade, which offer a meager living.

The precariousness of their position within modern states and their vulnerability in times of political instability feature predominantly in the life of all the pastoralist groups. Over the years, the pastoralists have taken charge of their own survival and moved around the region irrespective of imposed constraints and boundaries—not, however, without cost. As conflicts arouse border sensitivity, local and regional authorities on all sides create obstacles and are hostile toward or suspicious of peoples insensitive to what are, in geographical terms, artificial boundaries.

To the Eritrean pastoralist community, freedom means the right to live the life of their choice without interference. To the totalitarian regime that has taken control of the country, it means forcibly settling those who wish to remain unsettled. As an elderly pastoralist said in disdain, "I was part of the struggle for freedom, so that my goats could move back and forth freely, without any fear, in peace. Now my mobility is limited and my security is threatened. Where is my liberty?"

2 The People's Health Center: Building Primary Health Care in Bangladesh

Zafrullah Chowdhury and S. L. Bachman

In the spring of 1972, nearly two dozen young men and women drove along a two-lane highway through a dry landscape scattered with slender date palms and sturdy jackfruit trees. The small group parked beside the highway and pitched three rugged canvas army tents in which they would live and work during the coming months.

Recent years had been filled with violence and political turmoil. When the men and women were young children, the British ended their colonial rule in India and the Indian subcontinent was divided into Pakistan and India. Pakistan had two wings more than 1,000 miles apart, with the vast plains of India in between. The new capital of Pakistan was built in the west, even though more than half of Pakistan's total population lived in the east. East Pakistan had rich agriculture and many rivers. Although the East Pakistanis had their own language (*Bangla*), political history, and culture, the military regime of West Pakistan ruled the country and exploited East Pakistan in the name of "Islamic unity." For more than two decades, the people of East Pakistan struggled to make their voices heard in Pakistani politics, with no result.

Then a chain of events began that would rapidly lead to a civil war. In 1970, a cyclone in the southern region of East Pakistan killed over 250,000 people. At that time, the president of Pakistan was in Dhaka, the capital of East Pakistan, but he did not bother to visit the cyclone-devastated area.

Soon after the cyclone, Pakistan had a national election. The Awami League of East Pakistan under the leadership of Sheikh Mujibur Rahman won an absolute majority, which entitled him to become the prime minister of Pakistan. West Pakistani leaders, however, blocked him from taking office or implementing a plan for East Pakistan's autonomy. Protests were held all over East Pakistan. In March 1971, the Pakistan Army attacked the people of East Pakistan, slaughtering thousands. East Pakistanis fought back and declared independence. The liberation war lasted until December 16, 1971, when Pakistan was defeated and Bangladesh was born.

The small group of men and women had participated in the war, and now, as their country was healing and starting over, they decided also to heal. On that dry patch of land, they would build a hospital and village health center as part of a health service incorporating paramedic workers—a generation before such workers became common in developed countries such as the United States and United Kingdom.

If you come to Gonoshasthaya Kendra[i] (GK) in Savar today, what you'll see will look nothing like the desolate place it was in 1972. Instead, there is a brick wall beside a busy highway, a gate guarded by women in khaki uniforms, tall trees and flower gardens, and a four-story hospital with 150 beds. Inside are vaccination clinics, a pathology lab, and more. In addition to doctors and paramedics, you will see dentists, physiotherapists, and student doctors studying at the community-oriented medical college, which is part of the private university started by GK.

See the palm, mango, mahogany, arjun, and teak trees that surround the hospital? We planted those trees. See the brick driveways and paths running from one building to the next? We set each of those bricks in place. See the vegetable fields? GK doctors, paramedics, and other workers pulled ploughs, or drove teams of water buffalo, or chopped the mud with small shovels to level the fields so that we could plant green rice seedlings and spread vegetable seeds on the red soil. In 1974, government mismanagement, more natural disasters, and the war's aftermath caused a famine in Bangladesh. To this day, some 60% of all Bangladeshi children are malnourished. Our staff was determined to do what we could to supply ourselves with food. It was unusual for Bangladeshi doctors to work in agriculture fields, but GK doctors worked alongside all other GK staff members to produce as much as we could.

When you visit GK today, you may see a few cars, trucks, and three-wheeled delivery vans starting their engines in the small parking lot beside the hospital, waiting to pick up doctors, paramedics, and workers going to one of GK's other satellite health centers or GK's six-story urban hospital in Dhaka city. Some trucks might be going to the textile factory in Sirajganj to the west, or to distribute milk for GK's Tulip Dairy. Early every morning, you'll still see doctors, paramedics, teachers, and others weeding and doing other agricultural work.

A bit later in the day, walking out of the main gate in the morning light, you'll see the paramedics again. Most are young women, each carrying a shoulder bag containing medicine, a blood pressure cuff, a stethoscope, a thermometer, a diagnostic set, measuring tape, testing kits for examining urine albumin and sugar, and a nail cutter. The paramedics are also carrying cards for families that are part of GK's Community Health Insurance scheme, as well as family information cards and blank receipts to be filled out when the paramedics sell one of the medicines they are allowed to dispense in the villages. The paramedics dress like normal middle-class professionals in colorful salwar kameez[ii] or sarees or pants and shirts. Most ride bicycles. Some walk in single file at the roadside. They are headed toward the villages, where they will go from house to house delivering preventive and curative health care to the community—especially to pregnant mothers, newborn babies, and elderly and disabled people.

A DAY IN THE LIFE OF A PARAMEDIC

One of the paramedics, Nahar Akhter, a young woman about 19 years of age, breaks away from the group and walks down a dusty village path.

Nahar Akhter weaves between houses of mud and corrugated metal, heading toward a village, her scarf billowing from her shoulder. She steps into a tiny mud-floored courtyard in front of a small corrugated-metal hut barely tall enough to stand in. She first stops to see a young man who has lived there every day of his 6 weeks of life. Now is the time for his checkup.

"How is the new baby?" Nahar coos.

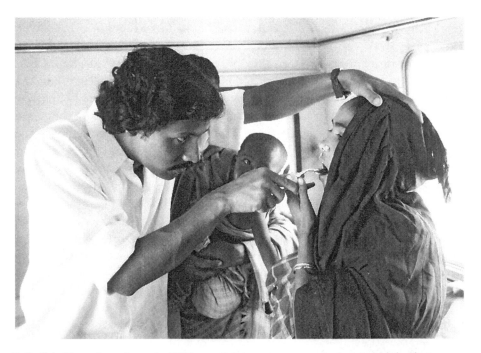

Zafrullah Chowdhury in early 1977 examining a woman patient at a mobile clinic run by Gonoshasthya Kendra. (Photo: Steve Jones.)

The baby's mother, her saree loosely wrapped around her body, hands over the child and begins to prepare food for the afternoon meal, which is the big meal of the day. The washing of rice and raw lentils, cutting up of vegetables, and cooking will last for at least 2 hours. In stray moments, she will breast-feed her son.

Nahar records the boy's weight, the circumference of his upper arm, and his body temperature. She reaches into her vaccine carrier and pulls out a vial of DPT (diphtheria/pertussis/tetanus) vaccine. After injecting the vaccine into the baby's left thigh, she helps the baby open his mouth and places oral polio vaccine drops onto his tongue. Then she injects a dose of bacille Calmette-Guérin (antituberculosis) vaccine into the baby's arm and a hepatitis B vaccine into the baby's right thigh. Nahar fills out the vaccination card and gives it to the mother with a reminder to keep it in a safe place. Finally, Nahar records the vaccines and everything else she has done with the baby on the yellow GK family card. She then turns her attention to the baby's grandparents.

"Nana,"[iii] she addresses the grandfather, who has been weaving a floor mat from strips of palm fronds, "Put away your mat for a moment and come sit by me."

Nahar takes his blood pressure and records it on the family card. She reaches into the bag again and pulls out a small nail clipper. Gently, she holds the old man's hands and feet and clips his nails while explaining the importance of keeping toenails and fingernails short and clean.

For the rest of the day, Nahar visits more homes in the village. On her last stop, she examines a pregnant woman. Nahar pushes the woman's saree away from her belly and presses a stethoscope against it to listen to the baby's heartbeat. She also measures the woman's ankle to check for swelling. She tests the expectant mother's blood hemoglobin and checks her urine for traces of protein, to determine whether the woman has preeclampsia.

Preeclampsia, which is a hypertensive disorder, is a sign of a very high risk pregnancy. Eclampsia causes convulsions before, during, or after labor and can lead to death. Any patient with preeclampsia becomes a high priority. One sign of preeclampsia is traces of protein in urine. Paramedics check for protein, in the pathology lab or even in a home by holding a vial of a pregnant woman's urine over the flame of a small spirit (alcohol) lamp. The heat will cause any protein to coagulate. If the pregnant woman did have preeclampsia, the paramedic would tell her that it was a sign of danger and needs special attention, therefore referring her to the maternal outpatient department at GK's health center to consult a medical doctor. If the woman and her family have not yet enrolled in GK's health insurance program, the paramedic will explain its benefits.

When Nahar's work for the day is finished, she walks back to GK. If we had been with her on other days, we might have seen her working with a team of paramedics—vaccinating children for polio, talking to mothers-in-law, collecting blood to ascertain the blood groups of pregnant women (in case one such woman should hemorrhage and require an emergency blood transfusion), or treating patients in the hospital.

Nahar eats lunch in a big dining hall, and then returns to her room for a bath and rest. In the evening, she and other paramedics walk down a brick path from their dormitory to the hospital for the nightly meeting—known as the reflection meeting. Here, she and her fellow paramedics will tell their supervisors about the patients they encountered during the day and discuss any questions or complications.

You might wonder what took place between 1972 and today—what was involved in the creation of all this. The answer is a lot. It involved, among other things, a book, a change of heart, my mother, hundreds of Bengali men and women— *especially* the women—a war, a military ruler with a university education, an arson, and a murder.

BEFORE THE WAR

I am a son of the middle class. In Third World countries, sons of the middle class are ambitious. They harvest the benefits that their countries accrue from the hard work and the sweat of the toiling masses. When I was a young man, I heard that plastic surgery paid well. I moved to Britain to study postgraduate medicine. But Pakistan already had one plastic surgeon, so I decided to become the first vascular surgeon. I worked hard to learn cardiovascular surgery, and I got good results. I also took an interest in investing in the stock market, driving fancy cars, and learning to fly in my spare time.

Then, I read *Away with All Pests*, a book by a British surgeon who had worked in China after the revolution. The book's message was that one must help the common people first. They are the lifeline of any society. If they survive and prosper, the country will prosper. *Away with All Pests* had a significant impact on the way I thought of my role in life. I asked myself, "What am I doing living a nice life in England? Why are poor people around the world, and in my country, not getting basic medical care?" Finally, I met Prof. Joshua Horn, the book's author. Talking with him, I was further inspired to work for the people who have the least.

When the civil war broke out in Pakistan, I was still living in England. East Pakistani students living overseas, like me, had been agitating for independence for years and wanted to help. Within 2 weeks, we had formed the Bangladesh Medical Association in the United Kingdom. I was elected the organization's general secretary. In early May, my friend Dr. M. A. Mobin and I arrived in India to join the freedom struggle of Bangladesh.

BANGLADESH FIELD HOSPITAL

During our first meeting with the Mukhti Bahini[iv] commanders, we explained who we were and that we had come to provide medical care for the wounded freedom fighters and refugees.

The commander in charge said, "I don't need doctors and medicines. I only need soldiers and weapons. Go and join the guerillas."

We were disappointed, but, as it happened, I had trained during my student days with the University Officers Training Corps (UOTC) in Dhaka in the late 1950s. I had also received voluntary training with the British Territorial Reserve Army in England and I had acquired a provisional private pilot's license for flying small planes.

As weeks passed and many people in senior positions were wounded, the commanders changed their minds. A group of us started searching for land on which to build a makeshift hospital.

We were helped by Mr. Habul Banerjee, an old Indian freedom fighter, who had fought along with Netaji Subhash Bose against the British. Mr. Banerjee offered us a few acres of land in Melaghar, 30 kilometers from Agartala, the capital of Tripura, an Indian state on East Pakistan's eastern border.

Once we had the land, we built, with the help of the local people, a simple, basic hospital: walls of woven bamboo slats, roof of a bamboo mat covered by grass thatch, and a floor of pounded earth. The operating theater was a small, clean room, lit by kerosene lamps and torchlights.

Once we had our hospital, we realized that we needed nurses. Surgeons are key, but nurses are the most important. Health care, like sports, requires teamwork. We sought permission from the Provisional Government of Bangladesh to bring British nurses—who had excellent education, training, skill, and dedication—to our hospital.

The political leaders were horrified. They said, "We cannot guarantee their safety. They could be killed in battle; they might write back to their homes about how many casualties we have."

So Mobin and I began looking around, trying to think of what to do. People were dying, and our hospital was severely understaffed.

Meanwhile, hundreds of girls were living in our refugee camps in India, and all of them wanted to join the freedom struggle to fight the Pakistani Army. The provisional government and army leadership did not want to take them. Thousands of women were being raped in occupied East Pakistan by Pakistani troops and their Bengali collaborators. The Bangladeshi leaders did not want to expose any more of our women to the risk of rape and other dangers.

I began to think of the girls in the camps in a different way. Their lives reminded me of my mother's younger life. She had always been clever, but her father, a Muslim religious leader, refused to let her attend school.

I also remembered *Away with All Pests*, which described "barefoot doctors," ordinary people trained in basic health care, when China had very few medical doctors and surgeons. We started to realize that the more education you have, the more you will think that education is needed to do the simplest things. This is one way we close the door to the poor. To be a doctor, you need 20 years of education and training; it takes 3 or 4 years after 10 years of basic schooling to be a nurse.

Poor people are seldom able to pursue many years of schooling, and by requiring that, we do not allow them to enter into our professional arena.

Together, Mobin and I convinced the leaders to give the girls a chance. True, they were young and inexperienced, but they were brave.

We began to train the girls almost immediately.

Even though they had never worked in a medical clinic, every girl quickly mastered every task, from simply counting the pulse to giving intravenous fluid in a vein.

The girls and young women—Gita Kar, Ira Kar, Gita Chakrabarty, Khuku, Nilima, Padma, Dalia, Tulu, Lulu, and many others—did phenomenal work, helping us in all realms of medical care. Soon, we sent for more girls, until hundreds were trained. We worked during the days and trained them at night, so that their knowledge—of selecting and administering medications, assessing patients' symptoms, and evaluating pathology and blood tests—was constantly growing.

The war was a great time of unity, and the women were happy that they were doing something purposeful. Men and women worked together. Hindus and Muslims worked together. It was revolutionary to have young, unmarried Hindu women with only basic medical training tending to the wounds and illnesses of young, unmarried Muslim male fighters. In peacetime, many people would have been shocked.

The hospital grew—in size and in reputation as well as in numbers of doctors, medical students, and volunteers—until we had 480 beds. One morning, when I looked across the hospital at all the newly trained women and girls now working as nurses, I realized that Mobin and I did not build and operate the hospital ourselves as we had planned to do. Hundreds of girls had done everything. We were delighted, but even then we did not realize that we had been so innovative—we had experimented with a new cadre of health workers who would not only transform Third World health systems but also influence health care systems in the western world.

BUILDING GONOSHASTHAYA KENDRA

The war ended very quickly, after only 9 months. The other doctors and I had just begun to learn how well we could train people and how much we could learn from them. After the war was over, most of the doctors wanted to live in the cities, even though most people who needed medical care lived in villages. Village life was difficult: there were few roads, no clean water, no electricity. Doctors had to operate on patients by lantern light. To live an easier life, many doctors left for Britain and other countries.

I could have gone back to a country that was rich and prosperous and had a nice life, or I could have stayed in my country and helped build it. There would not be money in Bangladesh, but there was already so much opportunity. I stayed. Mobin became disgusted with the new government administration and left. He is now an orthopedic and casualty surgeon in the U.K.

The remaining doctors and the young health workers we had trained moved to Dhaka. Gradually, we decided we needed to build a real hospital and health program in the villages. We were joined by Dr. Abul Qasem Chowdhury one of my friends from Dhaka Medical College; we share a common last name, but he is from a different family. Another friend's family donated a piece of land 22 miles outside of the city, in Savar subdistrict. The land was located next to the main road going west toward India.

In those days, there were a few two-lane highways, and many smaller dirt roads that led to villages. The traffic then was moderate, and before our hospital was built, Qasem and I, along with the men and women who joined the new organization, lived in tents near a jackfruit tree by the road.

Savar is hot and dry. Although rivers flow through it and green trees and palms grow in the villages, the heat and lack of rain mean that farmers who cannot irrigate their crops can harvest only once a year, compared to two or three harvests in other parts of Bangladesh. That is one reason why, when we first arrived in Savar, the people there were very poor.

Our first months were difficult. Immediately after the war, there was famine. Nothing was growing on the land we had been given. One of the first things we did was clear the bushes and weeds to plant vegetables and dig paddy fields to grow rice. We named our clinic in Savar the Bangladesh Hospital in remembrance of our Bangladesh Field Hospital in Tripura. The government's health secretary objected, because the name sounded like that of a government hospital. We consulted Bangladesh's new prime minister, Sheikh Mujibur Rahman. He chose the name Gonoshasthaya Kendra, the People's Health Center. We put up a sign with our new name by our tents. We held our first health clinics under the jackfruit tree, as tall as a house with thick leaves that offered a deep shade. Hundreds of people came with common complaints: diarrhea, scabies, upper respiratory disease, peptic ulcer, constipation, gallbladder pain, common eye problems, skin diseases, renal colic. Many of their symptoms were complications of poverty and hunger.

We also began taking a census of the local villages and talking with people about their needs, hopes, and desires. We quickly decided that holding clinics in fixed locations was not enough. We needed to send health workers from house to house, especially to help the poor women and children whose health problems made up the bulk of our work. The women we had trained in the field hospital began going to the villages, and GK began training more volunteers to become paramedics.

LIFE IN THE VILLAGE

Living outside of the city, in a village, helped us learn about the people we wanted to help. Sometimes—actually, quite often—we thought we were helping when really we were showing our ignorance.

Here is a typical story.

In the very early morning, in a village, around 4 A.M., you will find the farmers singing and plowing the land. They sing to keep themselves company and also to keep up their strength while doing hard work.

Their singing used to keep me awake. Finally one morning I got out of bed and walked to the rice field right next to my hut. The farmers were surprised when they saw me. One asked if they had disturbed my sleep.

I said, "Of course you did! When are you going to be civilized? Why can't you come after having your breakfast at 8 or 9 o'clock? Work in the daytime and in the afternoons, then go back and be with your families."

They were silent. I continued on like a high priest giving a sermon. When I paused for breath, one man, who looked old because of undernourishment and hard work said, "Doctor, have you ever worked in the sun?"

I said, "Well, haven't you seen me? Every day I go to the village to educate your people, your children. I work hard. I take my breakfast and then at 9 o'clock, I go to your village."

The man said, "Yes, we have seen you with your shoes and umbrella. But have you ever cut paddy or dug earth, while the sun shines on the top of your head?"

Now this was my time of silence. The farmer started giving me a bigger lecture. He said, "If you had ever done that, then you would understand why we come to work so early in the morning or past midnight when the moon shines and the air is cool, when it is easy to work. Later in the day, when the sun is hot, it is more difficult to plow. By noon, when the sun is starting to beat on our heads, we have finished plowing or planting. We are done with the work. Then we go back with our families and children, go to the pond, take a bath, take our lunch, and then in the afternoon we go to a nearby market to sell our products. What is wrong with that?"

That was the day I realized that if I wanted to be of use, I would have to adjust myself to their schedule. I told myself: Don't expect 74 million people to change for you.[v]

At this time, GK was growing. We began to take on local young people and train them as health workers. At first we took both boys and girls, but we soon discovered that girls had an advantage. They could enter the family quarters at any time and examine pregnant women and women with gynecological problems without embarrassing the patients or their husbands.

Every night, we would gather around a lantern and talk for hours. We shared stories from our day in the villages, our concerns, and our ideas. We'd then lecture on topics that came up in these discussions, using a blackboard to illustrate concepts and providing the health-care workers with a steady stream of information.

Gradually, we learned that if we wanted to do anything in the community, we would need a large number of people to do the job. The trainers and doctors grew to understand that the paramedics and nurses were not their assistants—they were their partners and team members. Without them, we would not have a strong health care system. They are professionals in their own right.

One night when we were discussing the development of an agriculture program, Qasem returned from a village with this story.

He was observing a paramedic giving an injection, when a farmer spoke to him. He said, "Doctor, do you believe that you are doing a good thing?"

Qasem said, "Yes, I am helping teach a paramedic how to give a vaccination. The vaccination will help keep your children healthy and living."

The man said, "Yes, I believe that the vaccinations work. The children will not become sick and they will live longer. But when they are adults, they will curse you."

Qasem was startled. "Curse me for what?"

The man said, "They will curse you for keeping them alive! You will have kept them from getting a disease, but you will not have solved the bigger problem, and that is hunger."

Qasem was silent.

The man said, "I tell you, doctor. If you invent a vaccination against hunger, you will be able to come here at 5:30 in the morning and find a line of people one kilometer long, waiting for your vaccine."

When Qasem went back to GK that night, he told the story. Soon, we started helping farmers to install deep tube wells for irrigation,[vi] distributing more vegetable seeds, and helping develop agriculture and employment, especially for women, in various other ways.

THE IMPORTANCE OF PARAMEDICS

The paramedics at GK do everything from basic health care to family planning to surgical operations. Because most of our health workers are from the community, they know the local language, dialects, and pronunciations. They also understand how the community mind works. As a result, they are often more effective in the field than doctors.

I learned this from experience.

One day, at a clinic, a mother complained to me that the medicine a doctor had prescribed had not gotten rid of her child's intestinal worms. A health worker then gave the patient the same medicine. When the mother next returned she exclaimed, "Ten worms came out!"

I asked the paramedic what she had said or done differently, and she explained. She had asked her patient's mother to get a clean glass of water, then had handed the child the six pills.

"Take one," the paramedic began, and after she saw the child swallow, she continued. "Now, please, one more. And now, please one more . . . one more. . . ." She had known that the villagers would never accept such a big dose at once, so she made sure that the child swallowed all six tablets in her presence.

New paramedics spend the first 2 years training at the Savar campus or the training center in Sreepur. They are trained in the classroom, during house-to-house village visits, and in the hospital. Hospital training includes basics such as pathology and recognizing the wide variety of health problems that patients bring into the clinic.

Paramedics spend most of their days in the field, visiting pregnant women, children, and the elderly, who suffer from lack of attention and care. Unlike doctors, the paramedics focus on preventive care. Most children die from preventable diseases such as tetanus, whooping cough, diphtheria, and polio. Our paramedics give vaccines to prevent all these diseases. They also treat worms, diarrhea, pneumonia, and skin diseases, which, if not treated, can lead to the destruction of the kidneys.

After each day in the field, a paramedic will rest and then return to the hospital for a nighttime discussion with a supervisor about what was learned that day and what complications were seen. Senior GK paramedics learn specialized skills, such as simple surgery. Paramedics are also constantly retrained, to keep their skills fresh.

At GK, we stress the importance of teamwork. Paramedics know which symptoms they can treat on their own and when they should refer their patients to a doctor. Paramedics are trained to alert their colleagues in the hospital if any of their patents are expected to come for treatment. It is not uncommon to see one walking with a patient back to GK for further testing or treatment.

If the GK doctors do not have the necessary specialized medical skills to treat a patient, we refer him or her to the nearest specialized hospital. In this way, paramedics are part of a whole team of health workers, which includes the *dai* (or traditional birth attendant) in each village, the paramedic herself, the local nurses and doctors, and the specialists at the urban hospitals.

SEIZING OPPORTUNITIES

Often, we discovered that paramedics and women could do more than we thought simply because when they saw opportunities, they took them.

One day, a woman with obstructed labor came into the Savar hospital. The woman needed a cesarean operation immediately. No trained parasurgeons were around to help. Desperate, I looked at a paramedic in training who had been downgraded to the humble position of floor cleaner. We all thought she was unintelligent.

"I can help," she told me.

"Let's scrub up," I said.

As we stood side by side at the sink, I noticed that she was washing her hands in the same way that I was washing my own. I thought, "Well, she is a Muslim girl, and Muslims wash their hands before prayer." But she was washing her hands together, not separately, the way Muslims do when they avoid contact between the ritually clean right hand and the ritually unclean left hand. I was curious, but didn't have time to ask her.

The operation happened quickly. Soon, the baby came out and cried. I relaxed, thinking that I had just saved a life. As I began to sew up the incision, I began to ask the paramedic questions.

"How did you learn to scrub your hands so well?"

She said, "Every woman knows how to wash her hands. Moreover, I have seen you wash your hands many times."

"Well," I said. "How did you know what tools to hand me when I said, 'scissors,' 'artery forceps,' 'needles'?"

She laughed. "What woman hasn't seen scissors and needles? You use different English words but use signs as well and what you are doing now is just the kind of stitching which every woman does all her life."

I felt so small! Whatever I had done, there was no innovation in it. Every woman knows how to do it already. I wondered why, if she was so clever, she could not pass a test. Then I realized that she had never been to a school. She did not write notes or take written tests because she did not know how to write, not because she didn't understand what we had been teaching.

I asked her, "Would you like to do surgery?"

"Very much," she said, and she smiled.

So she learned how to do a minilaparotomy and other minor operations. She became news in Britain, where the headline of one of London's national dailies announced that she could not read or write but could operate as a parasurgeon.

Another time our paramedics made the most of their opportunities was when they began to ride bicycles.

One day in 1974, a young woman named Hosne Ara said she wanted to learn how to ride a bicycle. She said she was tired of walking to villages and it would be easier if she could ride a bike. So, on the brick path in front of the hospital, she practiced. Before long, she and all the other women paramedics joined the men in riding bicycles to the villages.

Village people were shocked at first. Men and women said, "GK paramedics are indecent!" They said it was against Islam to allow girls on a bicycle to pass through their villages. I went to the villages to face village leaders. I saw a village headman who had performed Haj (the pilgrimage to Mecca, Saudi Arabia). Some time back, I had sent his mother to Dhaka for an eye operation. I asked him about his mother's operation. The village leader replied that the operation had been successful and she had been well looked after in the hospital because of my letter.

I asked, "How did your mother go to Dhaka? Did she walk?" He replied, "Oh, no! Dhaka is far way. She went by bus and the bus was overcrowded."

In the overcrowded bus, the mother of the Haji had been touched and pushed by the male passengers. I said, "I hope that Allah will forgive you! But you know, if a girl rides a bicycle, she will not be touched by strange men. Moreover, during the wars fought by the Prophet Muhammad, he and his men were always nursed by women. If that was not 'indecent,' why do you say that these paramedics are indecent?"

After that, the Haji always supported our paramedics.

Gradually, other village people agreed with the Haji, and more paramedics became eager to learn how to ride a bike. Women on bicycles gained acceptance around Bangladesh, but not in all places or all at once: One paramedic riding a bicycle died after a truck pushed her off the side of the road. To show the nation that women on bicycles could work and maintain their dignity, we planned a combination of celebration and demonstration.

In 1977, on May 1, International Labor Day, 22 GK women workers, including a woman doctor, rode their bicycles all the way from GK's Savar campus to the Shaheed Minar in central Dhaka—22 miles! The Shaheed Minar is a monument to the students killed in 1952 during the preindependence movement to establish Bangla as an official language of Pakistan. Riding to the Shaheed Minar identified the women as Bangladeshi patriots. The next day, the newspapers had big headlines and photographs of the GK paramedics riding bicycles.

Today you can see women workers all over Bangladesh riding bicycles and motor scooters. You will also see a few woman professional drivers, and you can be sure that most of them were trained by GK in the nation's first professional driving program for women.

GONOSHASTHAYA PHARMACEUTICALS, LTD.

On your visit to the GK campus in Savar, you must not forget to visit the factory, Gonoshasthaya Pharmaceuticals Ltd. (GPL). To find GPL, you must leave the busy crowd at the hospital and walk halfway around the campus to a quiet area with a small gate. A woman guard will let you in. Once inside the gate, you will find a modest but pretty garden. You will also see a two-story building in the same brick-and-concrete style as the hospital. The air inside is cool, and the factory is simple and clean. Women in white coats and sandals that are worn only inside the building peer through microscopes, measure and mix pharmaceutical ingredients, fill capsules, manufacture tablets, and so on. Where the work is dusty, they wear white masks to cover the nose and mouth. The atmosphere is very serene.

GPL's history, though, is full of struggle.

From the start, we were shocked by how much drugs cost. They were so expensive that entire families became poor when one member got sick. When an earning member—the father, for example—became ill or injured, the family often had to take out loans or sell assets to buy medicine. They were left with huge debts. And there was corruption, too. The transnational corporations were, and are to this day, run as businesses and are willing to do almost anything to sell a product, even if the product is not safe or useful for patients.

In 1981, therefore, we started GPL to manufacture medicines on the WHO's (World Health Organization) list of "essential" medicines. It took 7 years to start the factory because of direct and indirect obstacles placed by the multinational companies as well as government bureaucratic inefficiency and corruption. Our first two products were the painkiller paracetamol and the antibiotic ampicillin.

At first, GPL had a very good share of the market. We were manufacturing much-needed drugs and selling them at half the previous market prices, something we thought would benefit not only the well-being of Bangladeshi people but also the integrity of the medical community. To our dismay, medical associations vehemently opposed GPL, and from 1982 to 1995, the doctors in the Bangladesh Medical Association (BMA) boycotted GPL products. This was for purely selfish reasons: Many of the doctors had links to pharmaceutical companies, and they profited from their investments. The president and other important members of the BMA had substantial shares in multinational drug companies. The then-secretary general of the BMA, Dr. Sarwar Ali, was also the medical director of Pfizer-Bangladesh, the local affiliate of the giant multinational Pfizer.

At first, our amoxicillin sold very well, and then it did not. We heard rumors that doctors were telling their patients that GPL products were inexpensive because they were no good. The truth was, they were inexpensive because we did not make much profit. But some doctors found tricks to fool their patients. For instance, they said GPL amoxicillin caused diarrhea, although diarrhea is a common side effect of amoxicillin from any manufacturer.

Our hard times continued. In 1984, the GPL factory was attacked by more than 2,000 hooligans who tried to set fire to the building. GK workers resisted; as a result, 63 female workers and 21 male workers were severely wounded. The factory remained open, but for months we endured written attacks in the newspapers. In 1990, another group of hooligans attacked and burned the Dhaka GPL office, stores, and vehicles.

NATIONAL DRUG POLICY

You may be wondering why people would be angry enough to act so violently and go to such great lengths to try to ruin GPL. Well, the answer is that they were angry with the military ruler who ran the country because they had been misled by doctors and politicians about policies he wanted to adopt, and they were angry with me for working with the government. Many thought the formulation of a pro-people drug policy might give the military ruler a good name.

In 1982, General H. M. Ershad became Bangladesh's military ruler. Although he was a military man, he had attended university and was well-read, and he wanted to do something good for the people.

General Ershad contacted me and proposed that Bangladesh should limit the drugs for sale in the marketplace to those that were essential or had therapeutic value. He called on me to formulate a national drug policy (NDP).

Initially, I did not want to work with him. What business did I have working with a dictator? I turned him down, but he was persistent. Some of my family and friends cautioned against working with a dictator; some were hopeful that I might be able to do some good.

Finally, I warned him that a pro-people drug policy would be opposed by the United States, the United Kingdom, and many other western governments. In 1974, for instance, after Sri Lanka adopted a policy limiting sales of some pharmaceutical formulations, the U.S. government threatened to cut off government aid. I told General Ershad that I would help him on one condition: If the new NDP faced opposition, he would make the policy's supporters and opponents face each other and he would act as a judge to decide himself whether to continue the plan or not.

General Ershad appointed an expert committee composed of some of Bangladesh's most famous doctors (and including me), which drew up a list of essential medicines to be retained and bad drugs to be discarded. General Ershad declared the policy effective beginning June 12, 1982. It accomplished a few things: it banned the sale of approximately 1,800 harmful, inappropriately formulated, or therapeutically ineffective drugs. It limited drug preparations and unnecessary combinations, which raise the price of formulations. It also limited drug prices to the cost of raw materials and assembly plus a reasonable maximum profit.

We knew there would be opposition, but we did not know just how far-reaching and powerful it would be. The leaders of industrialized countries became involved. The U.S. ambassador, Jane Coon, called on General Ershad and threatened him with a reduction of U.S. aid to Bangladesh. Then, when her threats proved ineffective, President Ronald Reagan invited General Ershad to visit Washington D.C., which for the president of Bangladesh is a very big honor. He went, and the Reagan administration tried to persuade him to scrap the drug policy.[vii]

Soon after the NDP was implemented, opponents insisted that we cancel it. General Ershad lived up to his gentlemen's agreement with me and called the members of the expert committee, which formulated the NDP, and NDP opponents to his office for a debate. We arrived in the afternoon. We waited outside for 5 hours as our opposition—represented by army doctors holding a brief prepared by experts belonging to the multinational corporations—argued their position. Through the door, we could hear arguing. Our opponents spoke mainly against me and against GK. We watched the light change and the sky become dark. Finally, I heard him say, "All right. You have told me what a terrible man Zafrullah is. Let him come in and speak for himself."

So we went in, armed with manuals, literature, slides, and documentation of facts and figures about various products. After some negotiating, the opponents agreed to allow the discussion of each banned formulation one at a time. Each time the opponents said that a formulation was perfectly safe, we would refer to a page of a manual or the literature we had brought with us and name a problem, reveal a side effect, or cite official information on how ineffective or harmful the drug was.

This went on for hours.

The last drug we discussed was clioquinol, popularly known by the brand name Enterovioform. It was used very commonly, especially by army physicians, to combat diarrhea.

The drug policy's opponents said that the drug was perfectly safe.

I referred to the manual in front of me, and said, "But General Ershad, do you know about the side effects?"

"No."

"Have you ever taken that drug?"

"Yes, of course many times. The army physicians prescribe it all the time. And I have had no problem." We thought that we had lost the case, and we remained silent for a minute or two while looking for the proper response.

Suddenly, I noticed General Ershad take off his spectacles. I asked him if he had been wearing glasses for a long time, even before taking clioquinol, or had his eyesight deteriorated since he had taken the drug.

"Did your ophthalmologist ask you whether you had used clioquinol?" I asked.

Gen. Ershad answered that he had used the drugs for many years but his eyesight had deteriorated only recently.

I showed him the current literature, which said that prolonged use of clioquinol had been linked to ocular degeneration and optic neuropathy. Now, safer alternatives are available.

"That is enough for me," he said. "The drug policy stands."

Today, local pharmaceutical manufacturers are grateful. The policy we set in place requires that certain medications be made only in Bangladesh, a guideline that has strengthened local companies. But the multinational companies and their allies have picked away at the policy, piece by piece. About 60% of the original policy remains, and we have had to sacrifice in order to hold onto this much. When the expert committee formulated the original NDP, we had hopes that a national health policy would fall into place beside it. Such a policy would, for instance, have banned private practice by government doctors, many of whom collect both their government salaries and the fees paid by private patients they see in their own clinics, often on government time. Together, the two policies would have reduced the cost and improved the quality of all health care.

The BMA and other medical organizations opposed the health policy as vehemently as they had the drug policy. In 1990, when General Ershad was driven from power and an interim government took over, the national health policy was canceled for good.

CHALLENGES REMAIN

Behind the four-story hostel where the paramedics in training stay, several tall trees shade two graves. The graves are low, rectangular brick walls surrounding patches of bare soil. In front of each one is a waist-high pillar of brick, topped with a marble tablet etched with names, dates, and other information in Bengali lettering.

One is the grave of an agricultural worker who was killed when GK staff members defended GK land from encroachment by another landowner. The other is the grave of a health worker who was killed by assassins hired by a corrupt local political leader and an influential village doctor who feared that GK's services for the poor would cut into his business and increase people's awareness of local corruption.[viii]

Death is a big price to pay for helping the poor. We have carried on in the spirit of building our nation.

Today, GK works in almost 600 villages of Bangladesh, providing health care for a population of over a million people, which makes it one of the largest service providers in the health sector outside of the national government. We have also trained thousands of health workers for nongovernmental organizations throughout the country and some abroad and have helped to shape government policy. The employment, development, and emergency projects around the nation that we operate are too numerous to mention.

About half of GK's recurrent expenditures are covered by money generated by its activities, such as its health insurance scheme and service fee. The other half is covered by its business ventures (e.g., the pharmaceutical factory) and other funding sources.

GK's insurance system classifies people into four categories and charges them enrollment and service fees accordingly. The destitute and very poor are charged an enrollment fee in Taka that comes to no more than US $0.10 per year per family.[ix] For the next class, the poor, the enrollment fee is about US $0.20 cents per year per family. Patients in the middle-class category are charged an enrollment fee of less than US $1 per year per family, and for people in the wealthier class, the enrollment fee is the equivalent of about US $1.20 per year per family. (Fees are higher for smokers.)

Patients also pay a fee, on a sliding scale according to their insurance category, for each visit to the clinic. When they purchase prescribed medicines, the fee also is calculated on a sliding scale.

GK's health statistics are better than those in the rest of Bangladesh. That is both good news and bad news: GK has demonstrated ways of reducing maternal mortality and morbidity, helping women survive pregnancy and childbirth, and helping their babies thrive. How long will it take before these measures are adopted throughout Bangladesh?

Despite the poverty of the areas served by GK, data for the last decade in GK's service areas show steady and significant declines in perinatal, neonatal, and infant mortality rates. The maternal mortality ratio (MMR) in GK's service area is considerably lower than the national MMR—by at least 42%.[x]

How can this success be explained?

First, every single pregnant woman in GK's service area receives antenatal care services during her pregnancy, compared with less than half for the country as a whole. Also, 97% of pregnant women in the GK service area received tetanus tox-oid vaccinations, compared with 70% for the country as a whole.

Second, starting from the very first moment a woman is identified as being pregnant, GK health workers determine whether she is at high risk for complications. GK workers closely monitor the health status of all pregnant women, and especially high-risk mothers, providing follow-up services that include treatment and the timely referral of complicated cases to specialist health facilities.

Third, when a woman dies, GK personnel attend her funeral ceremony and then conduct a verbal autopsy with an independent team headed by a GK doctor and a government medical officer. After finalizing the verbal autopsy report, a discussion meeting is called, under the authority of the local government in the village of the deceased woman, to discuss the cause of death. The local Ministry of Health official is invited to attend, as are teachers, religious leaders, and other members of the Village Health Committee, which GK organizes in each village. A detailed discussion is conducted with these officials as well as with the community as a whole to determine the possible cause of maternal death. Together with the community and the *dai* or traditional birth attendant (TBA), the group explores whether or not this death could have been avoided, and if so, how. This has a huge social awakening impact.[xi]

Fourth, over 90% of births/deliveries in the GK service area take place at home, but most (87%) of them are attended by TBAs and closely supervised by trained paramedics, compared with only 24% at the national level. GK strongly believes in the TBAs and tries to ensure that TBAs are recognized for their skills and the important role they play in maintaining a community's health. By working with TBAs, GK tries to help the community take responsibility for its own health while also helping community members trust their own ability to learn.

Additionally, our paramedics and GK-trained TBAs have brought down the infant mortality rate by following a program of several steps, all of which help to create a healthy home. The program includes (1) promptly identifying babies (within 12 hours of birth) with pneumonia, diarrhea, or other illnesses and ensuring their proper treatment; (2) promoting breast-feeding and appropriate supplementary feeding; (3) ensuring easy access to safe drinking water, which is critical to reduce the incidence of childhood diarrhea; (4) launching a vigorous campaign against smoking; and (5) persuading families to limit their family size, thus encouraging them to give more attention, food, and care to each child.

We are constantly trying to improve the way we help our community by adopting new ideas, equipment, or techniques. Paramedics today, for instance, are trained to use auroscopes (for examining ears), fetal monitors, and an oxygen-supply machine. They are trained in blood grouping, collecting blood for transfusions, and in blood cross-matching. They also can use some 20 essential medicines.

The spread of mobile phones into every village in Bangladesh has allowed patients, especially pregnant women, to contact us whenever they have questions or concerns. The mobile phones of the paramedics' supervisors ring day and night with calls from pregnant women and their families. Depending on the situation, the supervisors send paramedics or doctors to check on patients in their village homes, or, in an emergency, send an ambulance.

Often, a TBA will call with news of a birth. GK medical personnel must see every newborn baby within 12 hours of birth.

GK has tried to keep alive the unity built during the war, but we still have a long path to travel and many obstacles to overcome.

Although China's "barefoot" doctors are still perhaps the most famous paraprofessional medical workers in modern times, health systems around the world depend on paraprofessionals today—and GK was in the vanguard of incorporating them into a complete health service. What GK started by training paraprofessionals in the 1970s, the American health system picked up the idea in the late 1980s through physician assistant and nurse practitioner programs. In the 1990s, the British Royal College of Physicians recommended a new type of health service provider similar to GK's paramedics. In 1994, the British Health Ministry allowed nurses to take more curative responsibilities, including the prescription of certain drugs.

Both the United States and the U.K. acted after a developing country had led the way. We shall continue developing and improving the model of a health system that incorporates paraprofessionals in a whole team of health workers, from the village *dai* to the paramedic herself to the local nurses and doctors and finally to the specialists at the urban hospitals.

There will surely be obstacles ahead—we only hope that there will be no more murders or arsons—but we will persevere, as we have in the past, and we shall win.

NOTES

i. *Gonoshasthaya Kendra* is a Bangla phrase. *Gono* means "people," *Shasthaya* means "health," and *Kendra* stands for "center"—People's Health Center.
ii. A *salwar kameez* is a knee-length tunic combined with long, loose pants, which are worn by men and women in many parts of South Asia. Women add a long scarf, called an *orna* or *dupatta*.
iii. *Nana* means maternal grandfather and is one of several words used for old men, whether or not related to the speaker.
iv. *Mukhti Bahini* means "freedom brothers" but is usually translated as "freedom fighters."
v. Bangladesh's population is now more than 150 million.
vi. In the 1990s, arsenic was discovered in well water in many places in Bangladesh. Fortunately, most of the GK program areas were spared this problem. An exception is Kashinathpur. There, GK is trying to raise community awareness and is supporting a variety of medical treatments for arsenic-associated medical conditions, including the use of arsenic filters and homeopathy.

vii. For details, please see *The Politics of Essential Medicines* (London: Zed Press, 1995).

viii. The paramedic who died after a truck pushed her and her bicycle off the road is buried elsewhere, at her family's request.

ix. Using an exchange rate of Taka 60 to US $1.

x. The MMR in GK's service area is 186 per 100,000 deliveries in 2002–2005 (the most recent data available). See Rafiqul Huda Chaudhury, Zafrullah Chowdhury, Achieving the millennium development goal on maternal mortality: Gonoshasthaya Kendra's experience in rural Bangladesh. Dhaka: *Gonoprokashani*, April 2007, p. xiv).The national MMR rate in 2001 (the most recent data available) was 320 deaths per 100,000. www.unfpa-bangladesh.org/php/about_bangladesh.php, and "Health, Nutrition & Population Programme Proposal (HNPPP), July 2003–June 2010," January 2005, www.mohfw.gov.bd/hnppp.htm, accessed June 7, 1007.

xi. Paramedics and immediate supervisors must also prepare detailed case reports explaining why cases of maternal or neonatal/infant death were not prevented. Each case report, which must be prepared within 72 hours and preferably 24 hours, is verified in a field visit by the next higher level of health supervisor. A GK doctor investigates death reports on random selection.

3 The Whole Is Greater: How Polio Was Eradicated from the Western Hemisphere

Ciro A. de Quadros

FIRST STEPS: SMALLPOX, 1960–1977

The DC3 plane rattled its way through low-lying clouds, carrying a full load of passengers, supplies, and me to the remote town of Altamira in Brazil. I drew the back of my hand across my forehead and it came back damp from sweat. Having grown up in the southern part of the country, I was unfamiliar with this kind of heat. We approached the landing strip, and I caught a view of the Xingu River weaving through the Amazon River Valley, long, slow, and blue against the bright greens of the jungle. Despite its proximity to the river, Altamira could not be reached by boat, as it was upstream of a large waterfall and when I arrived, no roads had yet been built.

After landing, I went immediately to the health center compound, where I was to work as the head doctor. The center was constructed, like many other buildings in the Amazon basin, of thick cement, brick, and wood, with openings on the top to allow heat to escape. Mango trees shaded the compound, and everywhere I walked there were fruit and vegetable plants growing.

I had just finished my medical studies then, in 1966, and although I had never been in charge of an assignment like this, I was full of energy and ambition to do good work. Inside the health center, I found the small staff already assembled: a community nurse, a sanitary inspector, a lab technician, an administrator, and a janitor. After briefly introducing myself to them and receiving their equally brief introductions, I launched into my purpose for being there.

"We've been given clear objectives," I said to them. "Patient visits, vaccination targets, the building of latrines, and the formation of clean water lines to connect to the houses." I spoke loudly and clearly, and paused to let the objectives sink in. Then I asked, "How are we going to get this done?"

The staff sat silently for a moment. I stood in front of them waiting for their ideas. Soon, the community nurse spoke.

"Vaccinationsⁱ can happen here at the clinic. We can do outreach, schedule appointments with each family, and then track the families so we know that everyone's been vaccinated." I nodded.

The lab technician spoke up next: "The traditional birth attendants could help us."

"How so?" I asked.

"They could direct us to the homes of the newborns they've delivered."

For the next few hours, the health center staff and I worked together to create a comprehensive program for addressing local health-care needs. I took a tour of the compound, assessing our resources. My role as head doctor meant much more than diagnosing and treating patients; if I wanted to help the people of Altamira, I needed to learn about the community itself. By familiarizing myself with what infrastructure already existed politically and socially, I would be able to develop ways to work with that structure to meet our objectives.

So, in the days that followed, I found myself fast becoming a part of the brain trust of the town, connecting with local authorities, agricultural cooperatives, bank managers, and community leaders. Twice a week, the community nurse and the sanitary inspector conducted home visits, looking for children who failed to come to scheduled appointments, and then referred their mothers back to the clinic for vaccination. When we visited patients in their homes, we were always welcomed. They offered us coffee, food, whatever they had to give. We made small talk about the garden, whether water and latrines had been set up already, if the children and other household members were well.

Our community-based efforts proved very effective. At that time, in most of Brazil and other developing countries, immunization rates were well below 10%. In contrast, by the end of our year of hard work and careful planning, immunization rates in Altamira had reached almost 100%.

After I received my master's degree from the National School of Public Health in Rio de Janeiro in 1968, I took on the task of coordinating smallpox eradication activities in the state of Paraná, Brazil. I knew that with the right strategy, we could help to eliminate smallpox. This disease is spread by respiratory droplets and is relatively easy to diagnose. All carriers show symptoms, which start with a rash that develops into pustules; it is transferred only from person to person. All I had learned in Altamira proved useful on this broader scale. My team and I worked with the state secretariat of health to contact doctors at all clinics and mayors of all municipalities. With their cooperation, we established a weekly surveillance reporting system. The plan was to give each clinic 52 aerograms and ask them to mail one every week to tell us if they had seen or not seen any cases of suspected smallpox. When reports of smallpox reached us, whether by phone or mail, we would find the infected patients and vaccinate everyone with whom they had been in contact. In this way, we would trace and effectively interrupt the chain of smallpox transmission.

In April, the first aerogram arrived at our office. The message read: "Smallpox outbreak identified in Telemaco Borba municipality. Five suspected cases. Direction and assistance requested."

Because the smallpox vaccine did not require any refrigeration or special care in transport, a nurse, a driver, and I were able to mobilize and pack our supplies very quickly. Once we arrived in Telemaco Borba, we entered the home of a family with a child showing the signs of smallpox: fever, fatigue, headache, and blisters. I knelt down next to their other children and brought out my supplies in order to vaccinate the other family members in the house. As I vaccinated them, my nurse asked if they had seen anyone else with similar symptoms.

"The neighbors," they said, nodding to the house next door, which I could see through the broken planks of the wooden walls around us. "They have the skin marks too, and have been sick."

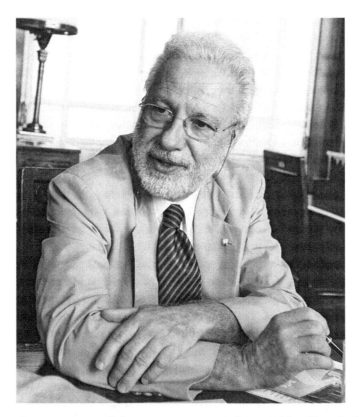

Ciro de Quadros signing a collaborative agreement – between the Albert B. Sabin Vaccine Institute (of which he is now the Executive Vice-President) and the Oswaldo Cruz Foundation – to carry out a clinical trial of a vaccine against hookworm.

After we had finished vaccinating the members of the household who were not yet sick, we packed our supplies. It pained me to leave the small child who was already sick, but smallpox is an untreatable disease, so we knew that we needed to vaccinate everyone who was not yet infected—and quickly. We walked next door, my nurse and I leading the way, our driver kicking up dust with his boots behind us. I asked this family the same question.

"Us? Oh, our neighbors also have it."

"Yes, we have seen them already," I said.

The father shook his head. "No, no, not those neighbors. *Those* neighbors," he said, pointing across the dirt roadway, over a hill, clearly indicating a village some distance away. My nurse's brow furrowed—whether with worry or determination, I couldn't tell. But our driver went straight to the car and started the engine, ready to enter the next village.

In this way, our travels followed the stories of the people we met. We traced the chain of transmission of the outbreak and vaccinated those that had been in contact with the patients. Their knowledge of the area and their ability to identify who had been showing symptoms created our road map for containing and interrupting the spread of the disease.

During our travels, we came upon an entire village infected with smallpox. I had never seen anything like it. From house to house we went, finally realizing that every person in the village was in some stage of being exposed to, fighting, or recovering from smallpox. Whole families with smallpox; a whole village sick.

I walked outside and looked up at clouds gathering in the Brazilian sky. How could this be? A whole town with smallpox? We found children whose faces and arms were covered in pustules, and babies in pain. We had no choice but to leave them there, suffering, knowing that the best we could do was cover as much ground as we could, administering the containment vaccinations in order to ensure that others would not have to suffer in this way. There was much more work before us, as we would have to track the chain of transmission back to the link that had exposed this village to the disease in the first place. Since smallpox was easily recognizable on the skin, even by people with no medical training, villagers could inform us of where they had first encountered the disease.

Using these techniques, in 8 months our team of three people managed to uncover over 1,000 cases of smallpox, trace the chains of transmission, and vaccinate about 30,000 people who had had contact with smallpox patients. This strategy of "surveillance and containment," which had been recommended by the World Health Organization (WHO) and consisted of selectively vaccinating people who had been in contact with infected patients, later became central to the global eradication of the disease.

Near the end of my work in Paraná, D. A. Henderson (known as D. A.), the leader of the WHO's Intensified Smallpox Eradication Program, came to visit us. A medical doctor who had been trained at the University of Rochester, he was a tall, squarely built man with a charming demeanor; I liked him immediately. He came out to the field and spoke to the vaccinators with the same respect, curiosity, and authority as he did with high officials from the Ministry of Health. A few months after his visit to Paraná, he invited me to join the global program. Gladly, I accepted my second smallpox eradication assignment—I was to be the head epidemiologist in what was then the empire of Ethiopia.

In Ethiopia, I was given a small eradication team—only 30 people for a population of about 25 million. At the time, the Ethiopian government considered smallpox less of a threat than rampant measles and outbreaks of malaria. When D. A. first initiated the program, most people thought that smallpox was not common in Ethiopia. This misconception led to concerns that any resources devoted to smallpox would only take away from efforts to attend to pressing health needs targeted by other health programs. Yet to our astonishment, in the first 3 months of the program we found over 3,000 cases of smallpox. After reporting these cases to the WHO headquarters in Geneva. D. A. called, skeptical about the numbers.

"It's true," I said. "There are that many cases, and, by the look of it, many more. We have very good documentation, with a case investigation for every single one. We have an epidemiological storm on our hands."

During our first year in Ethiopia, we uncovered about 26,000 cases of smallpox, which helped reframe smallpox as an immediate rather than a remote concern. Because there were few roads and we had only five cars, we had, for the first four years of the six-year program, to walk through the mountains for days at a time to reach a single village. Adding to the challenges of limited resources and difficult terrain, we found that many people did not want to be vaccinated, particularly in the highlands. Most of the highlanders were Christian Coptic, and they thought that we were Muslims trying to convert them with our vaccine. As we approach their homes, they would throw sticks and stones to get us to leave.

Once, in the border region of Sudan and Ethiopia, south of the Blue Nile, we had a report of an outbreak. We walked for about 26 days in that area, just tracing the chains of transmission. This was a desert area, very hot, where we had to dig holes in the bed of a dry river in order to get water. During those long walks I thought, "When I get back to Addis Ababa I'm going to call D. A. and resign." But then, after we returned to Addis Ababa and I had had a good shower, eaten a satisfying meal, and looked back on the work we had done, the people we had met, and the kindness and thankfulness they showed us, I knew that I would never resign from the project.

At the outset of our work, we learned that an international health organization had just given 30 vehicles to the Ethiopian malaria program. D. A. decided to ask the leaders of the malaria program to help us.

The officials of the malaria program told D. A. that they were sorry, but the cars never arrived. This was strange but the cars were not seen out front, and it was understood how unstable the delivery of resources could be on these kinds of projects. We resigned ourselves to the resources we had at hand. A few months later, a WHO staff involved in the malaria program confided, "No, they had cars. But they hid them in Nazareth."[ii]

That the Ethiopia malaria program felt that their cars had to be hidden from our smallpox initiative troubled me, but heightened my awareness of the competition between health programs for scarce resources. Despite our shared goal of delivering health services to those who needed them, the structure of our two programs, separate and parallel, resulted in competition rather than cooperation.

Despite the challenges that the terrain, distrustful patients, and fellow health workers presented, the surveillance and containment program worked again, as it had in Paraná. By the time our work in Ethiopia was complete, the importance of strong leadership and effective coordination through surveillance and containment programs had been sufficiently recognized and put into effect to ensure smallpox eradication worldwide. By the late 1970s, smallpox was eradicated around the globe. The last case in Ethiopia appeared in August 1976, and the last case in the world appeared in Somalia a year later, in August 1977.

NEVER AGAIN?

I stood in the lobby of the Pan American Health Organization (PAHO) headquarters in Washington, D.C., getting a cocktail during the reception of the annual minister's of health meeting in 1977. Halfdan Mahler, who was then director general of the WHO, approached me. He pointed to a small pin on my suit jacket—a bifurcated needle that I had been awarded by WHO for my participation in the eradication of smallpox.

"Never again," he said, "will such a program be promoted by the World Health Organization."

Speechless, I listened as he said that the malaria and smallpox eradication campaigns represented vertical, top-down programming that would detract from comprehensive community-based initiatives and did nothing to help communities develop their own primary health care infrastructure.

I did not want to argue with a man in his position, but my mind was full of things I would have liked to say to him. He might have been right about the malaria eradication program, but was he aware of all the work we did on the ground during the smallpox vaccination campaigns? In Paraná and Ethiopia we worked in conjunction with local people—doctors, nurses, mayors. We held community meetings and did house-to-house outreach. We worked with existing infrastructures in Ethiopia and Paraná to establish communication and reporting systems. We took advantage of every possible opportunity to work with the communities we were helping.

I looked down into my drink instead of at his face. I felt as I had when I first debarked the plane in Altamira, preparing to prove my abilities as a leader. But I should not have had to feel that way now. My experience with smallpox eradication had shown that success occurs through strong management and proper coordination and that vertical programming can result in strengthened health-care infrastructures. This was the only proven way I knew of achieving global eradication of a vaccine-preventable disease.

Three years later, an international symposium on polio control was held at the PAHO. Polio is a destructive and often elusive disease. The virus can go undetected in many patients yet still spread easily to others, especially in areas with poor sanitation. Symptoms range from headaches and diarrhea, to the paralysis of limbs, to the inability to speak, swallow, or breathe, eventually leading to death.

The symposium concluded that the technology to eradicate polio was available, yet the lack of political and social will blocked implementation of a plan of action. So how were we to begin? I still held the conviction that what we had achieved with smallpox was possible with other vaccine-preventable diseases, which were eradicable, but I remembered Mahler's statement that such a campaign would never happen again.

Then, in 1983, a new director arrived at PAHO. Carlyle Guerra de Macedo, a Brazilian like me, was a strong advocate for immunization efforts and the goal of universal childhood immunization by 1990. The policy pendulum was beginning to swing back from comprehensive programs to those with carefully chosen and achievable objectives. In December 1984, he called me into his office to meet with James Grant, then the charismatic executive director of the United Nations' Children's Fund (UNICEF).

When I entered Carlyle's office at PAHO headquarters in Washington, D.C., he offered me a seat at the round conference table. Jim Grant occupied the chair across from me, dressed in a suit and tie, sitting comfortably behind a stack of papers, a note pad ready and a pen in hand. We started the meeting discussing the shifting political climate around health-care initiatives, but before long Grant got right to the point.

"Be straight with me, Carlyle," he said, leaning forward to look the man hard in the eye. "Can the goal of universal childhood immunization by 1990 be reached in the Americas?"

Carlyle looked toward me. "Ciro," he asked, "What's your opinion?"

I sat back in my chair. As I contemplated this question, I felt the tension building in the room as both the men waited for my answer.

"It's possible," I said.

Then, secretly thrilled by the opportunity, I added, "If we had a 'banner disease,' something that would gain the public's attention and rally support for the program, it could be a great success."

Jim and Carlyle exchanged glances. I could tell they were receptive to my idea. "We could start with polio," I continued. "It would revitalize interest in immunization, particularly in surveillance, and we could use similar initiatives as we did for smallpox. The immunization days in Brazil show that this can work if we have the resources behind us to get it done."

"This will require a lot of resources," Grant said. "The technical pieces are much more challenging than with smallpox."

"That's true," I answered. "But the national immunization days in Brazil had such positive results: 20 million children under the age of 5 vaccinated in 2 days, polio incidence plummeting from 200 or more cases per month to fewer than 20, viral transmission halted in several Brazilian states, and no new cases. Their work is a road map for us to follow if we can get the resources moving in the right direction."

"How do we get the resources, and those who hold access to them, behind the initiative?" Carlyle asked.

I remembered my previous work with smallpox—success resulted from coordinating resources and implementing strategies using existing structures.

"We need strong leadership and proper coordination," I said. "We'll share what we know, bring people and groups together, give them a chance to hear the purpose behind the initiative. We'll get them on board."

I left Carlyle's office with the feeling that finally momentum was building toward a broad-based polio eradication campaign.

I was right. On May 14, 1985, 30 years after the first live polio vaccination trial, Carlyle announced the goal of polio eradication in the Americas by 1990. The proposal was brought to the PAHO directing council in September 1985, where it was accepted.

CHALLENGES AND INNOVATIONS

As the chief advisor for immunizations at PAHO, I was the head of the team in charge of technical cooperation for the polio eradication campaign. The challenges were monumental: millions of people in both rural and urban settings, unstable national governments in Peru and several countries in Central America, a vaccine that required constant refrigeration, a disease that was difficult to diagnose without proper and efficient lab work. On my first day as chief advisor I wrote a list of goals and challenges and taped it to the top of my desk. Every morning when I arrived at work, it greeted me. Depending upon our progress and on my mood, the list seemed either daunting or energizing.

1. Obtain funding, but from where?
2. Develop a method to carry a vaccine that requires a cold chain.
3. Target whole communities for vaccination, because disease carriers often show no signs of infection.
4. Organize an efficient surveillance system for acute flaccid paralysis.[iii]
5. Organize a network of virology labs for confirming diagnoses.
6. Get national, regional, and international agencies to work together behind one goal.

The first goal I was able to check off owing to a fortunate coincidence: Rotary International had been looking for a global target to be achieved by the centennial of its foundation in 2005, and Albert Sabin suggested the global eradication of polio.

Rotary's enthusiastic fund-raising efforts brought in over $200 million in less than 2 years, of which about $30 million was eventually utilized in the Americas. We also received funds from UNICEF and the InterAmerican Development Bank. Our largest supporter was the U.S. Agency for International Development (USAID). We were fortunate to receive funds from these disparate organizations, but they did not come without complications. I knew that what we needed now was cooperation, but the agencies involved represented very diverse priorities and decades of separate efforts. Therefore the sixth goal on my list proved to be the most challenging.

In an attempt to unify the agencies, we established a regional interagency committee where representatives of the agencies met frequently to develop a plan of action. As the agencies jostled for position, each fighting for its own agenda, those of us from PAHO worried. For the first 2 years, my time was devoted to mediating disputes between the organizations. Intra-agency conflicts were just as difficult. Working with the members of UNICEF was particularly challenging, because they were decentralized to the extent that no one member was more powerful than any other. It made it nearly impossible for us to allocate resources the way we wanted to, and eventually we began to wonder if we would ever be able to come to an agreement.

During that time, other operational obstacles were cropping up everywhere, most dramatically in the forms of the civil war in El Salvador and the Shining Path, an extremist revolutionary movement, in Peru. In El Salvador, the implementation of national immunization days required negotiating a cease-fire between government and guerilla forces. The process was painstaking and involved PAHO, UNICEF, the Red Cross, and the Catholic Church. It also meant meeting individually with leaders from the guerrilla movement, a task I was more than willing to take on.

I returned to Washington, D.C., to meet with a representative from the political arm of the guerilla movement in El Salvador. We were to meet at a pub on K Street, and I had been preparing for this meeting for weeks, knowing that gaining the support of his movement was crucial.

When I entered the pub, the leader greeted me warmly, but after we ordered our lunch, we fell into a mutual silence. He sat across from me at the table, his hand wrapped around a white coffee cup. The waiter brought us each a glass of cold water. I took a sip, looked at the man across the table, and began trying to convince him that he should support the eradication movement.

"This disease is ruthless, and totally democratic. It can attack anyone," I said. "And those who suffer from it do so unnecessarily."

He sipped his coffee, then responded. "We're working for similar things, the health of the people," he said. "But these people that you vaccinate, they often have no other medical attention. What should I say to them when they ask me, 'why welcome vaccinators who don't help us with dehydration? With our children dying from malaria?' What we really need are more doctors on the ground, doctors who stay—not health workers who come through once a year and vaccinate for a disease that no one in the village has ever seen." His frown was interrupted only by the waiter delivering our food.

He took a bite of his burger and I took the opportunity to argue my side. "Every day that goes by without vaccinations leaves more room for an outbreak. And it's not just about polio. A broad-based vaccination campaign strengthens community health centers, improves people's overall quality of life. We need cease-fire days in order to make this work." We spent the next few hours discussing our program and the importance of polio eradication.

Our conversation ended later that afternoon without a firm agreement. At first I was disappointed, but at the same time I knew that he had to communicate the information he had gathered to the field commanders. Several months later, "days of tranquility" were established for the vaccination of children. Gradually, the program proceeded, until El Salvador held 3 days of tranquility each year. This arrangement lasted until the country achieved peace in the early 1990s.

On the immunization days, government and guerilla members collaborated to accomplish the vaccinations. Once, when one of our epidemiologists and his team of vaccinators returned from the field at the end of the day, they were stopped by a group of guerilla fighters. At first, the epidemiologist was terrified, but he quickly realized that they wanted the team to return to a village that had accidentally been skipped! El Salvador's days of tranquility became a symbol of cooperation in health and prompted a wider initiative in Central America that became known as Health as a Bridge for Peace. They also set a global example; for instance, in Lebanon and, later, several other countries in states of civil war, including Angola and the Democratic Republic of Congo, where days of tranquility were also implemented to ensure a pause in the war in order to vaccinate children.

Months passed and UNICEF's representatives were still at a standstill. Finally, in 1987, I called James Grant for help, hoping that he would be as invested in our vaccination efforts as he had been when I had met him in Carlyle's office. Grant then invited me to a gathering of all UNICEF representatives of the countries of the Americas at their headquarters, then located in Bogotá, Colombia.

Grant, the members of UNICEF, and I assembled in a conference room in the morning. All the representatives from the different countries sat around a long table and I stood at one end, feeling the pressure of their expectations.

When they had stopped talking among themselves and had become settled, I began: "Here is the strategy for the campaign."

I flipped on an overhead projector and explained the first steps over the machine's hum. "We'll have routine immunizations, supplemented by national immunization days twice a year, targeting all children under age 5." I removed my first overhead sheet and replaced it with my second. "Each country will implement a reporting system, starting with local health units, connecting all the way up to the international effort. . . ." I explained the reporting system in depth and then detailed the process for identifying cases of polio.

"Any case of acute flaccid paralysis in a child under age 15 must be seen within 48 hours by a trained epidemiologist for a thorough investigation." I drew a line on my overhead diagram from a small figure that represented a potential patient to the small house that served as the sign for a local health care center. Then I continued to the next step. "Diagnosis of probable poliomyelitis requires two stool samples, collected 24 hours apart and sent to a diagnostic laboratory." Here, I sketched another line from the health center on the overhead to an icon representing a centralized lab for the country.

The representative from Peru interrupted.

"How will this occur? Many of our villages can't be reached easily, and the Shining Path controls several areas of the country. I can't see how we'll make that time line and do so without contaminating the sample."

Another representative argued that the national immunization days would divert resources from other health priorities.

"It's true, the technical requirements for testing are massive," I said. "That's why cooperation on every level is vital. The national immunization days, if properly organized, will help strengthen the health infrastructure in each country." I returned my attention to the screen, circling the different key portions of the campaign and the surveillance plan as I spoke. "We need your help in tackling these logistics— you know best how to make this work within the current health-care infrastructure in the country in which you are working.

I looked out at the group of UNICEF representatives, waiting for further questions. When none came, I continued explaining the program.

For the next 4 hours, I outlined the technical aspects of the strategies we planned to implement and the support required on the ground to make our program happen. As I spoke, I watched the over 30 people gathered around the table, shifting in their chairs, their faces full of questions and doubts. Many times they interrupted my presentation, asking for more information about the intention behind a particular strategy and, more often then not, casting doubt on whether the plan I presented would work or was in the best interest of their countries.

"Who will administer the vaccinations?" A representative sitting in the back asked.

"This will be the responsibility of health professionals from all health-care facilities in the country. That is what they are there for: to protect the health of the population. We can also train volunteers to administer the vaccine," I said. "J. B. Risi's work in Brazil proved that national immunization days can be very successful."

"Local health-care workers tell us that polio isn't their major concern," he responded. "How can we address that?"

"It was the same with smallpox—we had to spend time with each of the health ministers explaining the importance of the project. We'll do that with local organizations, village leaders, and each mother and father if we have to."

For each of their concerns, I had a careful response, but I was growing increasingly frustrated. The fluorescent lights in the room, combined with the lack of windows and fresh air, left me with a headache. I felt I'd been over each of these issues time and again, and still the national heads of UNICEF came up with reasons to hesitate and challenge the program. I watched as the UNICEF officials argued over where funds would best be spent and suggested that their particular countries required more funds or that they had more effective strategies for initiating the campaign. Each time, I offered what information I could about the polio eradication campaign. After I had answered another set of questions, a moment of silence ensued. I looked at James Grant, who had spent the whole day listening both to the concerns raised by the national leaders and to my answers. Finally, he leaned forward and spoke.

"Okay, then, this will be the strategy for UNICEF, is that clear?" He pointed to the explanatory materials I had given to the group. He held up one of the pieces of literature, and said, "This is what UNICEF is going to do. The plan is clear and well thought out and depends on everyone's cooperation. We need you to back the initiative. If any of you have any problems with this initiative or do not want to cooperate, I will accept your resignation."

A hush spread across the room, and I wondered whether anyone would raise further questions. As it turned out, no one seemed to have any problems; in fact, after this moment of tension, they worked together as great partners. By the end of that year, all potentially endemic countries had national vaccination days as part of their basic immunization strategies. James Grant became a major player in moving the program from the Americas to the rest of the world. Grant worked to convince the WHO, which was still opposed to "top-down" programs, to embrace the polio eradication initiative internationally.

EPIDEMIOLOGICAL TECHNIQUES

Our reporting system developed at a rapid pace; soon, over 20,000 health institutions throughout Latin America and the Caribbean were reporting the presence or absence of polio cases on a regular basis. However, many patients came to the health facilities days or weeks after the onset of paralysis, tragically too late to prevent infection from the virus and too late for the appropriate collection of stool specimens.

Then, one day in 1988, one of my colleagues burst into my office.

"These just came in now," she said, sliding a stack of reports on my desk. "New outbreaks of polio in the northeastern states of Brazil." I thumbed through the reports, startled to find that despite an effective program of vaccination, cases of the disease had reappeared in sizable numbers in certain parts of Brazil.

"Looks as though there might be a problem with the vaccine," I suggested.

I rubbed my forehead, trying to relieve the pressure that was building. The challenges of accurate and timely diagnosis were large enough without adding an unreliable vaccine into the equation.

"We'll discuss this with the national health authorities, take a look at our field data again, make sure our reporting systems are solid, and test for the potency of the vaccine," I decided. "In the meantime, we'd better begin a mop-up campaign."

Contrasted with my experience of detecting smallpox outbreaks, where it was relatively easy to track the paths of infection, with polio, only 1 out of every 200 or more infected children experienced paralysis. With so many asymptomatic carriers, the only way to contain an outbreak was through sweeping, broad-based efforts—what we called "mop-up campaigns." They supplemented the national immunization days and involved the house-to-house vaccination of all persons living in an extensive area, sometimes including several states or provinces.

In the ensuing months, we learned that the vaccine had begun to fail because of a low concentration of the Type 3 component. The vaccine contains the three types of poliovirus responsible to cause the disease—Types 1, 2, and 3—and this outbreak was caused by the third type. After we learned that the concentration of the Type 3 in the vaccine was too low, we immediately asked the manufacturer to double the concentration of that component. Once the newly formulated vaccine was utilized, no more Type 3 outbreaks occurred—with the exception of the last outbreak in Mexico in 1990. There again, the vaccine had a low concentration of the Type 3 component. The Mexican minister of health fired two national health officers for this oversight. The WHO took another 3 years to recommend increasing Type 3 virus components in oral polio vaccine at the global level.

Our hurdles were not only technical. While we had been successful in establishing immunization days in El Salvador, we had less luck in Peru. There, the situation was far more complicated because there was no guerrilla leadership structure with whom a cease-fire could be negotiated. The Ministry of Health vaccination teams could reach certain areas and populations with the permission of local leaders, only to be refused passage by guerrillas who controlled the roads that led to neighboring villages. If the vaccination teams found themselves stuck overnight without access to refrigeration, the vaccine would lose its potency. The fragile nature of the oral vaccine meant that there was no time, once on the ground, to negotiate these kinds of stalemates. In Peru, transmission of polio, though curtailed, was still active in many places.

Then came the Peruvian cholera outbreak of 1990, which spread to other countries in the region. As with Ethiopia, swamped with malaria in some areas and measles in others during the smallpox campaign, Peru could not prioritize the movement to eradicate a disease that was not an immediate priority while thousands of their people were suffering from and spreading cholera.

Yet even with the cholera crisis in Peru, I knew that there was opportunity to combine efforts, something that had not occurred when I worked in Ethiopia on smallpox eradication.

I took a look at the schedule for Peru polio eradication efforts and realized that we could use that same network to detect cholera. We already had vaccinators visiting each household during house-to-house visits, administering polio vaccine to children. Because cholera and polio are both oral-fecal diseases, we could train vaccinators to give out information about preventing cholera at the same time that they were consulting with families about polio.

The Peruvian officials agreed.

The presence of our strong surveillance network eventually became a major element in detecting cholera cases. Searches for cases of paralysis and suspected cholera were carried out at the same time. Our years of effort to integrate resources, combine initiatives, and ensure increased health services to the most marginalized populations were producing positive results.

As we researched the historical data on outbreaks in Latin America, we found that they repeatedly began in the same geographic areas—usually in crowded communities with poor sanitary conditions—and then spread to other areas of the country. Targeting these traditional strongholds of the virus sped its final eradication. Results were dramatic and transmission declined steadily.

THE END OF POLIO IN THE WESTERN HEMISPHERE

When a child with paralysis in Junin, Peru, was detected, we knew that he could very well be one of the last cases in Peru, possibly in all of the Western Hemisphere. In response, we made every effort to vaccinate the entire country in what became the most comprehensive mop-up campaign in the history of the program. Of the 3 million households we wanted to visit over the span of 1 week, many were in areas where the Shining Path was particularly aggressive. We knew that if the guerrillas did not want to cooperate, the mop-up would be disastrous. Unfortunately no means of negotiation existed. Using mass media was risky, because the Shining Path could choose to disrupt the immunization campaign in a show of power, but we had no other option. We held press conferences to inform everybody that the Junin case could be the last polio case in the Americas, but only with the support of every individual in the country. Then we went to work.

I put Peter Carrasco in charge of the activities for this final effort in Peru. He was one of our best field epidemiologists and a veteran of the smallpox eradication efforts in Ethiopia as a Peace Corps volunteer; I was confident that he could handle the job. For the Peru campaign we needed about 10 tons of ice to keep the vaccine cold—and that was just for Lima. The Ministry of Health could not produce that amount in such a short time; they simply lacked the facilities. So every night of the campaign, health workers used the refrigerators of individuals in the community to freeze the cold packs for the next day. Vaccination teams visited nearly 3 million households and vaccinated about as many children under the age of 5 in a week, with no disturbances, and repeated the same operation 6 weeks later.

A few months later, the government of Peru launched a major offensive against the Shining Path and arrested its main leader as well as several high commanders and guerrilla fighters. We discovered that several of those arrested had worked as vaccinators or assistants during the mop-up campaign. At the time, no one had suspected that even the most brutal guerrilla group in the Americas had assisted with the polio eradication program.

In August 1994, the International Certification Commission, chaired by the Nobelist Frederick C. Robbins, met in Washington, D.C., with the presidents of the national certification commissions. After review and analysis, the commission declared the Americas free of wild poliovirus. The declaration was made public in September 1994 at the meeting of the Pan American Sanitary Conference, with the ministers of health of the Americas present. I remember the day clearly. Here again we were gathered to hold a press conference, to make a monumental announcement. This time, we had reason to celebrate. Dr. Robbins, the president of the International Certification Commission, made the announcement:

"Based on the impressive evidence presented, we conclude that wild poliovirus transmission has been interrupted in the Americas."

The crowd erupted in applause at receiving this confirmation of eradication in the Americas. People were in tears. I looked around at those who had been involved in the effort, at the faces of the many people behind the on-the-ground campaigns from Argentina to Mexico to Peru. We had taken a bold idea and turned it into a reality, a reality that would protect thousands of children from the devastating effects of a vaccine-preventable disease and that would serve as an example to other health initiatives in the future.

The experiences of the Americas were vital for the launching of the initiative for the global eradication of polio by the year 2000. Owing to a chronic lack of resources coupled with lack of leadership in many regions and countries, the target was not achieved as planned and the completion of the initiative is still under way. By mid-2007, polio transmission was still prevalent in a few countries in Asia and Africa, particularly India, Pakistan, Afghanistan, and Nigeria. Countries that previously had interrupted transmission—such as Bangladesh, Ethiopia, Somalia, Angola, and the Democratic Republic of Congo—have experienced reintroduction of the virus and suffered outbreaks.

However, the new director general of the WHO, Dr. Margaret Chan, has injected energy in the initiative and called upon the global community to make a final effort to interrupt polio transmission worldwide. If resources are forthcoming, polio could be once and for all eradicated from the world within 2 to 3 years.

The eradication of polio in the Americas was the result of vision, leadership, and appropriate coordination of resources from the various international agencies that supported the program, including civil society. Furthermore, it was based on a clear and technically sound strategy that was implemented by a superb group of technical staff at PAHO, with whom I was proud to be associated. This group provided the technical support to the national leadership of the program in the various countries, who inspired the thousands of health workers in the field and who finally got the job done. If Dr. Chan provides a similar scenario at the global level and in the endemic countries, polio will join smallpox in the pantheon of conquests of medicine and public health.

NOTES

    i. For diphtheria, tetanus, pertussis, polio, and tuberculosis.

   ii. A town about 100 miles southeast of Addis-Ababa.

  iii. Acute flaccid paralysis is a non-injury-related floppy paralysis that suddenly appears in the arms or legs of a child under 15 years of age. It is the signal condition for polio.

4 An Orphan Disease in Mozambique

Julie Cliff

THE MYSTERY

To anyone working in infectious diseases, the message seemed common enough: a telex in from the northern province of Nampula reporting a polio epidemic. My head of department, Ana Novoa, passed it to me with a "this could be interesting" look, and we studied the message together. Around 30 cases was a lot, but it was two words in the staccato message that grabbed our attention: *increased reflexes*. In polio, the reflexes disappear.

My path to Mozambique had seemed an inevitable one—a neat conjunction of a professional interest in tropical medicine, a political commitment nurtured in the solidarity movements of the 1970s, and a desire to do good, which had motivated me to study medicine in my native Australia in the first place.

I had been teaching at the medical school in Dar es Salaam, Tanzania, when neighboring Mozambique gained independence from Portugal in 1975. Under the Portuguese, few Mozambicans had been educated. The medical school in the capital was mostly for Portuguese students, and only a handful of African doctors had been trained. At independence, Portuguese doctors abandoned Mozambique en masse, leaving just 80 doctors for a population of around 10 million. The Frente da Libertação de Moçambique (FRELIMO), the liberation movement that had fought a decade-long war for independence, took power. The new government recruited health workers from the solidarity movement to help build a new health service and fill the gap left by the departing Portuguese. I joined this group of idealistic health workers.

After several years as head of infectious diseases in the central teaching hospital in Maputo, the national capital, I decided to move to prevention and public health. Seeing large numbers of children die from measles and neonatal tetanus, both easily preventable through vaccination, impelled me to move from clinical medicine. I left for London to study for a master's degree in community health and, on my return, moved to the Ministry of Health to work on disease prevention and control.

The telex from Nampula arrived soon after.

The year was 1981, the date was August 13. On learning of the telex, the minister of health, an obstetrician who had come back to Mozambique at independence after many years in exile, called an emergency meeting—whether polio or not, the outbreak needed investigating and controlling. He decided to send a team to the field, an unlikely trio of an astute Bulgarian neurologist, Dr. Nicolai Kulinski; a lively Italian microbiologist, Dr. Antonio Martelli; and myself. None of us had any real experience in epidemic investigation in rural Africa, and we barely knew each other. But we were confident—in my case, with all the certainty of youth. I had clinical experience, and here was a chance to put my recently acquired knowledge in public health into practice. I had been longing to get to the field.

In the provincial capital, our three-person team met in the health department offices, located in an old block of flats that had been taken over by the government. There, I was surprised and relieved to find a familiar face: Antonio Esteves, an immensely capable nurse who had moved from the central hospital in Maputo to work in community health in Nampula. The provincial health authorities were experienced in investigating epidemics and had already worked out a strategy. Together with Antonio Esteves and a provincial team, we traveled toward the coast to Nacala, a crumbling wreck of a city. Thrown up by the Portuguese during the last years of the colonial war, rows of jerry-built flats, now occupied by the poor, were rapidly deteriorating in the tropical climate.

After arriving at the local hospital in Nacala, we met a pair of dedicated Swedish doctors, Hans Rosling and Anders Molin, who had been laboring under difficult conditions. They had done a preliminary investigation and concluded what Ana and I had suspected—the disease was not polio. However, the number of cases was rapidly increasing. Most were in the remote district of Memba, which was drought-prone and had a low rainfall. A particularly severe drought had gripped Memba and neighboring districts for 2 years running.

We set off for Memba, accompanied by Anders Molin. Our first stop was a small health center en route, which was filled with patients, mostly young women and children with paralyzed limbs. A young woman dressed in a local cloth, its normally bright colors faded by wear, described falling suddenly as she walked back from the long trip to collect water. Now she could not speak properly and her vision was blurred. A couple of days later, her son had suddenly fallen while playing. Our examination of the nervous system showed a monotonous picture, spastic weakness of the legs with increased reflexes. The weakness varied from mild to severe. Some complained of fever, diarrhea, and headache before the onset of paralysis.

We set up base in the small district capital. Like many towns on the East African coast, Memba is astonishingly beautiful. It is set on a spectacular bay; coconut palms wave on a distant sandy shore while baobabs dot the dry coastline. A central grid of four blocks of empty-shelved shops, abandoned by their Portuguese owners, testified that the town was once an important trading post. Anywhere else, Memba would be a tourist destination, and indeed, in Portuguese colonial times, settlers had come from the interior to relax by the beach. We crammed into one of their old abandoned beach cottages and began work.

The hospital was set on a hill overlooking the bay, providing periodic glimpses of the sea. Despite the spaciousness and high ceilings of the old colonial wards, they now seemed to overflow with paralyzed women and children. We began the tiring task of methodically taking histories and examining the patients. We did not have long, as we needed to get out to the field the next day. By the time we reached the last patients, it was already dark, and we struggled to see by the light of kerosene lamps. We found that the disease was indeed monotonous; it mostly varied in

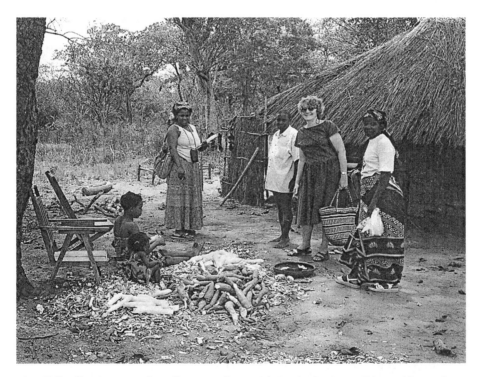

Julie Cliff collecting samples of cassava flour with Paula Cardoso. (Photo: Howard Bradbury.)

severity, as some of the worst cases also had paralyzed arms, were blind, and had difficulty hearing. I became so absorbed in examining the nervous system that I completely failed to notice that one young woman was heavily pregnant and about to go into labor. To everyone's amusement (except perhaps hers), she delivered almost immediately after my examination.

Each day we journeyed further from the district capital and deeper into the interior of the country. The endless vistas of the African savanna lay before us, parched by the drought—normally green lush trees now bore only a few dry leaves. In more inhabited areas, the fields were bare, with only dry twigs of cassava poking out of the ground. Cashew trees, the main cash crop, provided isolated splashes of green. Most people lived scattered through the bush, but every now and then we would come across a village. The houses there were attractive, built of mud brick with thatched roofs and set in neatly swept yards. Women sat around in groups on woven fiber mats outside their houses, often peeling piles of cassava roots. Cut cassava roots and smaller piles of tiny pieces of cassava were laid out to dry around the houses on roofs, mats, and rocks, wherever they could catch light and heat. Piles of peel lay crinkling in the sun. The women explained that food was so short that some families were forced to eat the peel, for the first time in memory. Occasionally, we would glimpse women energetically pounding the dried roots into flour, using large wooden pestles and mortars. Some were busy stirring pots of flour and water to form *chima*, the stiff porridge that was their staple food.

Our first stop was Cavá mission, where a smiling Italian nun, Sister Lucia, greeted us warmly. Children crowded around her plump figure, and she radiated compassion. Dozens of patients had come into the mission to receive food and physiotherapy. A tailor had clearly been busy, as the children were all dressed in beautiful new red tunics. We watched as they determinedly tried to kick a football around a dusty field. Owing to the spastic paralysis they were suffering, their legs were crossed and they were forced to run on tiptoes, often falling as they ran. Sister Lucia was a mine of information about the disease. She confirmed the sudden onset and also said that some children improved, went home, and came back with a second or even third attack.

We traveled further into the interior, along an appalling road, our hearts sometimes in our mouths as we crossed flimsy bridges straddling ravines, to the small administrative post of Mazua. Here we found both men and women exercising on parallel bars. One young muscled man struggled to walk the length of the bars. As with almost everyone else, the paralysis had struck quickly for him, as he was tilling his fields. He was determined to walk again.

In the villages, we stopped in central places, often the schools, where children studied outdoors, sitting cross-legged on the ground. Usually between 5 and 20 patients were waiting, clustered with their families under a shady tree. Local community leaders ran to get rudimentary chairs and mats from their houses and a curious crowd of children and men quickly gathered around us. Other patients struggled in. All had the characteristic scissors gait, instantly recognizable, of spastic paralysis.

Family members supported them, or they used crudely fashioned sticks. While Dr. Kulinski and I examined the patients, Antonio Martelli took blood in hopes of determining the cause of the disease.

Sometimes we would walk through the bush to a house. For the first time, I experienced the different perceptions of distance between city and rural dwellers. We trudged through the bush in single file, with the sun beating down, always with the promise that the house would be just around the corner. When we finally arrived, we often found the worst cases, those who had not been able to make it to the village center. On the outskirts of one village, we found a blind and paralyzed mother lying on a mat, her muscles wasted. Her two paralyzed children lay beside her. Often we found children with callused knees, a telltale sign that they had been crawling.

We had many meetings with community leaders. We would sit down under a tree while a group of men, mostly elderly, all thin, all in ragged clothing, would express their concern about this new disease that they had never seen before. The drought was the worst in their memory and had now lasted 2 years. Their staple crops of maize, sorghum, and sweet cassava and their cash crop of cashew had failed. Paid work was hard to find, and even when food was occasionally on sale, they had no money to buy it. Desperately short of food, they were living on bitter cassava and wild plants. The bitter cassava that had survived the drought was called Gurué, after its place of origin in a neighboring province. It had spread after independence because it was high-yielding and resistant to drought and attacks from wild animals. One elderly man blamed the cassava. I wrote his words in my notebook: "This disease has happened because the rain has not washed our cassava. The leaves have not developed." We noted the explanation but suspected an infectious cause.

After several days, we had gathered the basic information: an epidemic of spastic paralysis had begun around 2 months prior, and gradually worsened. New cases were still appearing—by the end of August there were 150. The disease appeared to be more common inland, with few cases on the coast and none in towns. It predominantly affected young women and children, often clustering in families. A severe drought formed a backdrop.

What was the cause? We approached the epidemic with an infectious diseases mindset; my experience and training was in infectious diseases and Antonio Martelli was a microbiologist. The presence of an epidemic and frequent clustering in families inclined us to believe that this disease was transferred by one family member to the next. Microbes often take advantage of extreme conditions, such as drought, and Africa was full of unknown viruses. We were scared that a failure to diagnose a potentially contagious virus could prove catastrophic if it spread further.

Soon we had run out of material to collect specimens, and we were anxious to get the specimens we had sent off for further analysis. We returned to Maputo to regroup and consult. We searched our medical textbooks. The only similar disease that we could find was lathyrism in India and Ethiopia, caused by eating the lathryus bean. As far as we knew, it did not exist in this area. But the similarities between the diseases made us question our position that the disease was an infectious one. After all, people were eating a variety of wild plants. Perhaps one of them was the culprit.

We also considered all we had heard about cassava. We knew that bitter cassava, the only staple to have survived the drought, contained cyanide, and our textbooks described two nervous system diseases associated with cyanide. One was a degeneration of the optic nerve in smokers. The other, called "tropical ataxic neuropathy," was nearer to home, in Tanzania and Nigeria, and was attributed to cassava. Both men and women in middle and old age slowly developed difficulty in walking. The disease was very different from the sudden paralysis we were seeing.

At endless meetings in the Ministry of Health, we debated long and hard what to do next. Most of the experts there were also infectious disease specialists; they argued that we should pay more attention to the possibility of an insect vector. We added questions about the presence of insects to our questionnaire. Not surprisingly, mosquitoes bit everyone frequently every night, and every household was plagued by bedbugs. Some argued that we should set up a special ward in the provincial capital to investigate the patients. But we felt that the answer was in the field, in the houses of patients. Only by looking at the community context would we understand this epidemic.

We contacted the World Health Organization by telex and received a quick reply, advising us to send our specimens to a virus laboratory in Glasgow to test for enteroviruses, a group of viruses with neurotoxic properties. We sent off the first samples and the results came back a few weeks later: there was no evidence of a viral infection. We were puzzled, but thought perhaps it was a new virus. We also received the opinion of a leading viral expert at Porton Down in the U.K. No particular virus had been described as giving these symptoms, although an unusual manifestation of an arbovirus (viruses spread by insects) could be a possibility. We began to think more seriously of a toxin, either a wild plant or cyanide from cassava, or possibly a vitamin and amino acid deficiency. We asked the Glasgow lab to test for toxins, including thiocyanate, a product of cyanide, and for vitamin and other nutritional deficiencies.

We continued to go back and forth to Nampula. By September 12, a total of 522 cases had been recorded. Our team expanded to include a methodical Dutch botanist, Paul Jansen, who patiently collected specimens of the plants that people were eating and pressed them in a book. The list was long, but there was no obvious candidate for the cause. He identified 12 cassava varieties, of which two were bitter, and took specimens back to Maputo for cyanide analysis.

We chose a communal village called Acordos de Lusaka for a more detailed study. After independence, the government had encouraged peasants to settle in villages so they that services could be provided more easily. Named after the peace agreement with the Portuguese, Acordos was at the center of one of the worst-hit areas: 28 of the 815 inhabitants had developed the paralysis. We compared families with the disease with their neighbors. A larger proportion of affected families ate dried, uncooked cassava. The noninfected families were more likely to have fish or meat in their diet and to be members of the Food Consumer Cooperative, which required a monetary contribution. This was a disease of the poorest families in the village.

On our way back through Nacala, we stopped at the hospital to see if Hans Rosling had heard anything from the Glasgow lab. He walked out eagerly and greeted us with the news—the results from our first blood samples had shown extremely high levels of thiocyanate.

The old man had been right. The probable cause was cyanide from insufficiently processed cassava.

CASSAVA

Cassava, a root native to South America, was introduced into Nampula province in the eighteenth century from the French colonies in the Indian Ocean. Its importance as a crop increased in the early twentieth century, when the Portuguese began to force peasants to grow cotton and cashew as cash crops. The cultivation of cassava, unlike that of cereals, did not coincide with that of cotton. Other staple food had to be bought, which reinforced the need to earn money from cash crops or manual labor. Cassava's importance as both a staple and a cash crop thus increased. Because of its toxicity, the Portuguese had attempted to control the cultivation of bitter cassava, but after independence, its cultivation spread rapidly in northern Mozambique, as peasants were now able to grow it freely.

The available evidence supported the causative role of cassava. People in the affected communities were living on a monotonous diet of bitter cassava, the only staple to survive the drought. We consulted agricultural textbooks and found that cyanide concentrations in cassava increase in drought. The laboratory results from Paul Jensen's cassava samples came back: both the roots and flour had high concentrations of cyanide. Fifty-five percent of the sweet root was extremely toxic and the remainder moderately so. Mean values were even higher for the roots of bitter varieties. We found a review of traditional processing methods; sun drying was ineffective in removing cyanide from cassava. Peel had a particularly high concentration of cyanide.

The community leaders had noticed that the bitter cassava tasted more bitter than usual and that the small quantities of sweet cassava that had survived the drought had turned bitter. Owing to the failure of other crops, they had been forced to begin harvesting the bitter cassava crop in June, earlier than the usual harvest month of August. Normally they would have stocks of well-dried cassava left from the previous year to tide them over through the harvest. This year, they were without stocks, and they were forced to eat the cassava before it was properly dry. The women were taking a shortcut to try and get rid of the poison in cassava, pounding or cutting it into smaller pieces and drying it for 1 to 2 days. They often suffered dizziness and palpitations after eating a cassava meal.

We could explain the relative sparing of the coast's inhabitants by the availability of fish, a good source of protein. In towns, which were also spared, commercial food was available. The predominance in young women and children could be due to the greater amounts of cassava in their diets. Men were served a cooked meal and their nutrition came first. Women and children possibly ate more raw and dried uncooked cassava during collection and processing. The affected women were in the reproductive age group, between 15 and 45 years of age. In rural Nampula, women bear an average of 6.5 living children and are constantly pregnant or lactating, with the associated increased nutritional demands. A local belief that raw cassava stimulates lactation may have led breast-feeding women to consume it. Even in good times, over 40% of children below age 5 in Nampula are chronically malnourished.

THE DISEASE HAS A NAME

We thought that we were describing a new disease and named it *Mantakassa*, the word for paralysis in the local Macua language. Those were the days before the Internet and rapid scientific communication, and Mozambique had no journal collection to speak of. I therefore decided to visit neighboring Zimbabwe, which had recently attained independence. South Africa, which was nearer, was still in the grip of apartheid[i] and out of bounds. For me, one of the delights of Zimbabwe's independence was to have a good library close by, with an excellent book and journal collection.

The library was part of a new medical school complex, built in the last days of white rule, in their 1950s time-warp style of unimaginative concrete and brick buildings. Sitting in the quiet modern library, I began with the more recent journals and could only find references to cassava and tropical ataxic neuropathy. I decided to go systematically back through the articles, reading every one. The first clue came in a reference to an article written in 1952, describing a paralytic disease in the Belgian Congo back in the 1930s. It, in turn, referred to the original report, written in French by Trolli in 1938. I noted it down on my list of items to look up in the catalogue. I did not expect to find it. When I had completed my list, I walked to the library catalogue and looked under T.

To my surprise and excitement, there it was. I rushed to the shelves and found the precious document: *Paraplégie spastique épidémique, "konzo" des indigenes du Kwango*.

The document contained a description of an identical disease in the then Belgian Congo (later Zaire and now the Democratic Republic of Congo). Trolli, an Italian doctor, who was head of Belgian medical support there, had gathered information from district medical officers, who described epidemics of spastic paralysis beginning in 1928. Old cases with onset 30 to 50 years previous were also reported; in the epidemic of 1936 to 1937, there were more than 1,000 cases.

I knew that we were seeing the same disease. The disease we had been studying so closely already had a name. *Konzo.*

TRADE

The konzo epidemic ran until the end of October 1981. Eventually 1,102 cases would be reported, spread over five districts in a total population of around 500,000. In the worst-affected villages, 1 in 30 people had the disease.

Now we knew the probable cause of the paralysis, we knew that it had a history, and we knew that if the people could stop their dependence on bitter cassava, there would be no more cases.

But it was not a problem we could easily solve, because cassava was tied to the fundamental economics of the region. Ruth First, an outstanding South African scholar and antiapartheid activist, had come from exile in England to lead research at a newly established Center for African Studies. From Ruth and her colleagues, I rapidly learned the basics of agricultural economics. These were not purely subsistence peasants, living in economic isolation. They also grew cassava and other crops for cash and were integrated into the global economy. The significance of the empty shelves in Memba and the ragged clothes became clear—rural trade had collapsed, and this collapse had also contributed to the epidemic.

The collapse was partly due to government agricultural policies that had promoted state farms and ignored the peasantry. Huge tracts of fertile land had been left empty by departing Portuguese, and the new socialist government concentrated on developing them into state farms, with the support of agronomists from socialist countries. These state farms were to be the motor of agricultural development. Peasants living in the poorest rural areas were of low priority to the new government except as cash-crop producers. The new government's attempts to promote voluntary production were ineffectual, especially as rural trade had dissolved with the departure of the Portuguese traders. Cashew trees became diseased and peasants burnt them in anger, as there was no longer a market for the nuts. Family sector cash-crop production plummeted.

In 1982, Ruth First was assassinated by the South African apartheid government when she opened a parcel containing a bomb in her university office. I was devastated, but I also became more determined to publish the story of konzo.

THE WAR

By 1984, we could no longer work on konzo, as travel out of the provincial capital had become too dangerous. The South African government had launched war against Mozambique. The independence of Mozambique had allowed the African National Congress to establish a presence close to South Africa, while the Soweto uprising in 1976 provided a whole new generation of recruits. At the same time, Mozambique became the key rear base for the Zimbabweans fighting for their independence. The Rhodesian government retaliated by forming a Mozambican rebel movement. When Zimbabwe gained independence in 1980, the South African government took over the rebel movement[ii] and soon almost the whole country was involved in the brutal war. By the time the war ended in 1992, the balance was around 1 million dead and 3 million displaced out of a population of 12 million.

Reports of smaller konzo epidemics came sporadically. In 1990, I ventured to the site of a recent outbreak, just off a main road. It was a hair-raising journey. At regular intervals, trenches had been dug across the asphalt road, a reminder from the rebels that traveling was not safe. We arrived at the village from which cases had been reported and stopped short in shock. The village was deserted and the air was heavy with smoke. Before us, houses still smoldered from a rebel attack.

PEACE

When apartheid ended in South Africa, a peace accord in Mozambique followed swiftly. I had by this time left the Ministry of Health to teach full-time in the Faculty of Medicine. Nine months later, in July 1993, I was back in Nampula with a group of medical students to investigate an epidemic of konzo. The epidemic had begun during the war the year before, this time centered in Mogincual district. The war had been particularly fierce in Mogincual and most of the residents had fled to towns and small settlements. When the war ended, they had rushed back to their homes.

We drove south from the capital along a narrow strip of dirt road, accompanied by a doctor from Médecins Sans Frontières (MSF), the international non governmental organization (NGO). The forest crowded in, and occasionally, a troupe of large monkeys ran across our path. The few small roadside shops bore the signs of war, their contents plundered and roofs removed. We stopped at a small settlement on the way for a toilet break, where I met an Australian engineer friend who was working for MSF, rebuilding hospitals that had been targeted by the rebels. From him, I learned my first postwar lesson. As I set off to cross the yard, he said, matter-of-factly, "Don't go that way, it's mined."

We arrived at our destination of Liupo, the small district capital, just as the sun was setting. We could barely make out what looked like a ghost town—ruined buildings with crumbling walls lining an overgrown main street. We were greeted by a familiar face—Domingos Nicala, the head of physiotherapy in the province, who had been my companion on the earlier trip down the scarred road.

For a week, we shared our lives with the konzo patients in the surrounding tents. We woke to the sound of children playing on the exercise bars that Domingos Nicala had constructed from local timber. The most impressive sight was the mass exercise class, where a community activist, shouting shrilly in the high tones of Macua, drilled a large group of women. Bravely, they raised their weak legs, trying to outdo each other.

We traveled out of Liupo to the rural areas where people were busy resettling. The normally busy yards looked curiously empty; the everyday things that accumulate with settlement—mats, chickens, tools—were all absent. We spoke to groups of men and women, relatively well dressed in western clothes. (The worldwide system of secondhand clothing distribution had reached this far.) Their message was uniform: they were struggling to survive and needed seeds and tools. During the war, they had switched to farming bitter cassava, as it was more productive. Back home again, they had been forced to harvest it early, as they had no other crops. They complained about the monkeys, who had gained the upper hand in the fields and competed for food. Fortunately, the monkeys avoided bitter cassava. Cases of konzo were increasing again, coinciding with the cassava harvest. Eventually, over 600 cases were notified in Mogincual and surrounding districts.

We went on to Memba, able to travel safely there for the first time in 10 years. The once spacious colonial hospital was no more; there was only a gaping hole where the rebel mortar had hit. We drove into the village of Acordos de Lusaka, which, remarkably, looked just the same. To our surprise, many of the old konzo patients had survived the war. The small children we had tended to were now adults. The neurological signs in their legs were still present—the lesions of konzo were permanent. As we entered the schoolyard, the children disappeared in a flash, running in all directions. We were greeted by the smiling village health worker, who explained that the children were still fearful from the days of rebel attacks and were conditioned to run away as fast as they could when approached by strangers. He had survived the war, but he explained sadly that he had slowly developed a chronic paralysis, with the all-too-familiar signs of konzo.

In both Memba and Mogincual, we found that a proportion of apparently healthy schoolchildren had signs of subclinical nervous system damage. We sent urine samples off to Hans Rosling in Sweden. All the children had high thiocyanate concentrations, and concentrations were higher in those with signs of neurological damage.

Faced with the knowledge that rural communities were still in danger of konzo and cyanide poisoning, we were anxious to intervene. Sander Essers, a Dutch nutritionist, had worked in Nampula in the early 1980s and had lived in Acordos de Lusaka, trying to find a solution to konzo. Although the war halted his work in Nampula, he continued to work on cassava on his return to Holland and became an expert in processing techniques to remove cyanide. He provided an intervention in the form of a new processing method: grating. The cassava root contains both a precursor of cyanide (linamarin) and the enzyme that breaks it down (linamarase) in separate parts of the plant cell. Grating breaks down the divisions and allows the enzyme to work. The resulting mushy product is then squeezed and either roasted in a pan or sun-dried. Graters were supplied free and dozens of village activists were trained to spread the method through communities. At first, the method was greeted with enthusiasm. But the number of graters was insufficient, and they broke as women also used them for grating maize. The method, both laborious and time-consuming, was not adopted.

We needed to continue monitoring, but transporting the samples to Sweden was proving onerous. In 1995, the International Institute for Tropical Agriculture convened a meeting on cassava and human health in Ibadan, Nigeria. There I met a retired Australian chemist and root crop expert, Howard Bradbury, who asked if he could help in any way. I suggested that he develop field kits to enable us to measure cyanide levels in the field. Now there were more Mozambicans with scientific training, and we formed a new lab analysis team led by Mario Ernesto and Paula Cardoso. Mario had trained in chemistry in East Germany and was stationed in the food analysis laboratory in Nampula. Paula Cardoso had graduated in chemical engineering from Eduardo Mondlane University and worked in the central food analysis laboratory in Maputo. She came from Nampula Province and was a keen field worker. Soon, we were sitting in the hospital in Memba with a group of community activists. They watched, fascinated, as the picrate papers in the kit darkened from the cyanide gas evaporating from cassava flour.

The team continued to visit Memba and Mogincual. In the late 1990s, peasants showed us cut cassava roots, disfigured by an ugly brown mush and inedible. This was due to brown-streak virus. As it spread, cassava production plummeted. In Acordos, the mean urinary thiocyanate concentration in schoolchildren at the time of the harvest had fallen from 512 μmol/L in 1997 to 130 μmol/L in 2003. Famine had been averted for various reasons: family members migrated to the nearby booming port town of Nacala, rural trade was reestablished, farmers grew more alternative drought-resistant crops such as millet and sorghum, and food aid was more readily available. Memba received attention from the government after the war, partly because of its reputation as a district of disasters. But Memba also had people looking out for it. The dedicated nuns in the missions in the interior had also run schools, which produced a generation of educated children. After independence, the government gave some of them the opportunity to study further in Cuba and East Germany. They were now in positions of power, where they could help their district. In Memba, no new konzo cases were reported after 1999.

In 2001, we drove into Memba along a smooth new road lined by electric pylons bringing hydroelectric power to the district capital. Setting off the next day for Mazua in the interior, I anticipated a long journey, remembering the perilous road of 20 years ago. We sped along and were there in a flash, as solid new bridges traversed the once almost impassable ravines. Acordos de Lusaka now had a scattering of cement-block houses with tin roofs, built by those working in the cities. Maurício, our formerly skinny guide and informant, greeted us, looking plump and prosperous, dressed in immaculate white robes. He spent most of his time as a trader in the towns.

Over and over again, peasants explained to us that they would continue to grow bitter cassava, as it is more productive, drought-resistant, and unappealing to monkeys. We knew that the sun-drying method currently used to remove cyanide was inefficient and would never get concentrations down to safe levels. The short-cut, emergency method of pounding it into small pieces to dry quickly was even less efficient. The effective grating method had not been adopted.

In Mogincual, we had noticed that people used heap fermentation extensively in bad years. They heaped the cut and peeled cassava roots in a pile and covered it with grass. They then laid the resulting fermented roots out to dry in the sun. Lab measurements showed that the cyanide levels were half that in sun-dried cassava. We promoted the method, but thiocyanate levels in the community remained high and we found that the method was not practical for the bulk of the harvest.

Sporadic cases of konzo continued to appear in Mogincual, with 83 cases recorded between 1994 and 2003. Mean urinary thiocyanate concentrations in school-children remained consistently high during and just after the time of the cassava harvest. Initially we were encouraged by the signs of life that were returning. Domesticated guinea fowls now pecked in the earth around houses, and cassava lay out to dry on platforms. In the village of Terreni A, we found that peasants had begun to plant sweet cassava around their houses as conditions improved. We hoped that this heralded a switch back to sweet cassava. But they explained that they could grow sweet cassava only near their houses, where they could defend it from the monkeys. Further away, in their larger plots, they still had to grow bitter cassava. Unlike the case of Memba, postwar assistance to Mogincual had been minimal and the district appeared to be stagnating. In agriculture, the NGO tasked with giving assistance after the war concentrated their efforts on livestock reproduction. We saw goats and even some cattle close to the district capital, but not in the rural areas where konzo cases persisted.

On our most recent visit, we saw other changes. Before, the road to the worst-affected part of the district had been so narrow that we had to drive with the windows up in case a branch from the extremely irritant monkey bean brushed against us. Now the road was broad, opened up by loggers who were cutting down the forests. We saw large fields planted with cassava; the government had introduced block farming in an attempt to control monkey predation. Brown streak disease had also recently appeared and threatened to wipe out the cassava crop. If this happened, konzo might disappear, but the Mogincual district would be at serious risk for famine.

AN INVITATION

In 2002, an international NGO invited the team to monitor the thiocyanate concentrations in their project areas in the district of Erati. Erati had suffered two konzo epidemics—drought-associated in 1981 and war- and drought-associated in 1988. But no new case has been recorded since 1994. The NGO had received funding for a cassava and food security project; they could not work in the districts where konzo persisted, as the province was divided up between NGOs. The current konzo areas were no one's first choice.

We drove west from the district capital in the direction of Mount Erati, on the principle that konzo occurs in the most distant areas. But our team was also keen to visit the fabled mountain, a sacred site of pilgrimage. As we drove along, the sharp-eyed Domingos Nicala spotted a young man walking by the side of the road with the characteristic konzo gait. We stopped, curious, and soon learned that the neighboring houses were full of old konzo patients, children who had developed the disease in the 1980s and were now grown up. These cases had never been recorded and many of them were in bad shape, their legs contracted, as they had never benefited from physiotherapy. Most of the young women who had developed konzo had died, but one old woman determinedly crawled out to greet us, helped by her daughter, who also had konzo. One young boy who walked with the greatest difficulty, supported by sticks, took a medical student aside and shyly whispered in her ear. She relayed the question: He had gone as far as he could in his studies in the village and wanted to go on to boarding school. Could we help? We were able to fulfill his request and also gave him a tricycle. In the village itself, we set up a rehabilitation center made of local materials and supplied walking aids.

Erati had good agricultural potential, with good soil and rains. The district had benefited from postwar assistance and people were consuming a variety of staples. Locally grown beans were a predominant part of the diet. Mean urinary thiocyanate concentrations in schoolchildren were lower than in Mogincual. Konzo had disappeared, apparently owing to development.

By 2005, I was confident that konzo would fade as development continued. It had disappeared from Erati and Memba, and the last recorded case in Mogincual was in 2003.

HUNGER

Back in Mozambique in September 2005, after a break in Australia, I received a call from the Ministry of Health. An epidemic of paralysis in Zambézia province, initially notified as polio, had turned out to be konzo.

Zambézia was located to the south of Nampula. Apart from one small outbreak in 2000, konzo had never been reported there. Back on the road again, this time with colleagues from the Faculty of Medicine, I had assumed that we would be traveling the usual long distances. But our first stop was a rehabilitation center on the main road to Malawi, not far from the large district capital of Mocuba. Konzo patients, with their familiar gait, struggled around the yard. We walked to nearby houses where other patients sat, in sight of the main road. The fertile land amazed me. The soil was rich, the cassava plants green and leafy. Compared with the dry landscapes of Nampula, I found it hard to believe that this was the site of a konzo epidemic.

But the story was familiar. Community members explained that the drought had caused failure of other crops. They had earlier sold their surplus to Malawi and then were caught short when their own crops were hit by drought. They had nothing left to eat but bitter cassava. They knew it was poisonous, as they were suffering frequent symptoms of dizziness and headaches. But they had no alternative. Malawi had offered good prices for their crops, because it was suffering a severe food crisis, caused by a combination of drought and the HIV/AIDS epidemic.

At the same time, the provincial health department in Nampula was busy dealing with the reemergence of a dozen cases of konzo in the poor interior of Memba. New cases were reported from several other districts in the province. In Memba, cassava yields were low as a result of drought and brown-streak disease. People now had to buy cassava to feed themselves. Measurements showed that this purchased cassava was high in cyanide.

The persistence of konzo in Mogincual, the emergence in Zambézia, and the reemergence in Memba all highlight the fragility of peasant agriculture in the poor rural cassava-dependent areas of Mozambique. At the best of times, children suffer poisoning during the cassava harvest; a drought can easily tip them over into konzo.

This fragility is a result of economic and agricultural policies that have marginalized the poor. Over 20 years after the first konzo epidemic occurred under a socialist government, konzo is now occurring under the free-market policies of a firmly capitalist government. In 1987, Mozambique adopted an International Monetary Fund/World Bank economic structural adjustment package that relied heavily on market-based solutions. Government spending was cut as a result. After the war, Mozambique has recorded impressive economic growth and a fall in poverty levels. But the free-market economic policies led to increased inequity. While a rich elite grew rapidly in the capital and provincial towns, poor peasants were not allowed any subsidies for fertilizer and other inputs and therefore had to take all the risks of bad weather and market failure. The government has been blocked from setting up a rural development bank that might give them credit. Peasants increasingly grow cassava as a fallback and food security crop in case anything goes wrong. In Mozambique, more than 60% of farmers now grow cassava; in 2004, the cassava harvest was 6.4 million tons, compared to just over 2 million tons for cereals (maize, rice, millet, and sorghum).

Agricultural policies have promoted cash crops for trade, which have marginalized the poorest peasants. On a larger scale, potentially richer agricultural districts have been prioritized by both the government and NGOs in a search for quick results. On an even larger scale, with globalization, many cash crops grown by poor countries face falling prices, as selective protection is offered to richer economies. Agricultural subsidies to cash crops in developed countries artificially lower prices and give their farmers an unfair advantage over their counterparts in developing countries. Cash crops in poor countries such as Mozambique thus generate less money, leading to a deepening of rural poverty.

From 1970 to 1985, when konzo was reemerging, food production in Africa as a whole grew at half the population rate. Most countries in Africa are now net food importers. Investments in agriculture in Africa have been falling for many years; World Bank lending for agriculture fell from about 31% of its total lending in 1979–1981 to less than 10% in 1999–2000. Support mechanisms such as marketing boards and extension services have collapsed. In the last 20 years, Africa has borne the burden of the AIDS pandemic, which has cut a swath through the most productive part of the adult population. Konzo has now been reported from Tanzania, Cameroon, and the Central African Republic. It continues in the Democratic Republic of Congo, where it is often associated with war.

While most food production in Africa is dwindling, cassava cultivation is spreading rapidly; production nearly tripled between 1961 and 1999. Although much of this growth can be attributed to increasing use of cassava as a large-scale commercial cash crop in West Africa, poorer farmers have also turned to cassava as both a cash and subsistence crop. Wars, decreasing farm size, economic stagnation, erratic rainfall, and rapid population growth have contributed to the recent rapid spread of cassava. Today it is increasingly the basic staple of many poor rural communities. The move to cassava is likely to continue if current economic and agricultural policies are maintained. Farmers will increasingly use cassava as a crop to stave off hunger and famine in bad times. Yet by a bitter irony, in the worst of times, when it is most useful for food security, it can cause konzo. People are faced with a dilemma—they might be poisoned by their daily food, but without it they will starve.

It comes down to hunger.

AN ORPHAN DISEASE

The study of konzo has been my greatest professional success, meticulously documented and written up in scientific journals. But it has also been my greatest failure, because it still exists.

In 2004, I gave a lecture on konzo to a medical gathering in Australia. I began with a short movie clip that showed the konzo survivors in Acordos de Lusaka, struggling across the schoolyard. I then progressed with my lecture, dryly describing the results of our monitoring and showing images of new patients. Suddenly, the lecture was interrupted. An ethicist in the audience lept up and said, "I can't stand this any more." Offended by the images of human suffering and poverty, she could not imagine that konzo could not be prevented. Her interjection encapsulated my frustration—I had been working for over 20 years on a disease that I have been powerless to prevent. I believed that the answer lay in rural development, but the economic models now being pursued in Mozambique favor the rich rather than the rural poor. As a health worker, directing agricultural extension services to the rural poor lay outside my realm of action.

But could konzo have been prevented by targeted interventions? In the beginning, prevention seemed easy. The disease was due to a severe drought. Once the drought was over, konzo would disappear. Blame lay with bitter cassava. Replace it, and the problem would be solved. A priest devoted himself to the task of distributing cuttings of sweet cassava in Memba. Peasants called it Caritas, after the Roman Catholic charity.

The drought ended, urinary thiocyanate levels fell, and konzo did disappear from Memba. When we returned after the war, I asked if people were still growing Gurué. No, Maurício, of Acordos de Lusaka, grinned. Now we are growing an even more bitter variety, Makwela. And what about Caritas? Oh, it turned bitter along with the years.

Thiocyanate levels were up again.

Better processing to remove the cyanide had seemed an attractive alternative. But our efforts to introduce grating had failed. Howard Bradbury also joined in the search for a solution and came up with a brilliant piece of lateral thinking. In Mozambique, we had found that cyanide concentrations in flour fell over an extended time period. But in his Canberra laboratory, the concentrations remained high. Why? Could the difference lie in the humid climate of Mozambique compared to dry Australia? He wetted samples of flour from Mozambique and Indonesia; after 5 hours, the cyanide concentration had dropped by 85%. This exciting finding needed to be tested on more samples from Mozambique. Arnaldo Cumbana, a methodical Mozambican chemist, traveled to Mogincual to collect flour samples. In his laboratory in the city of Beira, he repeated the experiment. It worked, but he was still using only tiny samples. He decided to test a larger volume of flour in a single container so as to simulate real life. Cyanide levels remained high, as the gas could not escape. He spread the paste out and repeated the experiment. By the end of 5 hours, 85% of the cyanide had evaporated.

In 2005, I watched as a team from the Faculty of Medicine field-tested the method. Women in konzo-affected communities in Zambézia prepared *chima* with both dry and wetted flour. Amid laughter, curiosity, and scepticism that their *chima* would lose its usual strength, men and women lined up in two queues to do a blind taste test. There was no clear preference. The new method did not require special equipment or extra labor. The cyanide levels dropped. Could I dare to hope that we had found a solution? I was skeptical that konzo could be eliminated by such a simple measure, yet I had seen peasants readily experiment and change their habits on many occasions. And neonatal tetanus, the disease of poor communities that had marked my early career in Mozambique, had virtually disappeared with vaccination. Changing deeply ingrained food preparation habits seemed a tougher call. But I felt that we could not ignore this potential solution while still pressing for action on the longer haul of rural development. Now, 2 years later, people have yet to adopt the wetting method, but these things take time.

I realized early on that I had become an advocate for an orphan disease. Once the excitement and novelty of the big epidemics was over, few people were interested in konzo. Only those who had traveled to the remote rural areas of Africa and seen the victims were moved to act. Those who have not been there cannot understand us. Being an advocate for an orphan disease puts one out on a limb—as somehow not quite rational—in a world where there are too many competing priorities. Orphan diseases occur in the poorest rural communities and often persist unnoticed and ignored. They lack attention and advocates; they rarely make the list of priority diseases for prevention and treatment.

I continue to advocate for konzo because I cannot get the images of paralyzed women and children out of my mind. It may not rank high on the list of priorities in terms of numbers of cases, but konzo is an indicator of an unacceptable level of inequity. To starve or to be paralyzed by one's only food source—that is a choice no one in this world should have to face.

NOTES

i. Apartheid was a system of racial segregation enforced in South Africa from 1948 to 1994.
ii. The United States supported the South African government as part of its geopolitical Cold War strategy.

PART II

The Difference That Gender Makes

Daniel Perlman and Ananya Roy

Social scientists use the term *sex* to refer to the biology of reproductive differences and *gender* to the social construction of biological difference—the systems of symbols, practices, and discourses through which human societies give meaning to the categories of "man" and "woman." Gender also includes the power relations within these systems, which treat social hierarchies and unequal resource allocations as if they were natural rather than social phenomena.

Viewing gender as a social construct allows us to interrogate what was previously seen as "natural," and thus indisputable. It is revolutionary, for a gendered perspective allows many taken-for-granted meanings in societies, and thus in the domain of public health, to become unlocked. Provocative questions follow: Who constitutes the "public" in *public health?* And where do the boundaries of public domain fall? Who establishes, and polices, the divide between public and private, and where does the domestic arena lie? The arena of labor and the workforce? Is the family a private realm or is it a public one, a site of politics and struggle for resources and identities? Are the division of labor and the enactment of violence within the domestic sphere matters of private concern or public interest? These questions, among others, are frequently posed by feminist theorists and have enormous implications for the practice of public health.

Although the term "gender" is often used synonymously with "woman" in health care-related issues, it is evident that it encompasses much more than simply the conditions that affect women's bodies, such as cervical cancer. A gendered analysis allows for the boundaries of what constitutes "health" and "health care" to be reexamined. This is especially relevant when we consider reproductive health. Reproductive health is often equated with women's health—diminishing the equal weight with which issues of reproduction involve men and compartmentalizing it into the same specialized and marginalized side category where topics that pertain primarily to women's bodies are so often cast. Reproduction is more than simply the biological production of infants—it is also the reproducing of social mores, community traditions, and cultural beliefs. Feminists influenced by Marxist theory note that the social divisions of labor, both domestic and otherwise, are repeatedly reinstated and reinforced in society via reproduction within the family: nurturing a family, raising children, and laying the groundwork for roles to be adopted and held in the realms of economy, society, and state. This, in turn, eliminates the distinctions between a private household and a public world because the public world is shaped directly by the politics of the household. These theorists ask: If reproduction is social rather than biological, what is reproductive health? Is it gynecological care, or is it also, as Suneeta Krishnan's case in this section implies, the material realities and cruelties of backbreaking labor, both within and outside the household? The case suggests that silence on political issues involving women cannot be reconciled with the professional ethics of the health practitioner.

The accounts of Nuriye Nalan Sahin-Hodoglugil and Aruna Uprety pose an even more radical question: is not the issue of reproductive *rights* a fundamental element of good public health? The shift from *needs* to *rights* is radical because it repoliticizes the often depoliticized domains of family, women, and bodies. Discussing reproduction in terms of rights – the right to reproductive control, the right to choose – is powerful; it opens the hidden world of the family, it makes public the politics of the body, and it insists that the practice of health is not simply a professional or compassionate act but also a highly political one. This view suggests that a good doctor might have to be a social activist as well as a biological technician. When confronted by dying women, as was Aruna Uprety in her early days of medical practice in Nepal, she renders not only a medical diagnosis but also a social, political, and economic one. Nuriye Nalan Sahin-Hodoglugil stands up on the floor of the United Nations and calls for an end to honor crimes. Sandra Lane takes on the forces of urban renewal and welfare reform, inevitably racialized processes, in trying to make sense of teen pregnancies and infant mortality. These authors illustrate how medical issues cannot be distinguished from social and political ones in discussions of the health of women and children.

THE GLOBAL AGENDA: MAINSTREAMING GENDER

Development institutions had, since the 1950s, promoted policies for engaging "women in development," adhering to an ideology that endorsed modernization and proceeded on the belief that educating girls en masse and incorporating women into lines of economic production would improve individual livelihoods and increase childhood health and survival rates. During this period, population limitation policies focused largely on spreading contraceptive technology and convincing couples to use it. However, reasons for resistance to contraception proved more complex than the conservative religious beliefs that most development specialists imagined. The reasons included widespread misinformation about side effects and efficacy, lack of access to modern methods, economic issues such as the value of children's labor as opposed to the cost of educating them, as well as fears that contraception would empower women to engage in infidelity or allow them to take wider economic and political roles outside the household and outside the control of men in the family.

At the end of the twentieth century, a new approach emerged, known as "mainstreaming gender." In utilizing the terminology of "gender" rather than "women"; it made the case that gender was a system of social relations that had to be transformed in order to mitigate women's vulnerability, powerlessness, and ill health. Reproductive health was at the forefront of this new agenda. Beginning in 1987, the Safe Motherhood Initiative has sought to reduce the alarming numbers of deaths among women that occurred in relation to childbearing. When worldwide data were compiled on maternal death, it became clear just how many women were dying from unsafe abortions. At the same time, studies showed that women who did not have access to contraceptives were much more likely to die during pregnancy. Emphasis in family planning shifted from issues of access and of population limitation as a strategy to alleviate poverty and facilitate development to concerns about quality of care. This attention to quality of care made the individual woman, her health, and her dignity an important rationale for the provision of contraceptive care.

Gender was not the only global agenda of the 1990s. There were others: the environment, housing, microcredit. Each issue had its own global summit, organized by the United Nations. The gender summits were among the most visible of these. Three in particular are worth noting. In 1994, the United Nations Conference on Population and Development took place in Cairo; it was concerned with the crucial but controversial issues of population growth, family planning, reproduction, and contraception. The policy shift from family planning to a broader reproductive health framework—which included issues such as sexually transmitted diseases, infertility, abortion, reproductive cancers, gender hierarchies, inequalities, and divisions—was a central concern to the conference.

In 1995, the United Nations Fourth World Conference on Women was held in Beijing. Although there had been previous world conferences on women (between 1975 and 1985), the Beijing summit was large (in fact, the largest conference in the history of the United Nations), visible, and ambitious. It put forward a Platform of Action that sought to tackle the most entrenched forms of gender inequality. In 2000, the United Nations headquarters in New York hosted a special session of the General Assembly titled Women 2000: Gender Equality, Development and Peace for the Twenty-First Century. Known as the Beijing + 5 conference, this forum sought to develop the actions and initiatives necessary to implement the Beijing Platform for Action. Nuriye Nalan Sahin-Hodoglugil provides a firsthand account of the Beijing + 5 forum.

There are several hallmark features of the global agenda of "mainstreaming gender." The various summits were organized by the Division for the Advancement of Women (DAW) of the United Nations. However, the real energy lay elsewhere: in a global civil society comprising nongovernmental organizations (NGOs). Thousands of NGOs registered for these summits and helped shaped the very fundamentals of the gender agenda. This unleashing of civil society's energies indicated a new political field of development. But it did not mean that nation-states were no longer relevant actors. NGOs were embedded in the political economy of the nation in a variety of ways—from close collaboration with governments to negotiated status to oppositional social movements. In other words, nation-states continued to be important players in the gender summits, but "national interests" were now more fractured, divided, and fragmented, with multiple (albeit unofficial) representation of a nation and its citizenry. This contradiction was enshrined in the Beijing Declaration and Platform of Action, which sought to ensure "the participation and contribution of all actors of civil society, particularly women's groups and networks and other non-governmental organizations and community-based organizations, with full respect for their autonomy, in cooperation with governments." Could the autonomy of NGOs and community organizations be always reconciled with the cooperation of governments?

The gender summits were animated by ideas of equality and empowerment: to promote "women as equal participants and beneficiaries of sustainable development, peace and security, governance and human rights" (DAW). It is worth paying closer attention to this agenda. The Beijing Declaration and Platform for Action sought to expand the scope of gender mainstreaming not only by acknowledging poverty and economic deprivation but also by going well beyond this economic realm and including issues of access to power and decision making. This shift from poverty to inequality is significant because it marked a political imagination, one that was more ambitious than the inclusion of women in economic growth. This new imagination confronted the very relations of inequality and thus implied the redistribution of both material and political resources.

But there were some important paradoxes and dilemmas in such an agenda. The Beijing Declaration drew upon the 1945 United Nations Charter to assert the human dignity and human rights of women. But it dramatically expanded the scope of such rights by insisting "the explicit recognition and reaffirmation of the right of all women to control all aspects of their health, in particular their own fertility, is basic to their empowerment." In other words, the Beijing Declaration and Platform of Action not only asserted "women and health" as an important component of the "mainstreaming gender" agenda but also defined reproductive rights as a central element of this domain of good health. The Beijing Declaration and Platform of Action also asserted the right to religious belief as an equally central element of the empowerment and advancement of women: "the right to freedom of thought, conscience, religion and belief, thus contributing to the moral, ethical, spiritual and intellectual needs of women and men, individually or in community with others." Nuriye Nalan Sahin-Hodoglugil's provocative account of the Beijing + 5 forum demonstrates the clash of these various rights-based frameworks: reproductive rights versus the right to difference. The latter asserts cultural difference, recoding social practices and inequalities as "natural" and "traditional."

It is not surprising that by the time the "mainstreaming gender" agenda found its way into the Millennium Development Goals, gender equality and empowerment was confined to less controversial topics: maternal mortality, the vulnerability of women to HIV/AIDS, women's participation in parliaments and labor forces. The politics of the body had been set aside; the global agenda had been domesticated and tamed. Aruna Uprety's fiery narrative of medical practice in Nepal shows the disjunction between this domesticated global agenda and the very real politics of the body that exists in the extraordinary everyday world of doctors and dying women.

SOCIAL STRATIFICATIONS

In the global agenda of "mainstreaming gender," language plays an important role. Control over names and categories allow control over the agenda. Nalan Sahin-Hodoglugil illustrates these politics of knowledge and voice when she asks: "Who can speak, in what idiom, and with what authority and legitimacy on the floor of the United Nations?" Her account is complex because it points not only to issues of *international* authority and discourse but also to those at the national scale. Who represents Turkey? Did these women, all highly qualified and dedicated, speak for the heterogeneity of Turkey's women and men? Such issues also become central in Suneeta Krishnan's reflexive narrative of "doing good" in the villages of India. We see Krishnan challenge the traditions of the countryside by insisting that women from lower castes be able to work shoulder to shoulder with high-caste women. In doing so, her health work became undeniably activist, taking on a radical politics of the body: that those whose bodies had been deemed untouchable by the cruel, arbitrary rules and norms of religion and culture would now be in charge of healing all bodies. What are the frontiers and limits of such health activism? Is Krishnan the interfering, missionary, urbanized Indian do-gooder, seeking to catalyze social change? Or is she simply arguing that the professional ethics of inclusive health care required surpassing the barriers of gender, caste, race, ethnicity, and class?

There are no easy answers to these questions. Each of the cases indicates that the answers must be negotiated and struggled with in the crucible of geopolitics, community politics, and household politics. They also indicate that a gendered framework is much more than a concern with women's health. Gender is a system of relations between men and women. It involves practices and discourses. It is thus both mundane and esoteric. Gender as a social category of difference is also closely connected to other categories of difference. The category "women" is thus a highly differentiated social group with complex contours of access and risk. In Nepal, wealthy women do not shoulder the same burden of unsafe abortions as do poor women. In India, poor women, reliant on state-provided primary health care and its network of male doctors, are unable to voice their gynecological needs. Poor women from the lower castes are completely disenfranchised. In Syracuse, New York, distinctive and shocking vulnerabilities are associated with being poor, black, and a woman. The word *gender* condenses such social stratifications; it is shorthand for talking about power and inequality. It is also a powerful discourse for imagining change and imagining alternatives—for imagining an entirely different social calculus.

5   Beijing + 5: What Can International Conferences Achieve for Women's Health?

Nuriye Nalan Sahin Hodoglugil

According to the maps, the United Nations headquarters was only a few blocks from my hotel. Still, I set out early that day, and took my time strolling up First Avenue. As I drew closer, I caught sight of the immense skyscraper rising above the sea of other buildings. Although it was late spring and the sun was well above the horizon, the morning air was chilly, and I pulled my jacket close to my body as I walked. My stomach was jumping with nerves; to ignore it, I forced myself to look around at the city. The streets of Manhattan were just waking up along with me. If I were at home, in Ankara, I too would be moving with the throng of people, headed for the School of Public Health, consumed with my agenda for the day ahead. Being here felt very different as I watched men and women in spotless suits disappear into the tinted doors of office buildings—I had no idea what to expect from the upcoming morning.

I reached the entrance plaza and gardens within minutes. I shielded my eyes with my hand and looked up at the impossible building. It was so big that, up close, I could no longer see it all at once. Around me, tourists were snapping pictures. Moving through the wide glass entrance, I saw more of the same—they swarmed the lobby, and a long line had already gathered behind a small sign reading simply, "Tours." I drew a breath and squeezed by the line of people. Their guide, I had read, would lead them past the highlights of the building and through the common areas.

My destination was not so public. Following a discreet sign, I turned into a hallway which led me to a lower level of the building. Soon I turned and followed another hallway. I was now a few floors below the ground level. The walls were lined with a dark brown wood, and soft, low bulbs were placed every few feet, casting a dull, artificial light. This was in sharp contrast with the large windows and sunshine that had filled the main lobby.

People walking brusquely in both directions passed me by without a glance. They seemed to take no notice of the absence of light. Some were dressed in brightly colored traditional outfits and the rest wore business suits. My own outfit, in comparison, felt neutral and unimportant. I had tried my best to look both serious and professional, donning a black dress and black leather shoes, but despite the confidence I had felt when my mentor at the university, Dr. Meliha, had asked me to attend the meetings in her place, my insides had been a jumble of nerves ever since I had arrived in New York. Even my dress, at that moment, was a cause of anxiety.

As I continued down the hallway, I tried to quell my worries by reminding myself of my qualifications and of my initial excitement at accepting such an opportunity. As a physician and researcher in Turkey, I was certainly prepared to discuss women's health needs within my country. Having worked in family planning clinics, I had inserted thousands of IUDs and worked with countless married women to address their health needs.

Just then, I saw a small break in the wood paneling on my right. A placard, stationed next to a small gate, read "General Assembly Conference Room." The closed door was plain and unadorned, and I pushed it open quickly. The room that spread out in front of me made me catch my breath.

The room was split into two levels, the first of which was designed like an amphitheater. A polished stage stood in front, with the seats spreading outward in rows of semicircles, like the layers of a cinnamon roll. Tags for each country marked off sections of seats, moving along the rows in alphabetical order. Each country's section was equipped with a microphone and multiple sets of earphones for listening to the simultaneous translations.

I looked to the second level, which was divided from the first by a high wall and could only be accessed by a separate entrance. Later, I would learn that these seats were reserved for spectators, persons from nongovernmental organizations (NGOs) and others, who, since they were not named as official delegates, were forbidden from directly participating in the meetings. I walked slowly to the center of the amphitheater, searching for Turkey's tag. A few people sat casually in some of the seats, but the vast majority of the room was empty.

In 1995, when the Fourth World Conference for Women was held in Beijing, women came from all over the world to discuss pertinent issues such as health, economic and political power, and violence and oppression. The final document produced at this conference was the Platform for Action, which described the overall status of women internationally based on these issues. In very strong language, it outlined suggestions to improve gender equality. The Beijing +5 meetings, which would all take place in the huge room where I was standing, had been organized by the UN's Division for the Advancement of Women to assess the current situations of women globally and to make relevant changes to the Platform for Action while also reaffirming commitment to the original document.

I spotted my country's tag, between the signs for Trinidad and Tobago and Tuvalu. Our seats were empty; I was the first of my delegation to arrive. Instead of going directly to our section, I hovered in the center of the room, my head tilted back as I stared at the top rows of the second level. For a second, I wanted to scream "Can you hear me?" out into the vacant seats. As children, we would do this every time we visited one of the many ancient amphitheaters scattered along the Mediterranean coast. One would yell "Can you hear me?" to which someone else, poised at the top, would respond "Yes! I can hear you. . . ." The acoustics amazed us: after screaming the first time, we would drop our voices again and again until we were using only whispers, to see what could still be heard. The important thing was the sense that somebody was listening.

I made my way up the steps to await the arrival of my codelegates. After a few minutes, more and more people began filtering into the room, coming through the same unimposing doorway that I had used. I watched them file in, greeting each other, making their way to various sections. I noticed a group of three women making their way up the stairs, walking directly toward where I sat. They reached me quickly and before I could stand up, the leader, a short, heavy, dark-haired woman with large glasses, stepped forward and put out her hand, introducing herself as Cemile. She had a strong, clear voice and held herself in an authoritative

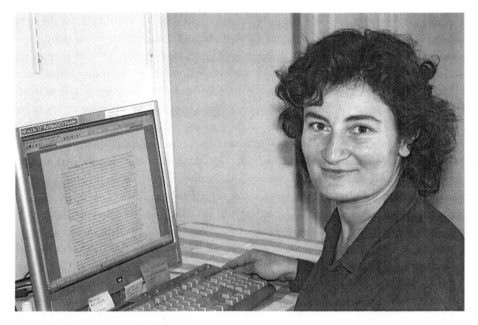

Nuriye Nalan Sahin Hodoglugil.

manner. It was obvious that she knew who I was, probably having been in contact with Dr. Meliha, because without waiting for an introduction, she used the cordial, official "Mrs. Nalan" to address me. I tried to shake her hand firmly but was struck by her impressive voice—she spoke with the formal emphasis of a government official or television newscaster, and her tone was very serious. She turned to the others and began introducing them, continuing to use the same formal voice.

Nuran was nearly Cemile's physical opposite—petite and blonde. She wore a light-colored suit and struck me as having a soothing, motherly attitude. Despite Cemile's command of the situation, Nuran was actually her supervisor at the General Directorate of Women's Status and Problems in Turkey. On the other side of Cemile was Sevgi, a woman who gave me a big smile. Although I did not know her, she was a teacher in the department of Gender and Women's Studies in Ankara. Behind Sevgi stood Aylin, whom Cemile introduced last. She was younger than the others, had dark, flashing eyes, and wore heavy lipstick.

We shook hands and greeted one another warmly. I smoothed my dress with my palms while the others set their bags down and filed past me into the seats of our section. These would be the women I would be working with, day and night, for the next few weeks.

Just then, a loud banging noise filled the room, and the static of a microphone turning on crackled over the speaker system. The five of us turned; on the polished stage at the center of the room stood a tall woman in a crisp gray suit, leaning into the podium and looking out at the rows of chairs expectantly. The banging noise had come from a long wooden gavel she held in one hand. She poised it over the podium and brought it down again, three staccato raps that amplified out over the audience. A hush fell over the room, followed by the sound of shuffling papers and bodies shifting in chairs. I looked out over the sections below us and craned my neck to see the rows behind. Most of the chairs were filled; however, there were some countries, such as Tuvalu, next to us, that had only empty seats. It was not until that evening, back in my hotel room, that I came to realize that this was because these countries were too impoverished to send delegates.

The woman cleared her throat into the microphone. Across the room, delegates lifted earphone sets and adjusted them on their heads. "Welcome," the woman began, "to the United Nations Beijing +5 Conference. . . ." While I listened to the opening remarks, I scanned the crowd. If I turned to the side, I could see into the higher sections, where the NGO participants sat leaning forward, some with their arms resting on the top of the dividing wall. We all had, I presumed, been given a copy of the draft outcome document, put out by the UN's Division for the Advancement of Women (DAW). DAW had asked all countries to submit an assessment of the past 5 years, describing their accomplishments, problem areas, and future plans of action for improving women's rights. These assessments were put together to create the Outcome Document for Beijing +5. This document would be the focal point for the entirety of the conference—after the World Women's

Conference in Beijing, 1995, DAW had taken suggestions from every country and added them to the old platform, coming up with a draft that would be debated and reworked throughout this conference, ending 5 years later. The specific changes each country had requested—most often, it had looked to me, to be deletions, additions, or simple rewording of phrases or single sentences—had been added in bold type.

I listened dutifully to the rest of the opening speech. Next to me, Aylin tapped her foot and shifted in her seat. I wondered what my codelegates had thought about the draft outcome document; we had not gotten that far in our chatting. Mentally, I recounted the changes in the draft that had been suggested by Turkey: honor crimes, abortion, etc. Most likely these changes were made directly by Cemile and Nuran's Office of Women's Status, which would have received the draft from DAW.

The woman at the podium began explaining the details of how the conference would be run. The draft document would be read aloud to the conference room, and each time a change had been suggested, the moderator would pause and open the floor for debate. The country that had suggested the change would speak first, followed by any other country that had input. If there was disagreement, the debate would continue until a consensus had been reached. To complicate things, DAW had allowed for additional changes to be suggested during the conference proceedings. The deadline for submitting these written changes, she announced loudly, was 2 days away. Oral changes, the woman continued, could be suggested by a country at any point during the conference. It dawned on me then that the number of potential changes that could be made—if each country had even more additions or deletions to the document—was staggering.

After the opening session had concluded, the five of us made our way to the cafeteria. Like the hallways, it was dim and poorly lit. We carried small trays of food and situated ourselves at one of the square tables. Around us, I saw that numerous other delegates, mostly middle-aged women in suits and formal attire, were doing the same thing. Interspersed were groups of regular UN employees, whom I quickly learned to recognize by the plastic badges hanging around their necks.

Cemile wasted no time. Without touching her sandwich, she moved her tray aside and dug into her briefcase, withdrawing her copy of the outcome document and a legal pad for notes. On one side of me Aylin lit a cigarette, setting the used match in an empty ashtray at the center of the table. I watched as Sevgi followed suit, pulling out a box from her purse and lighting up. She pulled deeply on the filter while she watched Cemile and waited.

Cemile spread the papers out in front of her and looked up. "We need to make a plan as soon as possible, so that we can begin working tonight and tomorrow." She ran her fingers along the first pages of the draft document, which was divided into 12 subjects: women and poverty, women and violence, women and health, women and the economy, etc. "We should split up the sections based on our specialties, and review them."

Aylin tapped her cigarette on the rim of the ashtray, and spoke up. "I agree." she said, leaning forward. "We should come up with a list of priorities from each section—those changes that are most important for Turkey to advocate for."

The smoke from the cigarettes snaked hazily up towards the ceiling. My eyes already felt parched and itchy. Until about a year before, I too, had been a smoker. When I started smoking, it had been a sign of being a liberal woman in Turkey—all of my activist friends were smokers. At the time, it was considered abnormal for women to smoke in public, and my friends and I would intentionally stand on the street and smoke in protest. It was a small form of activism for us. Now, however, I had grown unaccustomed to it, and I blinked as Aylin continued: "We have to act quickly, decide on the changes as soon as possible, in order to give the committee our written suggestions." At this she stubbed out her cigarette and pulled out her own copy of the platform draft. Cemile frowned.

"Yes," she said, "but we can submit our changes orally as well, for many of the subjects, during the meetings." I thought quickly back to the opening speaker's instructions. It was true, she had specified that new changes could be suggested both orally and in writing.

"If you don't write your suggestions down formally, they won't count," Aylin said, her voice full of authority. "If you want the changes to be taken *seriously*, you have to write them down. And the deadline being so soon, we should begin tonight."

Cemile shook her head. "We have to prioritize, Ms. Aylin. If we write something, we will have to argue for it orally during the meetings. There will be many, many arguments going on. Turkey does not need to participate in all of them, particularly the ones that are not pertinent to our country."

I looked around the table. Nuran was still reading, and Sevgi sat stonefaced. I felt myself torn between the two sides of the argument. Cemile's stubbornness reminded me of the attitude typical of Turkish officials and of how much of government seems to work: Don't poke your nose into things too much, go at the pace that is expected. However, we *were* dealing with a writing culture, and I understood Aylin's point about being taken seriously.

At Cemile's words, Aylin sat up straighter in her seat. "Yes, I understand that," she said, "but we should still try. No one will listen to an oral intervention, and it's important that we make a strong statement about Turkey's position on *all* the issues."

Cemile nodded curtly at her. "Of course your ideas on all the issues are important, Ms. Aylin. But we cannot focus on too many things at the same time, and we cannot go to extremes either. Turkey should have a lead role in supporting certain issues, such as reproductive rights, and in including the prevention of honor crimes. My General Directorate is also strongly supporting women's role in politics, and in relation to the economy. But that's all. For the rest, we can offer support if we like the idea, and withhold support if we don't. They are not directly related to us and our problems." She paused. "We should write, of course, but not on all issues. As the head of the delegation, I feel it is more important to focus on two or three issues that are most important to us."

Aylin opened her mouth to respond, but Cemile cut her off. "Ms. Aylin," she said, "we are losing time. Prepare as many written statements as *you* want to. Do you have a laptop?"

At this, Aylin looked, for the first time, hesitant. "No," she responded.

We decided to use the computer laboratory at the UN the following day, after each reading over the outcome document that evening. We quickly reviewed the 12 sections, then gathered our things to leave. As we cleaned the table, I looked at our trays. Most of the food remained untouched.

That night I read over the document again, paying special attention to the sections on women and health and violence against women. The subsections on reproductive health would be especially contentious. Throughout the section where birth control was mentioned, bold type suggested replacing *contraception* with *family planning*. The change had been suggested by the Holy See, the delegation from the Vatican.

Working in the field, in Turkey, my colleagues and I often used the two terms interchangeably. However, in the politics of population policy, *family planning* implies that birth control is only for a married male and female couple—not for adolescents and unmarried women. In Turkey, too, this is a difficult issue. Sex within the institution of marriage is celebrated in Islam, but anything outside of wedlock is considered unacceptable. I am constantly aware of this in my professional life: often, when teaching at the university or working in a clinic, I am approached by young, unmarried women seeking contraceptives or treatment for sexually transmitted diseases. Even within marriage, too many Turkish women do not have the means or resources to control the number of their pregnancies. I thought briefly of my sister's mother-in-law, who, like many women living in rural and Eastern Turkey, was a good example of this. When I met her she was 75 years old and told me "I was like a man, I did not menstruate for 30 years." A tiny woman from a small village in the east, she had delivered 10 children, 6 of whom survived. She spent 2 or 3 years breast-feeding each child, only to find that she was pregnant again before even restarting her menstrual cycle.

Abortion would be another important topic for Turkey. It has been legal for Turkish women since 1983 and is generally not considered a highly sensitive topic. It is, however, utilized as a method of contraception in place of birth control itself. I was proud that Turkey had been the country responsible for suggesting an important change on this part of the document. The draft platform read that women should have access to "safe, legal abortions in countries where it is not against the law." Turkey had suggested the deletion of the phrase "those countries where it is not against the law." Although my efforts as a reproductive health practitioner in Turkey were focused on contraception, my attitude, and the attitude of every colleague I know in Turkey, is that the matter of abortion is for each woman to decide independently. In fact, most educated professionals within Turkey seem to support this, making it appropriate for Turkey to assume a leadership role in advocating for safe and legal abortions in the international arena, such as the Beijing +5 conference.

I was surprised when I learned that things are very different in the United States, and abortion practitioners are sometimes murdered by those opposing legal abortions.

I carefully wrote out a persuasive argument to be submitted and also a draft of Turkey's oral argument for the issue's debate during the meetings. I tried to ignore the butterflies that flapped around in my gut at the thought of reading these arguments out loud in that gigantic room. Crumpled papers littered the floor of my hotel room. Surely we could drum up support for the recommendation of safe abortion practices even in places where it was still forbidden. As a doctor, I knew that despite a country's legal restrictions, women would still have abortions, and if there were no access to safe ones, they would resort to methods that often caused serious physical illness and death. I had detailed some of these as examples in my argument for the deletion, and I fervently hoped that these arguments would bloom to full fruition at the meetings, influencing the other delegates to agree with Turkey.

The last section I reviewed before the meetings began was the section entitled "Violence against Women," which referred to honor crimes. This change had been suggested by the European Union (EU) delegation, which included Turkey in its regional preparatory meetings because Turkey was a candidate for EU membership. Aylin had attended and had pushed for the EU's support on including the issue in the platform. The EU had agreed, and in the draft document it had been added in as follows:

> Develop, adopt, and fully implement laws and other measures, as appropriate, such as policies and educational programs, to eradicate harmful customary and traditional practices, including female genital mutilation, early and forced marriage, and so-called honor crimes, which are violations of the human rights of women and girls. . . .

Aylin had also taken the important step of making individual connections within the EU, people who would verbally support the inclusion of honor crimes when the issue arose for debate. As I read over this paragraph, I felt unsettled. As the document noted, honor crimes were considered a traditional practice; although I disagreed with it very strongly, I saw it differently than many western theorists seemed to. The western perspective often condemns honor crimes and "other harmful traditional practices" without having an understanding or sense of the tradition involved. I certainly did not approve of honor crimes, but the question for me was more "When does a traditional practice become coercive?" I set the document on my lap and looked out the window, remembering my year of compulsory service after medical school. I went to work in a tiny village and rented a room in an apartment building where there were several other professional women who were also doing their year of service in the same area. One of these women, whose name was Gulsum, had a long-term boyfriend from college with whom she had broken up. They had not seen one another in 3 or 4 years. However, one weekend while I was out of town, he showed up. He professed his love for her and promised marriage.

She slept with him then, the first time for her. He left, promising to come back, but disappeared. Only later did she find out that he was already married, with a child. Gulsum was devastated. She believed that the situation had been her fault and that she had lost her honor. I don't think that she will marry for the rest of her life. Furthermore, she can tell no one about her experience. She comes from a traditional family in Eastern Turkey. If she told anyone in her family what had happened, she would put both herself and the man in danger. Depending on the strength of her brother's reaction, the man could be beaten or killed, and if Gulsum was thought to have consented to the relationship, the same risks applied to her.

Certainly, it was important that honor crimes be recognized in the final document, and it seemed that Aylin had done an important service in bolstering support for Turkey's position. I wondered how the subject would go over during the debates. If honor crimes were to be included, the document would serve as recognition of the problem and as a point of reference for activists to advocate from. However, I could not help but wonder if the careful wording was unrelated to actually lowering the incidence of honor crimes. After all, the outcome document would not ensure that the governments of participating countries actually did anything about the issues included.

Within a few days, the debates were in full swing. By the middle of that first week, I had learned that the majority of my time as a delegate would be spent watching and waiting. The experience reminded me of the few baseball games I had attended: nothing of interest happened for long stretches of time and then, suddenly, some excitement. But here, instead of a home run, the excitement came in the form of an especially charged topic.

The session on women and the family exemplified this. For hours, most of the suggested changes had been set with no opposition or debate. Over and over again, when the moderator came to a suggested change in the draft, a delegate from the proposing country, or group of countries—as many nations were organized into groups—would stand and offer one or two sentences on why the change should be approved. The moderator would ask for opposing opinions, and receiving none, would declare the change accepted. This monotony suddenly shifted when, in the early afternoon, the moderator came to a paragraph of two sentences suggested for addition by the delegation from the Vatican, or the Holy See. The text read as follows:

> Women play a critical role in the family. The family is the basic unit of society and is a strong force for social cohesion and integration and, as such, should be strengthened. The inadequate support to women and insufficient protection and support to their respective families affect society as a whole and undermine efforts to achieve gender equality. In different cultural, political, and social systems the rights, capabilities, and responsibilities of family members must be respected. Women's social and economic contributions to the welfare of the family and the social obligation of maternity and paternity continue to be inadequately addressed. . . .

The Vatican had suggested these two sentences, which clearly took pains to emphasize the primary importance of the family. This was of no surprise to me; all morning the Vatican had proposed small additions that seemed intent on highlighting women's role within the family structure as much as possible.

After the moderator had finished, the lead delegate from the Vatican raised his hand to ask for the floor. He was a handsome, tall man, who wore a business suit, although the delegates on either side of him were dressed in heavy-looking religious robes. The moderator motioned, and said: "Holy See, you have the floor."

He gazed out at the audience before speaking. "We want to add these two sentences, because we believe that women's role in the family must be emphasized."

With that, he leaned back in his chair, away from the microphone. I was getting used to there being no in-depth discussion around a suggested change. Arguments both for and against a change were generally kept to one or two sentences, rather than the detailed orations I had expected. *Predictable*, I thought. But what happened next surprised me. Across the room, a representative from the EU motioned to speak. She was middle-aged and impeccably dressed. The energy in the room shifted noticeably as attention focused on her, and everyone waited.

"While we agree that women's role in the family is important, we are not here to introduce *new language* to the document, which this suggestion would be doing."

I was learning that this was a standard way of opposing an addition to the document—using the phrase *new language*—because the UN and DAW had clearly expressed, in premeeting informational materials and in the opening sessions, that we were not here to rewrite the Platform for Action, but to amend it in order to best address all women's needs. I had already, several times, heard a country use this argument to oppose a suggested change. The Holy See delegate looked neither surprised nor disappointed. After asking for permission to speak by again raising his hand, he responded.

"We insist that women's role in the family be emphasized. We would like to keep it in the document."

I looked quickly at the EU representative, but she, too, seemed void of any emotion on the matter, despite the stubbornness of the Vatican's representative. Without hesitation she leaned forward and spoke again.

"Yes, women do play a critical role in the family, and have for thousands of years, but do we really need to put it in this document?"

Titters of laughter could be heard throughout the room. Above us, in the NGO section, there were a few claps. I wondered why, with all the Holy See's suggestions on strengthening the wording of the section on family that morning, this was the one that the EU was choosing to oppose.

The man leaned forward again.

"We believe that the family, and women's role in it, must be emphasized. We all live in families, do we not? Is there an opposition to the role of the family at this conference?"

I wondered where this was going. In the front of the room, the moderator, an Indian man from India's permanent mission to the UN, said nothing but instead seemed to be waiting for a response from the EU.

The woman reached towards her microphone again. "We can accept the addition of these two sentences only if you add 'various forms of the family exist' after the phrase 'In different cultural, political, and social systems.' We have to respect families in *all* forms, such as single-parent families or same-sex couples."

Above me came more claps from the NGOs. I wanted very badly to applaud along with them—the EU had made several suggestions toward recognizing the rights of lesbian women in other sections of the document, and I admired the representative's decision to use the Vatican's suggestion in this paragraph as a bargaining spot. I turned towards Cemile at the same time as Aylin, sitting on the other side of her, did.

"We should say something in support, yes?" Aylin asked, leaning forward so that she was sitting on only the edge of her seat.

But Cemile seemed indifferent to the drama that was unfolding in front of us.

"No," she said, shaking her head slightly. "This doesn't concern us, Turkey, very much." Next to her, Nuran nodded her head in agreement.

I could see lines of frustration etched into Aylin's face, but there was no time for further discussion, because the Holy See delegate was leaning in to speak again. The room was silent as he turned to address the moderator.

"We will accept the addition suggested by the European Union contingent upon the acceptance of our original suggestion."

The moderator looked toward the section where EU delegates were spread out, but the woman did not motion to speak again. He nodded and made notes on the papers in front of him. Then, in the same steady voice, he began reading the next paragraph. . . .

The debates continued in this manner. They were intensely time-consuming, and one evening, Nuran, who had remained quiet during much of our time together as a group, commented that even DAW had not expected them to progress so slowly. Thus, it was not until a full week of meetings had passed that the section on women and health was finally read. By this time, the meetings were stretching late into the evening hours, and I had witnessed many more stubborn arguments similar to the one between the EU and the Vatican. Some of the most contentious subjects remained unresolved—the moderator, the same man from India, seemed willing to let an argument go back and forth for only so long. A few times, when there seemed to be no resolution in sight, he ended the discussion and left the section to remain in bold brackets on the document, which meant that it would be revisited later. However, time was running out before the meetings of the UN's General Assembly, which would be signing and certifying the document. It was therefore in our best interests to have as many changes decided upon as possible, because if they were left in brackets for a last-minute review, it was probable that they would be addressed hastily or possibly even dismissed.

Much to my disappointment, this happened very quickly to Turkey's suggested change on women's access to safe and legal abortions. As soon as the suggested addition was read by the moderator, many people raised their hands, wanting to offer both support and opposition. The moderator let the arguments go back and forth for a while, but when it became clear that the potential change would not be accepted or denied easily, because neither side was willing to concede, it was left in brackets. While Aylin and I were angry with this conclusion, Cemile, Nuran, and Sevgi were nonplussed. They had expected such a reaction and had known beforehand that the debate would not get very far. Earlier that week, I had spoken with many other women working in health care, and I was very worried that the Vatican's suggestion to replace the word *contraception* with *family planning* would also remain unresolved.

As the section on women and health continued, I grew increasingly nervous at the approach of this topic. Finally the moderator read the paragraph where the Holy See had inserted the suggestion. It was a spot that Turkey had agreed to speak on; my palms were sweating as I listened to the moderator read over the words: "increased knowledge and use of contraceptive methods as well as increased awareness among men of their responsibility in contraceptive methods and their use. . . ."

At the end of the paragraph he looked up.

"The Holy See has recommended deleting the word *contraceptive* and replacing it throughout with *family planning.*"

The tall and handsome man from the Vatican held his hand up. He was speaking for the Holy See on all matters. Earlier in the week, over dinner one night, Nuran had informed me that he was a businessman from California who regularly attended UN meetings on behalf of the Vatican.

"We would like to replace *contraception* with *family planning.* We believe that family planning more accurately describes the importance of addressing the health needs of families."

Across the room, a delegate from SLAC, which stood for Some Latin American Countries, a group of nations that were representing themselves collectively at the meetings, stood up.

"We oppose this change," the delegate, a tall woman with dark, bobbed hair, said in a loud voice. "We do not feel that *family planning* is either specific or inclusive."

She sat down in her seat. To my left, not far from Turkey's section, a woman from Uruguay's delegation stood.

"We support the change. Family planning will highlight the role of the family in matters of procreation."

While she was talking, Cemile turned toward me and gave me a little nod, indicating that my turn was next. I looked at Nuran, who sat next to her, and she gave me a warm, encouraging smile. I took a deep breath and raised my hand as soon as the woman from Uruguay finished her sentence. The moderator noticed me and said, "Turkey, you have the floor." Immediately, I could feel all the eyes in the room boring in on me.

"Turkey," I began, hearing my voice waver, "opposes this change. To use *family planning* instead of *contraception* implies that contraceptive methods are only for families, and we wish to include young people and people not in families."

I sank down gratefully in my seat and unclenched my hands, pleased that I had remembered exactly what I had planned to say. Aylin leaned forward in her seat and gave me a thumbs-up sign. Beyond her, the Holy See delegate was again waving his hand.

"We still want *family planning* included in this section of the document." He was displaying the same unrelenting stubbornness as before. I looked down at my hands, they were still shaking. Across the conference room, the woman from the EU raised her hand.

"Inserting *family planning* instead of *contraception* is akin to adding new language, and we oppose it."

The representative from SLAC began to hold up her hand again, but at that moment the moderator banged twice on the podium with his wooden gavel. *Oh no*, I thought. He was going to put the topic in brackets, just as we had feared. The SLAC representative remained holding her hand in midair but did not speak.

But instead of ending the topic, the moderator looked at the SLAC delegate and asked a question.

"Are you opposed to the words *family planning*, or are you opposed to the deletion of the word *contraception?*"

I felt momentarily confused, but the SLAC delegate did not miss a beat in answering him. "We are firmly opposed to the deletion of the word *contraception*," she said, loudly and clearly.

The moderator then looked at the section of seats where the Vatican's delegation sat.

"Can you accept the addition of *family planning* without the deletion of *contraception?*" he asked.

Without bothering to raise his hand, the businessman answered "We will accept this."

The moderator looked out to the rest of the room. "Is there any opposition to this agreement?" he asked, turning his head to address the span of delegates.

I glanced at Cemile, who in turn glanced at Nuran, who shook her head slightly, causing her blond hair to shimmy back and forth. The room was silent and no hands were raised.

"Accepted," announced the moderator.

As I sat and listened to the next paragraph begin, I felt conflicting emotions on this resolution. On the one hand, *contraception* would remain in the final document; on the other, the inclusion of *family planning* still managed to embed the implications I opposed. It was this kind of change that, in retrospect, seemed to weaken the language of the Platform for Action and hence to insist in less certain terms on rights and autonomy for women.

I looked across the room and wondered if the SLAC representative felt similarly conflicted. SLAC was, like the delegation representing the EU, one of the few converged groups of countries that were verbally supporting strong language in favor of women's health rights. Others, such as the G77 group, which included a large number of developing countries and China, were much more focused on issues of economics and finance in the document, and could not agree as a unified group to either support or oppose issues involving women and health. They had remained silent for much of this portion of the debates. In this way, Turkey was lucky—we were not bound to a coalition of countries, and could therefore decide as a small group which individual issues we wanted to speak on.

By the end of the second week, when the conference finally reached the section on women and violence, time was running out. Looking in the bathroom mirror one morning at my hotel, I was not surprised to find heavy bags under my eyes. The DAW had, for the past few days, been holding its meetings for almost 24 hours a day. More and more frequently, if a topic's change proved to be highly contested, it was put in brackets for the General Assembly to deal with.

The five of us tried to switch off attending the meetings, allowing each one to retreat for a few hours to sleep. We all went, in rotation, for a few hours to our respective hotels; however, it was very difficult for me to consider missing any of the section on women and violence. I very badly wanted to see that honor crimes would be included in the document. The end of the conference was only a day away, and the General Assembly would convene shortly after. Turkey's official representative in the General Assembly, a man named Mehmet, who was Turkey's Minister of Health, had already arrived in New York. The section on women and violence seemed to me one final opportunity to include an issue of high significance for Turkish women in the outcome document.

As I looked around the conference room that morning, it seemed that the other delegates were also feeling the fatigue of the relentless meetings. There was little chatter, a notable difference from the conference's beginning. Also, delegates seemed at all times to be coming and going—taking turns resting, I assumed, as we were doing.

Aylin, Nuran, Cemile, and I were present when the moderator read the paragraph that would potentially include honor crimes. His voice, I noticed, was an octave or so lower than it had been earlier in the week, and it broke as he read over some of the words. I felt a bit of relief at the knowledge that even he, such a high-level professional, used to this process, was feeling the strain.

We all swiveled our heads towards the EU section when he was done. As the same woman raised her hand, I saw that there were significantly less people in the chairs surrounding her. Even as she was speaking, another delegate scooted in front of her to leave.

"We wish to see the inclusion of so-called honor crimes in this section, because they are an important problem for many women, one that must be prevented."

The moderator looked over the conference room, and quickly asked "Are there any countries opposing this suggestion?"

The tone of his voice suggested that it was a mere formality; he did not expect there to be any arguments. I started to let out my breath in relief, but I had reacted too soon.

From the G77 section, a man stood up. I had not seen him speak previously; however, as the meetings progressed, more and more delegates from individual countries were standing up and speaking on specific issues, despite their allegiance to coalitions. All the procedures and guidelines surrounding this seemed to have dissipated.

The man wore a suit and had dark eyes and hair. "He is from somewhere in the Middle East," I thought. My stomach turned over as he spoke.

"We do not think it is necessary to add in honor crimes," he said, "because it is too localized and specific a problem. Honor crimes are never a problem in my country."

I felt my jaw drop as he sat down. Next to me, even Cemile and Nuram wore looks of shock. All of us knew that honor crimes, in fact, most certainly were a problem in his country, as the notion of a woman's honor is hugely important in many Middle Eastern and Muslim countries, not just in Turkey.

While the four of us quickly stuck our heads together, the EU representative spoke from her seat. "We would like to see it included," she said, but did not add more. The moderator nodded.

"We will put the issue in brackets and move on," he said.

Cemile listened to the moderator and then turned to us. She spoke to all of us but was looking at Nuran. "At this point, if we argue, he will see it as a confrontation and most likely will not back down."

Nuran was nodding her head in agreement. "We should wait and speak with Mehmet and see if he can approach the other Muslim countries for support privately, and then succeed in including it in the General Assembly," she said.

Aylin sighed. Mehmet was the Turkish diplomat of the Permanent Mission of the Republic of Turkey to the UN, which meant that it was his job to oversee all of the UN conferences and represent Turkey. Although he seemed to be a quite courteous and sensitive man personally, I suspected that the women's conference was not high on his list of priorities. I surmised that Aylin probably felt as I did, which was that although the desire to stand and argue with the G77 man was very strong, Cemile was probably right. Mehmet had worked with the General Assembly for a very long time, and most likely had personal relationships with the representatives of the other Muslim countries. I knew, too, that the man speaking from G77 could very well be opposing the inclusion just out of perceived Western pressure against traditional practices, because the suggestion was made officially by the EU.

And so it was done. I sat through the rest of that day listening to the hurried decisions on women and violence and thought about our delegation's successes and failures at the conference. The outcomes were not as black and white as I had expected; rather, two of our most important topics, abortion and honor crimes, were being left to the General Assembly to decide.

Later that day, when the meetings had adjourned for a lunch break, our group managed to hold a quick meeting with Mehmet in the hallway. He greeted Cemile and Nuran warmly, obviously familiar with both of them, but frowned as Cemile described what had happened during the honor crimes debate.

"I have been told," he began in a low voice, "that some of Turkey's allies in the Middle East are not pleased with our support of issues such as sexual orientation."

Cemile nodded and seemed unfazed. "Our support, for the most part on these issues, Mr. Mehmet, has been nonverbal." She paused. "I understand our need to please our allies. And if the issue comes up in any of the remaining debates today, Turkey will not offer an opinion."

Mehmet nodded, and spoke directly to Cemile. "Good," he said. "I will see what I can do to speak with the delegate who opposed the inclusion of honor crimes."

With that, he turned and walked down the hallway, on his way, no doubt, to one of the many meetings he had to attend. The Beijing +5 conference was only one of many of his concerns, therefore it made sense that he was more concerned with maintaining friendly relationships with Turkey's allies than with holding a brief on any one particular issue.

Mehmet must have been successful in speaking with the other Middle Eastern assembly members, because a few days later, as I was packing my belongings to catch an evening flight back to Ankara, came news that the document would, after all, include honor crimes. I smiled as Cemile, over the hotel phone, filled me in on what had been finalized at the General Assembly meetings. My smile faded, however, as she described what had happened with abortion. Nothing was changed, and the document would continue to read "in countries where it was safe and legal." The news was similar on a few other key issues which had been put in brackets.

As I set the phone back in its cradle, I thought that the wording on abortion might someday be a good indicator of women's progress—that things would have drastically changed for the better by the time "in countries where it is safe and legal" could finally be deleted. While I gathered my things, I wondered if such a time would ever really come. During the past few weeks I had felt that the conference was one of the most important things I would ever do, and yet at times I wondered if it mattered at all. I folded my clothing into neat piles and thought of my daughter—would conferences such as Beijing +5 make a significant difference in her life? In what ways would growing up female in Turkey be different for her and her peers than it was for me and mine?

6   Small Steps in a Long Journey in Nepal

Aruna Uprety

I spent the summer of 1998 traveling alone through the remote western region of Nepal. As I traveled, the same story was told to me over and over, by a gynecologist in a rural hospital whose voice trembled with emotion as she spoke, by hungry farm workers whose hands were rough from growing other people's vegetables, by bold headlines on newspapers that very few women knew how to read. The versions that I heard varied, as do all stories that are passed on and repeated, but here is the skeleton of the story, the bare events stripped of their color:

> A young woman's husband traveled south to India for work, leaving his wife with his parents and brother. While he was gone, the woman was raped repeatedly by her brother-in-law and became pregnant. When she discovered that she was pregnant, she had no one to turn to except her husband's brother, so she was forced to ask him for help terminating her pregnancy. First he brought her herbs, which he instructed her to take. When the herbs failed, he took her to an old medicine woman, who massaged her abdomen and inserted herbs into her vagina using a stick. At first, the treatment was successful: an abortion followed. However, the abortion was accompanied by bleeding and severe pain that lasted for days, until finally the woman fainted in front of her husband's mother and father. Her in-laws rushed her to the hospital, where doctors discovered that the stick the medicine woman had used perforated her uterus had wounded her intestines, filling them with pus. While the woman was in the hospital, beginning to show signs of recovery, her husband returned to Nepal. He went to the hospital but never went inside. He told people she was disgraced, that she had acted like a whore. Soon after, her condition worsened,

and despite her strides toward recovery, she died. Her husband's family retrieved her body and, in secret, threw her remains near the bank of a river. As
Hindus, forgoing cremation is a deep insult to the dead.

Because I am a doctor, an activist, and an educated Nepalese woman, I have
ways to disassemble and explain this story. For instance, as a doctor, I can defini-
tively say that this woman died of septicemia, which develops from untreated infections that poison the blood. I also know that septicemia often develops when
women undergo illegal and unsafe abortions and that it can lead to death within
24 hours. As an activist, I am aware of the woman's lack of options. Even in the
rare case that rapists are apprehended, very few end up being prosecuted or serving time. I also know that had she not had her abortion in secrecy, she would have
faced possible arrest and imprisonment for as many as 20 years. As a Nepalese
woman, I take in this story not as an account of a shocking aberration but as a
mere symptom of the standing of women, and especially poor women, in my
country. But even though I can explain this story and understand the technicalities
of how and why a woman's life ended this way, I cannot explain away the brutality
of it, the pure wastefulness and injustice of it.

This story, and hundreds of stories like it, have stayed with me throughout my
adult life. When I wake up and when I go to sleep, when I go to the market and
practice medicine, when I spend time with my children and love my husband and
simply exist as woman, these harsh realities surround me. There is no escaping that
a woman could be raped by her husband's brother, could be given no safer abortion procedure than that involving cow dung and a stick, could fall sick, and could
die in disgrace.

My grandfather was from the Brahmin caste, a very high caste, and that is why
he had the opportunity to study. He came to Katmandu about 80 years ago from a
far western region of Nepal where most of the people are still very poor and only
9% of women are literate. My family never had very much money, but our caste
gave us respect and enabled the men in my family to become successful. My grandfather was an advocate, or attorney. My father followed in his footsteps and also
became an advocate. He was instrumental in founding a college of law in Nepal.
My uncles also held high social positions: one was in politics, one became a government minister, one was an educator, and another was a diplomat and the ambassador to France. But the story of the women in my family is very different. My
grandmother was married to my grandfather when she was 5 years old, and even
though he was highly educated, he never thought to teach her how to read. She
took care of the home and bore 12 children, of whom only 6 survived. My father's
only sister received very little education and had an arranged marriage at 15.

My parents married when my mother was 10 and my father 16. When they met,
my mother was illiterate, but somehow, I am happy to say, she learned to read and
write. Still, domestic life was hard for her. Along with the other daughters-in-law,
she cooked and cleaned for the whole family. She worked in the fields, too, and

woke up at 4 A.M. every morning in order to have time to clean the house, milk our cow, fetch water, and make tea for everyone.

When my sister and I were old enough to help around the house, my mother would tell us sternly to help her in the kitchen—to clean and join the women in the household work. My sister listened and did as she was told. I, on the other hand, focused my attention on our only brother. My mother never asked him to help. Whenever there was any good, tasty food, she would give him much more than she gave to us. While my mother, my sister, and I scrubbed the pots, my brother played football. When we washed the clothes, my brother was nowhere to be found.

I would stand on the mud floor of our 100-year-old house, think hard about the extra fruit and chocolate my brother ate, the way he played while we worked, and declare, "If he's not cleaning, then I'm not cleaning either."

It was statements like these that tried my mother's patience. I would refuse to go along with something that I did not believe was right and she would tell me that I was the naughtiest baby in her family. Sometimes she would hit me with a

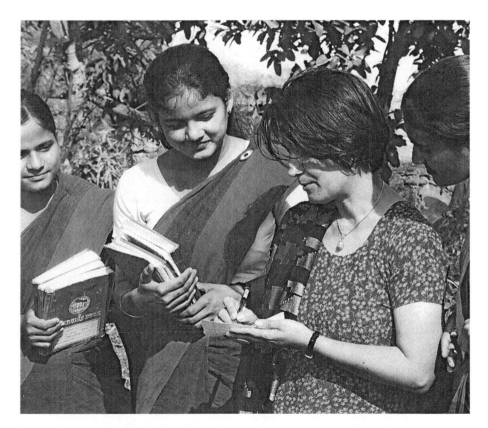

Aruna Uprety monitoring a health and education program at a high school in Pokhara (200 kilometers west of Kathmandu). (Photo: courtesy of the American Himalayan Foundation.)

stick. Angered, she would ask, "Why do you question this?" In our society girls were expected to keep mum and never to question.

Somehow my father got the idea that I should become a doctor, and in 1979 I applied for a scholarship to study medicine abroad. The pupils with the highest marks were sent to study in India and those with lower marks, including myself, received scholarships to study in Russia.

I packed everything I had: three pairs of pants, a few tops, and some toiletries. My parents gave me $50, which felt like a gold mine. They stood in the doorway of our home on the day I left, offering last words of advice.

"Be careful," my mother warned me, crying openly.

"Learn as much as you can," my father said.

"Don't talk to strangers."

"Write down your ideas and try to have them published."

I still remember the way they looked that day: my mother sobbing, my father standing proudly next to her. I was 18 years old and ready to go out into the world. They said goodbye and let me go.

My first 3 months in Russia were full of doubt and homesickness. I shuffled to and from my classes and my room and thought, "Okay, I don't want to be a doctor, I don't want to be anything. I just want to go home." But soon, it was as if the world were changing in front of my eyes, and I became too amazed, too involved with the people around me and the ideas we shared to feel that kind of doubt any longer.

Russia was a miracle. All around me were women. They were not confined to the home as they were in Nepal. Instead, the women outnumbered the men at our university; women were driving not only cars but buses and tractors; women were doing construction and engineering. Everywhere there were so many women.

In addition to myself and the other students from Nepal, there were students from Africa, India, and Latin America. We would all sit and talk together for hours, trying to understand our own societies in relation to the others. At night, my Nepalese classmates and I, as many as 15 of us at a time, would cram into sleeping rooms that were meant to fit only two students. We perched on the edge of the two small desks, sat side by side on the two twin beds, knelt on the floor, leaned against the doorframe. My friend Prakash, who later became a cardiologist, made curry and rice for us all, and we drank cupfuls of tea. Sometimes we sat silently, listening to radio broadcasts from America and the United Kingdom telling us what was happening in Nepal or South Asia, and after the broadcasts were over, we would thrash out our ideas.

"Why is our country so poor?" Prakash asked one night.

Ten of us were left in the room, and we would be staying up all night. It was past midnight, too late to leave the apartment. All of us were quiet, thinking our separate thoughts, waiting for another to answer.

Then one of my few female classmates said, "Because only people in high castes have access to education. As long as so many Nepalese are denied their basic rights, we will remain a poor country."

"Are any of us from a lower caste?" I asked.

"I'm not," she said.

"Me neither," said Prakash.

Everyone else responded the same way.

"Do any of you know of anyone who is studying here in Russia who is not from a high caste?" I asked.

No one did. Of 100 Nepalese students, not one was from a low caste. I lay on the floor that night, watching shadows move across the ceiling in the dim light, and for the first time in my life questioned the caste system. Before Russia, this would have been like questioning why there was rain or why there was nightfall—it seemed that much a natural part of life. I believed that people in the lower castes were poor because of "karma," because of what they had done in a previous life. I tried to remember the low-caste people who worked in our yard when I was a child, tried to envision their faces but could not. I realized that apart from my quick glimpses, I had never really looked at them, even though they worked right outside my home.

I was not the only person in the room lost in thought. Soon, the silence grew thick. My friend Udya got up from bed and stepped over me and another friend to reach his bag. He took out a notebook and began to read aloud. It was a poem he wrote about illness in Nepal and how so many people were sick because the government did not take care of the poor.

"No love poems?" Prakash asked when Udya had finished.

Without thinking, I blurted, "There is too much work to be done to write love poems."

In June of 1986 I returned to Nepal, and a month later I began a job as a medical officer in the main maternity hospital. I was placed in the outpatient department, where most of our patients were poor people from small village areas. Most of the women we treated were anemic because they did not have enough food to eat, even when they were pregnant.

On a September afternoon, at 5 o'clock, a man and his severely ill wife entered the hospital. She leaned on her husband for support; they both appeared to be exhausted. Later, I would learn that they had walked for 3 hours from their village and then taken a taxi to the hospital. The woman lay down on the examining table and her husband stood in the doorway, dressed in worn clothing. I could see pain in the woman's small eyes, and also fear. Even though I could tell that her skin was usually very dark, now it appeared pale, so pale that I immediately asked her husband to find some blood for us to give her. He headed to the blood bank. The woman's sari was thinning from age and wear, and the green jumper she wore beneath the sari was also old and ripped in several places. Her body smelled sour and strong.

I asked how old she was.

Weakly, she told me 38.

I remember writing the number on her chart. When I looked back at her, her eyes had closed and she began to moan. I told myself that she was going to be fine.

After all, I had just seen her walk. If she had been in any real danger, she would have been carried in by her husband or wheeled in on a stretcher. I tried to take her blood pressure but it was too low; I could not measure it at all. I tried to take her pulse but again felt nothing. Because I was straight out of medical school, and had never endured the loss of a patient, I was so sure of my abilities. I expected to see a patient, evaluate the symptoms, and know what was wrong, but here was this woman before me. She was not pregnant; she was not bleeding; nothing appeared to be wrong with her. I called a senior doctor for help, and while I waited for her, I bent down, put my mouth to the woman's, and tried to breathe her back to life. This was what I had been taught in school, and I had been taught that it worked, but it did not.

When I stood up again the doctor was at my side. Again I tried to feel the woman's pulse but felt nothing. The doctor tried after me and then said, "She's gone."

Just then, her husband returned, offering us the packet of blood he had traded his own for.

Now, so many years later, I clearly remember this woman's green jumper, her worn shoes, and her husband's reticence. I can almost feel the way her bones jutted out, the ridges of her ribs, the sharp points of collarbone and elbows. I had been so sure I could save her. I had been absolutely sure, that was the thing.

After she died, I sat with her husband in the waiting room. He told me that he and his wife already had 5 children; neither of them wanted a sixth. When they discovered that she was pregnant again, they turned to an old woman in a nearby village who was rumored to be able to get rid of unwanted pregnancies for very little money. With his head in his hands, looking weary and shaken, the husband told me that the healer had given his wife something to eat and then inserted a combination of herbs into her vagina with a stick. Within a day, the wife had expelled the fetus, but she also began bleeding profusely and running a high fever. The worried husband had traveled back to the old healer to see what was happening, to see what to do, but the old woman told him his wife would be fine in time. Three days after the abortion, however, his wife was only getting worse, and by the end of the third day she had lost consciousness along with a startling amount of blood. The man finally decided he had no choice but to bring his wife to the hospital.

The rest of my shift that night was a blur. I moved mechanically, unable to clear the husband's story from my mind. At the end of my shift, I found the senior doctor and asked her to step aside and talk to me. My medical training had not addressed this situation or any of the consequences of an unsafe abortion.

The doctor must have seen the urgency in my face. She said, "Aruna, you know, this is not unusual. We see three or four cases of this each month." She explained that most of the time, when women came in seeking care for a septic abortion, they were able to recover with treatment. "But in other cases," she added, "there is little we can do. Sometimes they die within an hour. And on occasion, they arrive here already dead."

The senior doctor left me in the hallway with my thoughts. I wondered how many women were too poor or too far away or too hopeless to seek post-abortion care in a city hospital. Even though abortion was illegal, post-abortion care was not, and it troubled me deeply to think of how many women must have lost their lives because they could not make it to the hospital in time.

As I had in Russia, I turned to writing to deal with my overwhelming thoughts and emotions. In the days that followed the woman's death, I penned an article that recounted her story and argued that abortion should be legalized so that such tragedies could be avoided. My pain over not being able to save the woman's life was still fresh, and I wrote passionately. I asked why so many women were dying this way. I argued that it was because they were poor, illiterate, and had no access to medical services or family planning. I challenged everyone—the readers of the article, the doctors, myself—to work together to make safe abortions available.

Raghu Panta, a publisher and member of a radical party, accepted my article for print in his small newspaper, and with its publication began my career as an activist. Soon after the article appeared, letter after letter came streaming into the newspaper's office, filled with shocking objections to my call for action. The letters were from schoolteachers and university professors, even many women. Several readers accused me of being a "western feminist." At this time in Nepal, western feminists were considered to be against men, religion, and cultural tradition; they were felt to have no place in our society. Other readers claimed that our country was a very Hindu country, a very religious and holy country, and if abortion were legalized, everything would be spoiled. They thought that to allow abortions would be to condone promiscuity.

At first I tried to reply to all the letters the newspaper received in response to my article. I was convinced that if people could witness what I had witnessed, they would retract their objections and change their beliefs. Soon though, with the help of the newspaper's editor, I realized that writing back to every person who wrote against my article was not the most effective way to change minds and laws, so I embarked on what would become an 18-year-long journey to change the Nepalese abortion law.

In the Nepali language, the word *abortion* means "murder of a fetus." Women who were prosecuted for having abortions could serve up to 20 years in jail, and according to Hindu beliefs, they would go to Hell after death. Abortion was considered highly unethical—so taboo that even as many women were dying from illegal abortions, no one had the courage to address the issue, especially under the monarchy.

For many months, it seemed that no one would be willing to help me contest the abortion laws. The government health officers would not speak out because they considered abortion to be a political issue rather than a health issue. Many gynecologists did not acknowledge the issue because as long as abortions were illegal, they were free to ask high prices to perform them. Religious leaders remained silent in their opposition. Even the few women's groups refused to address it, believing abortion to be too taboo a subject for public discussion.

Even with so many people against me, I kept trying to bring abortion issues to the spotlight. Only a handful of people were behind me, but slowly people began to talk. While all this was going on, I became concerned with another problem: the way junior doctors were mistreated. They often worked 72-hour weeks and were not given enough food or rest during their workdays. When I spoke out against these conditions, the senior doctors who were already unhappy with how vocal I was about abortion laws became even more displeased. As soon as my 1-year contract was up, I was told that they no longer needed me.

This was a great blow for many reasons. I had just been married and had my first child. My husband and I were responsible for providing for 15 members of our family. But also, apart from these practical reasons, I loved my work. It filled me with enthusiasm. I was proud of it. Getting sacked and then spending 7 months as an unemployed doctor was hard on my ego. My friends and family told me that I had brought this upon myself.

"You are suffering now because you've been problematic," they would tell me.

My husband tried to support me, but sometimes even he would say that I should not have spoken out as loudly and strongly as I had. It felt as though he were adding insult to injury. My 7 months of searching for work were difficult and dark.

When I finally found work again, it was with the government's Family Planning Department. I was responsible for traveling to rural areas and performing vasectomies for men and sterilizations for women. In the years that followed, my jobs as both a doctor and activist became inextricably intertwined. My work as a doctor taught me volumes about the status of women throughout Nepal and the links between law, culture, and the deaths of hundreds of women a year. I was educated in Nepal's unwritten abortion laws. Many women came to the traveling clinic and asked us to rid them of their pregnancies—a request that the head doctor would fulfill if the women agreed to permanent sterilization.

After our first abortion patient had been released, I asked him: "Is it legal to perform abortions in these settings?" I hoped that somehow along the way I had missed an important loophole in Nepalese abortion law.

His answer was not quite yes but not quite no. The government's unofficial policy was to provide the service if the pregnancy was not more than 10 weeks and the women wanted "permanent family planning," a euphemism for sterilization.

He explained, "It's done as a way to increase cases of family planning in the nation."

In other words, he was telling me that abortion was fine as long as it generated numbers that made the health ministry look good. When women came to our clinics asking for abortions, we were not allowed to provide them unless they were willing to be sterilized. It was a hard choice for many patients, and I knew that it was not a choice they should have been forced to make.

As in Russia, I again turned to writing. From 1987 to 1990 I wrote about the sterilizations, trying to bring this injustice to the attention of the public. I talked about how unattainable birth control was to women, how the decision regarding whether to use it was left entirely to their husbands. I also brought up issues of class, about how, while poor women were dying from illegal and unsafe abortions by the hundreds, wealthy women had the means to receive abortions at private clinics. There, doctors would see to it that women felt no pain during their procedures and that they left, 3 or 4 hours afterward, already on their way to complete recovery. Seldom was I able to publish these articles in newspapers that would reach many people, but I still tried to make these realities known, hoping that soon people would begin to take notice.

In 1990, a new and powerful movement erupted in Nepal. The people of our country grew tired of the king's autocratic regime. It was the twentieth century; we wanted the right to speak freely; we wanted a parliament, a cabinet, an open legal system. Doctors, lawyers, and people from various walks of life all took to the streets and came together to demand that Nepal become a democracy. While participating in the movement, I met doctors, lawyers, journalists, and many other people who would become allies in the struggle against unsafe abortions. Like me, they wanted to have a movement for women.

During this time of great change, I spoke at many prodemocracy meetings. One evening, in a room crammed with 400 people, I gave a speech stressing the importance of respecting a woman's right to abortion once we had won the struggle for democracy. I stated that it would be our responsibility to see to it that women would not die from unsafe procedures in the future. After I finished my speech, I took a seat near the front of the room, ready to listen to the next speaker. I watched as a tall, dark woman made her way to the front of the crowd. Even before she began to speak, I recognized intelligence, passion, and kindness in her face. Then her speech began, and I discovered that her words acted as an extension of my own. Eloquently, she argued that not only were women dying from illegal abortions but that many others were being held in prison.

"For these women, being prisoners is often worse than dying," she said. "They can be incarcerated for as many as 20 years, and even upon release they find themselves ostracized by their families and their society. They have nowhere to go."

Later on in the evening, I found her in the crowd. We connected immediately because we were talking about the same thing, but from two different perspectives. I was concerned with maternal health; she was concerned with a woman's right to control her body. She was 4 years younger than I, but was already a lawyer and the leader of her own organization, the Forum for Women, Law, and Development. Before we left the meeting, we had already committed to work together and planned a time to meet again. Her name was Sapana Malla. She was my first ally.

Our democracy movement was successful; the king agreed to a constitutional monarchy, and by the mid-1990s, the media in Nepal had been transformed. Before the establishment of democracy, the government controlled the media. The government had television; the government had radio; the government had its own newspaper. There were very few, only one or two, private newspapers at that time, and they were not very good. But after the restoration, many journalists started private newspapers, journals, magazines, and FM radio stations. People were eager for information, so these organizations thrived. Finally, I had open forums in which to discuss abortion rights and the ability to reach many people.

During the protests of the early 1990s, I met a journalist named Gunjraj who agreed with me on many issues. He worked on one of the new private newspapers with a wide readership. I wrote an article on abortion rights and he agreed to publish it. With his help, for the first time one of my articles achieved national recognition. From then on, abortion became something that was discussed—no longer a taboo issue. Gunjraj became an even more instrumental figure in our movement after that, sending his reporters to villages when he heard of abortion-related deaths.

Soon, we began to receive even more support for abortion rights. The Family Planning Association of Nepal was a respected and established group, led by Congress Party member Sunil Bhandari. Sunil had entered politics and was elected to parliament. Before that, he lived in the poor western part of Nepal. He was educated in local schools there and lived a very hard life. He had seen women die from abortion procedures, and had known women who were imprisoned because of them.

When Sunil came to Katmandu, he wanted to make dramatic changes to improve our society. He was inspired. Before he joined our cause, the Family Planning Association did not support us; parliament did not support us. In opposition to the rest of his Congress Party, he spoke out in favor of women's rights while other members vehemently opposed his ideas. This conflict amongst party members made good copy: here was a parliamentarian, a Congress Party member, a *man*, who claimed that abortion should be legalized!

With the help of discussions at the UN's Fifth International Conference on Population and Development, held in Cairo, Egypt in 1994, abortion rights became a charged public issue, at the forefront of political debates. Sapana and I often used radio to share our beliefs, because while newspapers were read primarily by the intelligencia and televisions were owned only by the middle class, everyone had a radio.

The first time I was on the radio, a man who worked for the station led me inside the building to a small air-conditioned room separated from the next room by a glass wall. He sat in one room, I sat in the other. He pressed a button and his voice came through the speakers, telling me that if anything went wrong with the sound or the recording, he would talk to me like this and tell me how to proceed. But technical difficulties did not concern me half as much as what I was about to do: condone "murder" on the radio. Of course, what I was really preparing to do was speak of the importance of *saving* lives, but as I have mentioned, the word *abortion*, in Nepalese, means "murder."

Soon it was time for me to begin, and I was forced to stop worrying about what I was going to say. I moved the microphone to my mouth and began with the story of my first experience with abortion-related death: the woman in the maternity hospital who took her last breath on my examination table. I followed this story with other stories about other women I had treated or heard about. Then I told my own story.

Six months after I gave birth to my first child, I became pregnant again. My husband and I both thought that it was too soon for us to have another baby, so I decided to have an abortion. The procedure was quick and painless. I told my gynecologist that I wanted the procedure done; it lasted 20 minutes. Afterwards, I rested in the clinic for half an hour. Then I went home. The procedure was so simple, so sterile, because I was a woman with money, with education, and with somewhere safe to go.

I recounted this scene from my life for my listeners, and then I declared: "If the government has the courage to come and arrest me, I will be glad to go. If it will not arrest a woman of my social status for having an abortion or performing abortions for other women, why will it arrest women from villages and spoil their lives?"

Many people considered my challenge to the government radical, and my first radio broadcast generated much discussion.

After that, I preferred talking on the radio to writing newspaper articles, because while writing articles requires hours of research and meticulous attention to detail, the radio was a forum that allowed me to speak from my heart. I gave examples from my clinical experience and from the communities, jails, and hospitals I had visited. I pointed out how men were suffering because their wives were dying, their sisters were dying, their mothers were dying. By bringing this to attention, I strove to make my listeners understand that this was a problem for all of society, not only for women.

A year after the conference in Cairo came the Fourth World Conference on Women in Beijing, also organized by the UN. I attended this conference as one of two doctors chosen by the government to appear as a Nepalese delegate. It was amazing—to think that I was fired from a hospital a few years before for vocalizing my views on abortion rights and now I was chosen to represent our country and share those same views.

In Beijing, however, one of my main opponents on the abortion issue was a woman from my country, Angurru Baba Doshi. She and I have similar views on many women's issues and I have great respect for her as a person. She is old now, 75, and her life is in many ways a conglomerate of tradition and progress. She was married at age 11 and became highly educated. She became the first woman principal in Nepal, then the head of a college. She established the first women's college in Nepal, has been around the world, and speaks three or four languages. She has done some remarkable things for women, and she and I have worked together on many issues.

However, having been raised in a very strict orthodox Hindu family, she believes that when a fetus is conceived it immediately has a soul. When I spoke for abortion rights in Beijing, she spoke out against them. After the speeches were over, she approached me.

She looked at me with intent, intelligent eyes. "Why are you raising your voice for abortion so much?" she asked me. "You shouldn't raise it."

I had been hearing this question from people for years, hearing the same shock and disapproval in their voices as they asked it. I should have been used to it by then, but hearing it from her pained me. Still, I told her the truth.

"Yes," I said. "We have to raise it. This is why we came here—to discuss reproductive rights."

She looked deeply disappointed in me, and I remembered seeing the same expression on my mother's face whenever I challenged the way she raised my brother or showed her my mediocre marks. Even as a woman, it was hard to feel disapproved of by someone so important to me, but I had learned as a girl how to stand up for what I knew was right.

I told her the truth: "I regret that this issue divides us."

She continued to look at me and I felt her waiting for something more. But I never apologized for what I believed.

Despite my radio challenges to the Nepalese government, I was not arrested. Instead, Sapana and I, with the help of a professor friend, Dr. Shanta, prepared for a seminar with members of parliament. We spent half a year traveling, gathering case studies, photographing, conducting polls, and learning from other countries where abortion was already legal.

In June of 1998, some 12 years into my struggle to make abortions safe and legal, I was traveling alone through western Nepal and heard the story of the woman who was raped by her brother-in-law and whose body was later discarded near the river. I was journeying from village to village, sometimes by plane, sometimes by bus, and sometimes by foot when my destinations were too remote. It took me 5 or 6 hours to walk to many of these places; a couple of trips took me 12. The gynecologist who told me the story was a senior doctor at the Lumbini District Hospital. When she finished telling me about the young wife's tragic death, she said, "There are so many women who come to us like this every month. The police don't catch the rapists, but they arrest the women who come here in need of medical attention."

In another case, Dr. Renu Rajbhandari, a Nepali Public health specialist, spoke of a woman she treated while working in Bharatpur Hospital, near the India-Nepal border. A village man had raped the woman while her husband was away, and the woman became pregnant. To rid herself of the evidence of the rape, she visited a traditional healer, who inserted something unidentified into her vagina. Two days later the fetus was expelled and the woman buried it near her home. Three days after the abortion, however, the woman began bleeding and developed a fever, symptoms so worrisome in their severity that she took herself to Bharatpur Hospital. By this time, however, a neighbor who had spied on the burial had complained to the local police of the woman's abortion. The police came to the hospital and asked Dr. Rajbhandari to write a report verifying the story. She told the police the woman had come to the hospital because of an infection, not an abortion. Dr. Rajbhandari spoke to me openly of her deception.

"Of course the report was not true medically," she said, "but I don't feel guilty about it. If I had written the truth, the police would have taken her. Her life would have been destroyed."

As I continued traveling, collecting information of abortion-related deaths from other doctors, Sapana compiled case studies of women who were imprisoned for having undergone abortions, and Dr. Shanta completed her survey of men and women in villages and towns all over Nepal. Soon, we met again and put all of our information together. The members of parliament, who liked to label Sapana and me as *city women*, unaware of life beyond Katmandu, would now understand that we were well informed and thorough in our research.

On the long-awaited first day of the seminar, we were thrilled when 70 members of parliament, out of 205 in all, attended. Secretly, we had been afraid that too few would choose to attend and that all our work would go unacknowledged. Raghu Panta, the journalist and parliamentarian who had helped me publish my first article about abortion, had worked hard for us, widely publicizing the seminar and rallying public support. The parliamentarians who attended were from all political parties, not only leftist ones. This in itself was a victory.

Over 3 days we encapsulated years of research and experience into our presentations. Sapana spoke of discriminatory laws and the effect they had on women's lives. She asked what we could all do to change them. I spoke of the abortion laws in surrounding countries, countries like India and Bangladesh, that were also very religious, and how giving the women this right had had a positive impact on women's health. I explained that in Bangladesh, in order to make abortion palatable to a wary public, it was referred to as "menstrual regulation." Following this example, we began to fight not for "safe abortion" but for the eradication of "unsafe illegal abortion." Dr. Shanta shared the results of her survey, which showed that 75% to 80% of the men and women in villages and towns wanted to see abortion legalized, and I shared the results of my research in 10 major hospitals, which documented that 60% to 80% of maternal deaths were caused by unsafe abortions.

To close the seminar, we offered detailed case studies, many times accompanied with photographs, of women who had died or been imprisoned because of illegal abortions. As we told these women's stories and passed around their pictures, we saw the parliamentarians' faces soften. Sapana, Dr. Shanta, and I discovered that our years of research, our linked passions and causes, our hard figures, and our case studies and photographs came together to form a pattern of the lack of reproductive rights, women's rights, and human rights. To our immense happiness, we learned that many of the parliamentarians who had entered the seminar in the belief that abortion was wrong had begun to change their minds.

For a long time after the seminar, Sapana, Dr. Shanta, friends from the parliament and the community, and I all worked together to draft a law that would make abortion legal. A special committee comprising parliamentarians from both the Communist and Congress Parties was developed to help formulate the draft.

When the draft went to Parliament for consideration, it contained many flaws. It stipulated, for example, that women could obtain abortions only if they had their husbands' permission. It also said that a woman could have access to abortion only if she or her fetus were mentally or physically unfit, if she were raped, or if she were a victim of incest. Many of us felt uneasy over these requirements, but our lawyers told us that once the bill was passed and legalized, we could make the necessary changes.

Still, many members of the Congress Party did not like the bill, and it was not passed.

In 1999, we tried again. Many parliamentarians wanted to keep the old draft and vote on it again, but we said, "Please, no, wait." We did not want a law that said women could have abortions only if their husbands allowed them to. What about the women whose husbands did not listen to them? What about the widows? What about women who were not married? After long discussions, a powerful member of parliament finally conceded. Our new draft stated that up to their 12th week of pregnancy, all women, regardless of their marital status, could be given an abortion. They did not need permission from anyone. If the pregnancy was a result of rape or if the woman or her fetus was mentally or physically unfit, she would have up to 18 weeks to undergo the procedure. The new draft took years of work, and in 2001, with great anxiety and immense hope, we presented it to parliament.

On a September night in 2002, I was watching the evening news in my room in the old house where I lived. The room was simply furnished, with my bed in one corner, the television in another, and books and papers strewn across the floor and the shelves.

Six months earlier, our women's rights bill had been passed by the vast majority of parliament. That was a joyous day for us. Sapana, Dr. Shanta, and I shared a good bottle of wine and then stayed up late with laughter and celebration. We thought that all that would be needed now was the king's signature, a formality really, and then the new laws would be put into action. Most of the time it takes about 2 weeks for the king to give his seal. But weeks passed, then a month, then 2 months, 3 months, and nothing.

But that night, as I sat in my room, watching the news at 7 o'clock as I usually did, the news I had been waiting for for 18 long years finally came: the king had signed the bill. I cried out in joy for the future, in sadness for the women whose lives had already been lost, and in relief at the realization that the moment we had been fighting for all these years had come.

All along, I have thought of this journey for women's rights as a long one with a thousand steps. I know that even though we have walked for so long, even taken a few leaps forward, there are still many, many steps ahead of us. Since the king signed the bill into law, not much has changed. When I travel through the western part of Nepal, most of the women I meet, even a lot of nurses, do not know that abortion is legal. If they do know, they think there are limitations in place that really are not.

A year ago, a small group of doctors and nurses told me, "We can only administer abortions to women who have permission from their husbands."

"No," I told them. "That is not the law."

"Yes," they said. "Yes, it is the law. We know."

I told them, "No." And then I took out the documentation and I showed it to them.

But in other cases, I have seen progress.

Throughout Nepal, the government and organizations like that of Marie Stropes have opened clinics to provide safe, legal abortions to women from rural areas. And in the maternity hospital, where 20 years earlier I had my first job, witnessed the first death of a patient, and raised my voice against illegal abortion for the first time, a special department has been opened; in it, 15 to 20 abortions are performed each day. In June of 2006, in front of the department for safe and legal abortions, a nurse approached me and said, "Dr. Uprety, you spoke out for safe abortions at a time when very few of us believed that abortions would ever be legalized. You and your friends have brought new opportunity to the women of Nepal."

Even though my friends and I have achieved so much, there is so much more left to do. Sapana is still fighting in the courts on behalf of women whose rights have been violated; Dr. Shanta is still gathering information to educate the public and the government; I am still writing articles for newspapers, talking on the radio, organizing meetings to let women in Katmandu and beyond know what their rights are. The challenge in coming years will be one of disseminating information about the new law and the facts about safe abortion to doctors, health workers, advocates, law enforcement officials, and politicians, and keeping their information as up to date as we possibly can. We need to make safe abortion and all health services affordable and accessible to all the population. I will need the support of my friends who work at the community level, the doctors who can educate the nurses and their patients, and the media to let the women who read the newspapers, watch the television, and listen to the radio know: you can go to the doctors, you can be safe.

7 Swasthya: The Politics of Women's Health in Rural South India

Suneeta Krishnan

In August 1997, three American students, including two of Indian origin, met at a newly opened cyber café in Bangalore city, India, to plan a women's health program in Vijaygiri,[1] a rural community 350 kilometers away. Rajiv, whose brainchild the program was and who had raised funds for it, did not turn up for the meeting. The others decided to go ahead with their trip to Vijaygiri anyway. So, at the height of the monsoon season, the trio traveled to Vijaygiri to conduct a needs assessment for the program. I heard of their plans through a friend. In search of inspiration for my dissertation research, I decided to tag along. My father had passed away recently, and the sudden loss had left me drifting. I needed to find an anchor, a focus.

At around 9 P.M., we boarded a "luxury" government bus that turned out to be anything but luxurious. Last-minute booking meant that we had the last row. After a few hours on a relatively straight highway, we started to climb up through the mountains. In the last row, even the most minor pothole tossed us high off our seats. And the rain! The rain came pouring down the whole night, leaking through the cracks around the edges of the windows. The next morning I stepped off the bus at the Vijaygiri bus stand damp and aching.

The bus stand was a patch of ground big enough to accommodate two buses and a few auto rickshaws. Coconut, arecanut, and other trees bordered the stand and houses crowded in on the sides. It was about 5 o'clock in the morning. Faint strains of the traditional Sanskrit morning chants played on a radio. A few auto drivers were standing around, yawning and stretching. Now that the rain had ended, the air was crisp, cold, and damp. Leaves on the trees were fresh with dew and rain. Ah, how peaceful, how idyllic were those first few moments in Vijaygiri after the hustle and bustle of Bangalore. "Perhaps here I will find a dissertation topic and peace after the turmoil of my father's death," I thought.

No one was there to meet us, so we approached an auto rickshaw driver and asked to be taken to the hospital. We drove through what looked like the main road of the town, up a hill and around a corner. There at the top of the hill was a sprawling pink building. To the left, by the side of the parking area, was a badminton court. People slowly moved about with toothbrushes, towels, and flasks. No one seemed to notice us. We wandered in through the main entrance and reached an inner courtyard with hallways going left and right and stairs going down. Just as I began to feel a bit frustrated, we saw a tall man, maybe in his fifties, walking toward us from the corridor on the left. He carried himself with an air of authority, but at the same time his smile was open, welcoming. He reminded me a bit of my grandfather. It was Dr. Vasan, the chief medical officer of the hospital.

Rajiv and the students I was with had worked out the broad goals of the project with Dr. Vasan. The idea was to extend the mobile clinics that the hospital was conducting to make outreach more regular and to recruit a group of local women to engage in health education. The initial mission was to "empower women with information and other tools to make and act upon health care decisions." I was wary of the fact that the project did not have an explicit ideological or theoretical orientation. Further, there had been no discussion about roles and responsibilities— of the student group, the hospital, or the health workers we would recruit. I was apprehensive that the undertaking might turn out to be a haphazard student project rather than a formal program and about being saddled with responsibilities that I had not had time to fully comprehend. I was already a year into my "all but dissertation" status in the doctoral program in epidemiology at the University of California, Berkeley, and was conscious of the need to stay focused on completing the dissertation. I was also committed to a project that would keep me linked to my childhood roots in India—a desire that had shaped the focus of my undergraduate and graduate studies in the United States. Thus, quite quickly, I became the group's point person.

Later that first morning, after we had showered and dressed, we met Dr. Vasan at the canteen, a low-roofed annex to the main hospital building. As we devoured the *iddlis* (steamed rice cakes), chutney, and sweet hot coffee served in 2-inch-high steel cups, a doctor who looked to be in his early thirties greeted Dr. Vasan with respect and then turned to us with an excited smile.

"So these are the Americans."

"This is Jagan," introduced Dr. Vasan. "He has been running the hospitals's nursing program and the community outreach."

Dr. Jagan seemed excited and enthusiastic about meeting people interested in his line of work. We began to discuss what our role at the hospital would be, and once our conversation was under way, Dr. Vasan excused himself to begin morning rounds and left us to our discussions with Jagan.

A few days later, in an airy, spacious office of the hospital, I met with Dr. Jagan and the honorary secretary of the hospital, an elderly, sprightly man who had retired from the banking sector. Jagan seemed far more relaxed in the presence of the secretary than in that of Dr. Vasan. In fact, he was in his element.

"What we need is mass education," he announced. "Now is the time to start. I have 20 girls finishing the nursing course this month." Dr. Jagan had been running a 1-year training program for nursing assistants, who were simply called nurses. If we did not move fast, we would lose the opportunity to recruit a few of the graduates. Most got hired by nursing homes and clinics in the district and neighboring districts. Once they got jobs, it would be difficult to recruit them for our project. And once we hired them, we would need to initiate training as well.

At first I was reluctant to rush to action, hoping instead to take our time in developing a solid plan. However, I caved in.

"We'll interview the candidates tomorrow," announced Dr. Jagan.

The secretary seconded the proposal. Dr. Jagan recognized the importance of identifying young women with a commitment to staying back in their home communities, with an interest in working on women's health. But I learned from him that in order to accomplish our goals, we had to work very strategically within the hospital. We had to bring on board the authorities, like the secretary, and the staff, like the head nurse, by trying to work on terms acceptable to them.

On one of my early trips, I drove back to Bangalore with Dr. Vasan and his wife, Dr. Sarojini. Dr. Vasan was in a nostalgic mood and eager to confide. We spoke

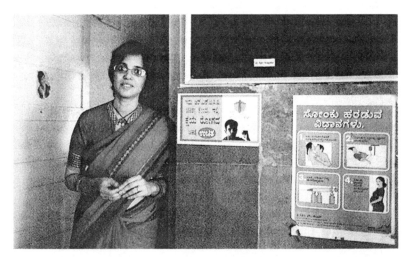

In her more recent work, Suneeta Krishnan has been operating out of urban clinics in Bangalore, India, interviewing young women about their marriages, economic situation, and sex lives. (Photo: Jason Taylor for *Time*.)

at length about the hospital during our ride to Bangalore—about the 10 years they had spent struggling to establish the hospital, and about Dr. Jagan. I learned that Jagan was a native of the town, trained in Ayurvedic medicine.

"We sent him to get training in anesthesia. The main problem with him is that he doesn't have confidence. He doesn't focus," Dr Vasan said.

"You know, for even a little thing, he will send people for an x-ray, an electrocardiogram," added Dr. Sarojini.

Dr. Vasan continued in a resigned voice, "I manage with him. His main strength is public relations. He will be good at helping you with the training of these health workers and talking to the panchayat [village council].ⁱⁱ He's good at handling politics. But I will come to the weekly clinics myself."

In contrast with what Dr. Vasan had told me, Dr. Jagan seemed very confident. As the project evolved, the student group and the community health workers (CHWs) relied on him to negotiate with the hospital authorities as well as with local village authorities like the panchayats and local landlords. He had the ability to connect with people and to speak in ways that they could identify with. I felt that ultimately it was Dr. Jagan who understood the project—and in many ways it was his project: it emerged as an extension of his nursing training program and his community outreach work. For years, before Dr. Vasan and Dr. Sarojini had joined the hospital, Jagan would hitch rides with taxis and jeeps going out to the villages to offer health care and information. He had a strong commitment to social service, which made him a natural leader for our project.

Our new recruits, the CHWs, participated in a 3-month training program in community health. During this time, Jagan lobbied with wealthy families and local panchayats to donate space for the CHWs' health centers. In January 1998, we launched health centers in six villages within a 30 kilometer radius of Vijaygiri. Jagan and Dr. Vasan planned a grand launch—a large multispecialty camp. Camps are a common strategy used in India to promote health-care access as well as utilization of particular kinds of health services such as sterilization or screening. A number of doctors we met at Vijaygiri and Bangalore who were involved in community health all felt that the most effective ways of establishing oneself in the community was by providing basic medical care through camps and outreach clinics. Dr. Vasan and Jagan too felt that this was crucial.

The day of the launch, Jagan was extremely tense but in charge. He paced up and down, checklist in hand, overseeing the packing of equipment and materials. We left the hospital as a convoy of four vehicles. The hospital van left at around 8:45 A.M. with a team of student nurses, laboratory technicians, and equipment. Jagan followed in his car with the CHWs, his wife Ila, his daughter Ashwini, and Ashwini's puppy Amitabh, named after a famous Bollywood actor. I followed in a jeep with Dr. Vasan and a few other doctors.

The first center, located in hilly estate country, was being launched at the village farthest away from the hospital. It consisted of two rooms within the village government office at the foot of a hill. Areca nut trees dripping with black pepper vines and sweet-smelling coffee bushes in bloom grew on the slopes. Closer to the summit were the neatly cropped tea plantations.

By the time we reached the site at about 10 A.M., at least 50 people had gathered. The majority were women, some with children. The panchayat officials, registers and pens in hand, seemed extremely organized, as did several community volunteers. There must have been a team of about 20 organizers and a total of about 8 clinical specialists at the camp. It was 10:15, and a festive atmosphere prevailed. Hindi pop music blared on the speakers. The panchayat officials decided it was time to begin.

The next thing I knew, the owner of a local tea estate who was sponsoring the day's program was announcing my name, and I was led to the stage by one of the camp volunteers.

With a dry mouth and a racing heart I walked to the microphone. Over 100 people had gathered by then. Dr. Jagan introduced me: "Now, Mrs. Suneeta Krishnan will say a few words about Swasthya. She is one of the dedicated students who has come all the way from America to work with us."

I reminded myself that I was the "laudable American" and could do no wrong. Braced by this thought, I launched into my speech, in English: "Today's program is a true representation of what Swasthya is trying to accomplish: local communities, the hospital, and the Swasthya team working together to promote health. We hope this partnership will be a long and successful one."

Dr. Jagan stepped up to translate and then launched into a few of his own remarks: "Our goal is to provide not merely treatment but also health education. Illness prevention is the goal." Throughout the life of the project, he would repeatedly emphasize this goal.

Finally, after what seemed to be an eternity, the speeches came to a close. The panchayat president (head of the village government) kicked off the camp by requesting all those who wanted a health checkup to register. In minutes, a long queue of men, women, and children formed at the registration desk in front of the panchayat office. Three young men, panchayat volunteers, sat at the registration desk and asked each individual to identify which specialists he or she wanted to consult. I watched the proceedings for a few minutes. There were many women in line—dressed in their holiday finest, with flowers in their hair and colorful glass bangles on their arms. Some had babies on their hips. A few were chatting and joking; others looked tense.

"Do you live here—in this village? It looks like the entire village is here!" I asked a group of women in broken Kannada, the local language, peppered with Tamil and Malayalam, the two languages that I spoke growing up in Kerala, another South Indian state.

"No, we are from the tea estates up over the hill behind you. We had to walk nearly 8 kilometers to get here," they replied. Behind me was a steep hill, crowded with tall, lanky silver oak trees whose leaves glistened like silver in the sun. The district had many large estates tucked away at the tops of remote hills. Some provided basic primary health care, but in general accessing care was a considerable challenge, given the terrain and the distances involved.

I was with another Indian-American student, Preeti, who was taking about 6 months off before starting medical school in the United States. For us, this first camp was an opportunity to begin understanding the range of health problems that women had, how they talked about them, what they did, and how local clinicians responded. We decided to split up, observe, and take notes.

I continued to stand by the registration desk to observe the requests being made. Once the women realized that I could speak a little Kannada, they started to talk.

"My two children and I walked 10 kilometers across the paddy fields over there," a woman told me, pointing to the valley down below the panchayat office. Green fields beginning to turn a golden brown, approaching the winter harvest, extended for several kilometers ahead. Near the horizon I could make out a settlement. At the camp, we learned how important the local terrain was in shaping women's access to care. This region is heavily forested and mountainous. Many villages are tucked into the hillsides and surrounded by dense vegetation. Because of heavy rainfall, there is extensive paddy cultivation in the valleys where "villages," consisting often of just a handful of homes, are separated by kilometers of fields. Distance and lack of transportation were therefore important barriers to healthcare access.

"We even missed a day's pay to come to the camp! Management is like that—they won't even give us a day off if we are sick," said one young woman.

"Sixty kilos we pluck. Is it any wonder that we have back pain and white discharge?!" questioned another.

Many of the large estates are mandated by law to provide basic amenities such as health care and primary education. However, most of these clinics are run by male doctors. Doctors and women are uncomfortable with physical exams; therefore, if a woman does seek care for a gynecological problem (which she may not), treatment is usually based only on reported symptoms. Without the estate doctor's permission, women would incur leave without pay if they needed a day off to seek gynecological care from a woman doctor, who might be anywhere from 10 to 30 kilometers away.

One woman explained, "When we to go to the town to see a lady doctor, we have to spend so much—5 rupees bus charge and another 50 rupees to the doctor. And then the medicines."

Even when health care was accessible, as in the case of our camp, the culture of silence around women's gynecological health was so pervasive that women would not reveal their problems. The fact that we were requiring everyone to publicly state which specialist they wanted to see was clearly not conducive to making women comfortable about indicating gynecological concerns. Further, we had young men sitting at the registration desk noting down this information. This did not strike me immediately. But as I stood there for 5, 10, 15 minutes and found that so few of the women were stating gynecological problems and seeking consultations with the gynecologist, I began to become suspicious.

My uneasiness was confirmed when I struck up a conversation with a tall, thin woman who looked to be in her thirties. She seemed tense and apprehensive, wringing the edge of her sari, scanning the crowd. I approached her with a smile and welcomed her to the inauguration of our new health center.

Bharati was her name. I described Swasthya's services and focus on women and I asked her what concerns brought her to the camp.

"Headaches," she said.

"Have you been having any other problems?" I asked as we waited for her turn to register.

"No," she said uncertainly. Given her hesitation, I engaged her in some lighter conversation. "So, how many children do you have?"

"Three—two girls and a boy."

"Have you brought them also for a checkup, or did you come on your own?"

"I came on my own."

"So tell me, how is your health? What kinds of problems do you have?"

She moved closer to me, and while keeping her eyes downcast, confided, "I have been bleeding a lot, more than what is my usual, and throughout the month."

I asked how long it had been happening.

"It's been more than half a year now. But the estate doctor said not to worry, he didn't even need to look at me. He said that it happens to women at my time of life and that it would stop soon. I am waiting, and yet I feel so weak. Every day is more difficult."

At 35, Bharati seemed young for menopause. I felt that her symptoms merited an examination, if not some extended treatment, and I was angry the estate doctor had not even examined her. I was sure she would benefit from an exam from the female gynecologist at our camp.

"Oh, there is really no need," she said, "I am sure I will be feeling better soon."

We had been speaking with a friendly rapport, but I reverted to playing the health professional role, and after a few more words of encouragement, Bharati nervously agreed to an exam. I completed her registration and then accompanied her to the line in front of the gynecologist's room. I returned to the main registration queue to continue talking to others.

I saw Jagan nearby: "You have to tell the men at the registration desk to ask all the women if they want to see a 'lady' doctor," I said anxiously. "The women are too shy to ask and they're going to miss out on an opportunity to see the gynecologist!"

I watched understanding flash across Jagan's face. Immediately, he headed to the registration desk to make our request. This approach worked much better. The doctors' consultations went on all day.

A typical exam took place like this: The doctor is sitting behind a wooden desk. The nurse is standing, attentive, by her elbow. The patient enters and stands, waiting to be acknowledged. She moves to sit on a stool by the side of the desk when the doctor motions her to do so. "So what is the problem?" the doctor asks, without lifting her eyes from the case sheet on the desk. The patient describes her symptoms and the doctor orders her to the examination table, chiding her if she does not cooperate by getting into the lithotomy position to facilitate a pelvic exam. Occasionally, if the patient resists out of fear, her legs are pried apart.

Later, we noticed the marked difference when doctors treated women whom they perceived to be their social "equals," that is women of an upper caste. Upper-caste women were welcomed into the consultation room with a smile. Eye contact would be made and explanations given. The women would be put at ease before the examinations began.

The most common problems that women at the camp reported were white discharge, excessive bleeding during menstruation, and missed periods. The doctors examined the women who complained of white discharge (some with a speculum and some without), but most of the time they could not find anything wrong and would either prescribe ayurvedic medications or order a blood test. The doctors did not offer much advice to the patients. Mostly, they simply prescribed medications.

The experience of Lakshmi, a thin, diminutive 28-year-old woman who worked on the tea estate, was illustrative of the lack of dialogue during medical consultations. She came to the gynecologist because she had still not started menstruating. Dr. Sarojini took her into an inner room for an examination. Shortly after, she returned to tell us that Lakshmi had poorly developed female sexual organs (immature breasts and poorly developed genitals), probably due to reduced production of female hormones. Dr. Sarojini told us that this problem should have been addressed when Lakshmi was much younger and that it was probably too late to do anything about it. While she explained all this to us in English, Lakshmi was standing patiently next to the desk, waiting for something to be conveyed to her in Kannada.

Dr. Sarojini asked her to come to the hospital at Vijaygiri on a day that doctors from the nearby teaching hospital visited for special consultations. Not surprising but telling was the fact that during the discussion with Lakshmi, Dr. Sarojini provided no information about her health problem or prospects for treatment.

About an hour later, I saw Bharati standing in a corner of the compound. The kohl she was wearing around her eyes was smudged down her cheeks. She was distraught and could barely speak.

"The doctor just said that I had to come to the hospital this week to have my uterus removed!"

"But didn't she tell you why?" I asked.

"No, she examined me and just said to come to the hospital to get my uterus removed." Fresh tears poured forth. "It's going to cost so much money. And I'm sure the doctor won't give me leave!"

I was confused. I had thought that Bharati was upset about having to undergo a surgery. "What do you mean—the doctor won't give you leave?"

Bharati explained that she needed to get a referral for the surgery from the estate doctor, otherwise she would not get sick leave or reimbursement for her expenses. I told her that I would go with her to talk to the estate doctor, who was also at the camp, and convince him to give her a referral to the hospital.

The doctor, a short, bespectacled man, was not someone I would see as an intimidating person. However, he clearly wielded great power over Bharati; she was even quieter in front of him, almost fearful. Later, while recounting the incident to Jagan, he explained that the estate doctors are quite powerful but also find themselves in the crossfire between estate workers and the management. Estate management wants the doctors to cut down costs and limit referrals and expensive procedures, but workers look to the doctors to help keep them in good health. The success of his job depends on his ability to establish good rapport with the workers and their families so that they follow his advice. This estate doctor seemed open to listening, and after I explained the situation to him, he agreed to give Bharati the referral letter she needed in order to get the estate's health insurance coverage for her surgery.

Bharati thanked me profusely for talking to the estate doctor and started to cry. I went to ask the gynecologist what was wrong with Bharati. She only had a moment between other examinations to inform me that Bharati had uterine fibroids and that a hysterectomy had therefore been recommended.

I returned to where Bharati was waiting and explained what a fibroid is and how it could be treated. Bharati told me that she had been experiencing bleeding for quite some time but had not been told by any of the doctors she had consulted why it was happening. The estate doctor, who had not examined her, had just given her some tablets for stomach pain and said that the problem would go away.

While I was describing fibroids to Bharati, a number of other women, also tea estate workers, gathered around us. One of them said that she was really very happy that we had come to her village: "We have no one to talk to about our health problems."

Yet another woman emphatically added, "It's very important for us to know more about diseases. Doctors never give any explanations." This lack of engagement on the part of doctors was brought up by several women, all of whom seemed eager for more information on health and illness.

Even as Bharati's health concerns had been dismissed by the doctor on the estate, her fears and anxieties and her right to information had been dismissed within the auspices of our own well-intentioned program. Clearly, there was more to offering health care to women than providing them with access to doctors.

Irked by these experiences at the camp, we began to conduct monthly outreach visits to one of the largest tea estates in the area. We also made several overnight trips during which the estate management would host us at their guest house— a cottage nestled in the center of the estate, surrounded by rolling hills of verdant tea plants. On our first trip, we walked down to the "lines" with Geeta, an estate worker whose husband was the president of the local panchayat. The lines typically consist of two long single-story buildings side by side. Each houses between 5 and

10 families. We went from door to door inviting women to join us outside for a discussion on health. Once we had invited all the women, we arranged ourselves in a circle on grass mats that the women had spread out on the ground in front of their homes and talked late into the night. Based on that night's discussion, we decided to conduct two more evening programs—one on hygiene and the other on body aches and pains. We divided the presentation by kinds of pain and explained each one and its remedy: stomach pain, back pain, shoulder and neck pain, chest pain, headache, and tired eyes. The premise of our work was that women could take charge of their lives, take their health into their own hands.

One evening, our Jeep did not turn up to take us to the lines. We walked along the winding, tarred road through the estate for several kilometers. The sun was setting and the silver oaks gently swayed in the breeze. Neither the estate nurse or the doctor attended and everyone seemed relaxed. Nearly 40 people—men, women, and children—had gathered and there was a festive atmosphere. We set up our battery-powered lamp (as there were no street lights) and our poster board. When it came time to demonstrate the exercises for relieving back pain (a common problem, particularly among women who plucked tea leaves), we asked the men to leave. We wanted the women to feel comfortable practicing the exercises we demonstrated. The men left reluctantly and then the party began. Amid fits of giggling and laughter, Saraswasthy, one of the CHWs, demonstrated the exercises. First, the younger women stepped forward to try them out. Then one by one the others joined in. Several different demonstration circles formed and half an hour later, women were dragging their friends to the circle and teaching them the exercises themselves!

There were these special moments when I would have a visceral understanding of the feminist texts that I read as an undergraduate at Barnard College. I drew inspiration from efforts like *Our Bodies, Ourselves* and an Indian equivalent called *Na shariram nadi* (My body is mine). During the CHW training, I drew extensively from these texts and from the literature on the women's health movement in the United States.

The CHWs were at first shy and merely giggled through these sessions. As, time went on, they not only became comfortable with the process but began to talk about how exciting it was to actually understand their bodies. This was the experience that we wanted to extend to other women in the community.

A combination of factors usually helped me establish an easy rapport with women—the fact that I had come all the way from America to work on women's health in Vijaygiri, that I could speak Kannada (within 4 to 6 months I was reasonably fluent), and that I was married and wore the local signs of marriage—a *mangalsutra* (a thread worn around the neck) and toe rings. One of the most inspiring aspects of the work that we did in Vijaygiri were these exchanges with women, when women opened up to us and shared their stories.

The Swasthya mission grew out of these encounters—we recognized that mere provision of medical consultations, the presence of health-care infrastructure in terms of a health center, a physician, a nurse, and medicines were insufficient and irrelevant if the quality of care was poor. An important aspect of quality of care is the nature of the interactions between health-care providers and individuals: to what extent are individuals' concerns and problems elicited? To what extent are the health-care providers' diagnoses actually communicated? How are they communicated? Do sensitivity and empathy imbue the interaction?

We began by setting up a network of women's health centers with a strong linkage to a referral hospital. With Dr. Vasan and Jagan at the hospital, we had assumed that care would be both appropriate and empathic. Dr. Vasan expected his junior colleagues to ask questions, observe, and follow by example. However, not all the junior doctors were sufficiently motivated and sensitive the way Jagan was. We, the volunteers and the CHWs, did not feel comfortable discussing these challenges with Dr. Vasan. Rather, we debriefed with Jagan about the insensitive and even discriminatory attitudes held by some of the junior doctors. But unfortunately, because Jagan had a degree in Ayurvedic medicine, few of the interns and junior resident doctors (practicing biomedicine) respected Jagan's style of health care provision and his openly expressed insistence on treating all people equally.

We tried to tackle this issue of empathy and sensitivity during our team's interpersonal interactions in a number of ways. In our training sessions with CHWs, we not only emphasized the importance of sharing information on health and disease but also worked on the more subtle aspects of the ways in which we shared information and the importance of recognizing and understanding the emotional and social dimensions of the interaction. *Pay attention to the emotional state of the person who has sought your advice or care. Acknowledge and facilitate discussion about their emotional state.* These were some of the guidelines we discussed in our training and that we tried to put into practice.

Such encounters led us to initiate the Well Woman Clinics. The main goal of these clinics was to provide empathic reproductive health care, including information, counseling, and clinical services to women. The CHWs were trained to take a comprehensive, broadly defined health history and provide pre-examination counseling to help women assess what kind of clinical consultation they required and become acquainted with routine examinations. Typically, the CHWs would offer to do a speculum examination (with visual inspection of the cervix to identify cervical abnormalities), a pelvic exam, and a breast exam. Then they would conduct a postexamination counseling session in which health promotion information and any other concerns (including the need to visit the hospital or our outreach clinic for further care from a physician) were addressed. The CHWs did not prescribe antibiotics. So, if such an examination indicated that a woman might have a reproductive tract infection, she would be referred to our outreach clinic or the hospital for further treatment. We also encouraged patients to help themselves by doing breast examinations and exercises.

Interpersonal dynamics in the health care setting were to a great extent shaped by caste and class. I was conscious of the existence of caste inequalities, perhaps in part because I had grown up privileged. My grandfather, whom everyone in our family referred to as Anna, had rejected caste and religious divides at a time when Kerala's rigid caste system was being challenged by lower caste–led social movements. To demonstrate his rejection, he dropped his caste surname, an act of defiance that few upper-caste Brahmins committed. Anna instilled in my father not only a nationalist spirit but a commitment to work against caste divides. My father often recalled how he would bring home a diverse group of friends, belonging to various religions and castes, and the ease with which my grandmother would feed them in her kitchen—a practice normally taboo in any caste-observant Brahmin home. Thus equality and respect were key values that imbued my formative years—a sense that all people are not only equal but have the right to be treated equally. However, the fact that my grandfather and father relinquished their caste name did not mean that we did not continue to benefit from our caste heritage. Neither I nor the other students, a few of whom had no awareness of their caste backgrounds, had expected to find that caste still remained central, particularly in rural communities like Vijaygiri.

Shantha belonged to the scheduled caste (also known as Dalits)—historically the most disadvantaged group within the Indian caste system, the majority of whom owned no land and were relegated to the role of menial laborers. She had finished 12 years of education at an English medium school, which is very unusual for any woman in Vijaygiri. The medium of instruction in most schools in the region is Kannada; it is only a very few who have the chance to study in schools where English is the medium of instruction. Although her parents were poor and had several children, they valued education and decided to send their youngest daughter to a "convent school." Shantha studied hard and did well. Moreover, she was acutely aware of the privilege she had enjoyed and was very interested in doing community health work.

The honorary secretary of the hospital, a devout Brahmin, recognized the importance of having a multicaste team. Further, Shantha was clearly very bright and ambitious, having earned scholarships all the way through her schooling. I was excited to find a Dalit woman with the qualifications to work for Swasthya, and I enthusiastically presented the idea to the other CHWs. Their response—total silence and, when repeatedly goaded, muted acceptance—surprised me. Although they did not openly refuse to accept Shantha as a colleague, there was marked hesitation and implicit resistance among them. Although the CHWs were all of the middle and upper castes, I did not expect a negative response from them, as they had been serving scheduled-caste clients up to this point without issue. Because of their excellent work, I assumed that they shared the Swasthya vision of equality.

For a week, there was a great deal of tension between me and the CHWs. We had the custom of beginning every meeting with a "check in," a 30-second sharing of our frame of mind, and ending with a "check out," another 30 second sharing about how we felt the meeting went. That week after I had communicated our interest in hiring Shanta, I felt that the check ins and check outs were strained, as though the women had something on their minds but could not say it. The situation finally became so intolerable that I decided to take the CHWs for a one-day re-treat to discuss the issue away from the day-to-day stress and rush of the hospital. We traveled outside the village to a lovely and tranquil bird sanctuary in the forest. Despite the serene beauty of the place, the tension between us remained thick. I was disappointed in their response to Shantha, and they felt defensive.

"I have no personal objections to this woman," said one of the health workers, who seemed unable to finish her thought.

"She is obviously well educated and willing to work hard," said another, filling in for the first, "but the truth is, if she comes into the field with us, she will not be permitted to enter the homes of higher-caste people. We will be scolded for bring-ing a scheduled-caste woman into their houses." She pointed out that this would especially be a problem amongst the Brahmins and Gowdas, the two main upper castes in Vijaygiri. The other CHWs murmured their agreement.

"I am afraid that upper-caste community members will complain to my par-ents," said another. There were more nods of assent. "My parents don't want me to be known as one who challenges the caste system," she continued, "In fact, I'm not even sure if they would appreciate my bringing Shantha to our own home." I could understand her concern, as she and three out of the four other health workers were unmarried at the time, and thus answerable to their parents.

"Swasthya is meant to meet the needs of the most disadvantaged individuals and families in Vijaygiri, and Shantha belongs to the scheduled castes, the most disadvantaged of all." I implored, "If we can't accept one of "them" as a colleague, then how can we possibly help them overcome the obstacles they face?" Yet even in that lovely, isolated place, away from the eyes of the village, we could not find a resolution.

Up to this point, I viewed my role as project director primarily as facilitator and coordinator. I would bring together resources that local women did not have access to, help to define the problems that we would address, and identify ways in which we could address them. From my perspective, the project fundamentally belonged to the CHWs and the other Vijaygiri women, not to me. However, the CHWs' resistance to taking Shantha on as a colleague challenged me: should I re-define my role and the nature of "ownership" over the project? My choice was to either accept their decision, going against my own convictions about the impor-tance of hiring Shantha in furthering the fundamental sociopolitical commitment of the project, or to assert authority and set aside the participatory principles that I hoped would underlie the organizational structure.

I decided to override the CHWs' resistance and hired Shantha. Further, I threat-ened to fire anyone who was not willing to work with her.

Back at the hospital the following Monday, I described my discussions with the CHWs at the bird sanctuary to Jagan. He was not only disappointed but incensed.

"No longer do we have untouchability in India!" he exclaimed. He marched over to our meeting room and launched into a tirade: "As long as you are in your uniforms, you are nurses—not individuals belonging to this or that caste. Caste should not enter into your professional activities."

I do not think this lecture changed the CHWs' attitudes. However, I realized how important it was that we critically examined the issue of caste and caste identity within our group. If it was this difficult for an educated Dalit woman to gain acceptance in a setting such as ours, I could hardly imagine the treatment she would get elsewhere.

In January 1999, Shantha enrolled in Jagan's nursing program to prepare for her work with Swasthya. In addition, we thought that Shantha could shadow the other CHWs while they engaged in community outreach. Thus, she would have the opportunity to learn by observing, and we would also be able to gauge community reactions to her. In the meantime, we had also initiated plans to set up a counseling service in the hospital, and since Shantha was being trained there, we decided that she would spend the majority of her hours outside of class working in the hospital as a counselor. So the issue of caste was sidestepped to some extent. On the infrequent occasions when Shantha did go into the community with her colleagues, they avoided the upper-caste neighborhoods. I still wonder whether or not this was the ideal situation.

A couple of months after Shantha began working with us, we conducted a door-to-door reproductive health survey in Vijaygiri. Initially, we were apprehensive about what would happen when Shantha attempted to recruit individuals for the survey, which did entail going into homes to conduct interviews. Yet we faced no problems. She was never once challenged and never saw any kind of negative reaction. In fact, community members respected her in her role as a Swasthya Community Health Worker, seeing her as a health worker rather than a scheduled-caste woman. Jagan's statement that caste was irrelevant once one donned the nurse's uniform seemed to finally have been established.

A number of months later, I saw Shantha at the hospital and we had the opportunity to talk about her experience thus far. "How did it go for you in the beginning?" I asked. Shantha did not answer my question. Instead, she told me, as she had many times before, how pleased and honored she was to have the job.

"Please, Shantha, it's important for me to know about your experiences, especially in the initial days."

Although reluctant to voice displeasure or discontent to me, she finally revealed the pain that she had experienced. "I was hurt," she said, "particularly by Anita." Anita is an upper-caste CHW with whom Shantha spent time in the field, and I had thought Anita would be a help to her. Shantha had been of the same mind.

"I thought Anita would be my greatest source of support, but she turned away from me, as did the others. Usually she would turn away when another was there; if one of the other CHWs was also present during outreach, the two of them would talk and walk together, leaving me out. At our weekly meeting days at the hospital, everyone would sit together and eat and talk, but no one would talk to me. I know they did not want me here."

Shantha had been hurt and sad but unable to talk to her parents. "I haven't talked to anyone about this until today. You know that my parents are old and my sister is always worried about me. I wanted them to think that I was happy here. And I am. I am so happy to have this job," Shantha said in her quiet, composed way. She was new to the hospital environment and did not have any friends or support in the hospital itself. I was the boss, and so she did not feel comfortable coming to me because she did not want to me to think that she was complaining. She had suffered silently, thankful for the position and determined to make the most of it.

"Things are getting better now," she said, "I am glad the survey went so well; I can feel that the others are beginning to trust me." But what struck me was the fact that I had not stopped to think of what the ordeal must have been like for her. Of course she knew that her caste status was an issue with the other CHWs, and they had made it clear to her, perhaps fueled by resentment at my insistence that they accept her.

At this point, we, the group of international students, decided to consciously confront caste inequality and build alliances with groups that were trying to promote the interest of the lower castes. Jagan, too, felt passionate about this need. His sensitivity and political commitments sometimes surprised the student group and always elicited respect from them. Jagan was born and brought up in Vijaygiri, steeped in the cultural milieu, yet he seemed acutely aware and unaccepting of these entrenched inequities. Jagan pursued connections with a Dalit group and a tribal development group. The tribal development group invited us to give a presentation at one of their festivals and printed pamphlets that had our names on them as among the invitees. Someone at the hospital saw the pamphlet and got very upset because the tribal group was engaged in political work. Hospital staff for the most part believed that their work was apolitical. Although a number of hospital staff engaged in politics in their personal time, their job was to provide health care to all, and therefore they felt that they should not take a political stand.

The hospital was set up by an ashram originally founded by Shankracharya, a Sanskrit scholar who lived in the eleventh century. He was responsible for the revival of Brahmanical Hinduism in South India at a time when Buddhism and Jainism were gaining popularity. Brahmanical Hinduism is a more conservative form of Hinduism in which Brahmins dominated. The ashram is a very old, powerful Brahmin institution. It runs a Sanskrit school for Brahmin boys and trains them to be priests. About 20 years ago, the leader of the ashram, the Swamiji, who was committed to serving the local community, founded this hospital. The hospital administration was willing to accept our work to promote women's health and even, to a certain extent, our efforts to promote women's leadership. But they were unwilling to accept a collaboration with a group that was explicitly political. This posed another dilemma, whether to distance ourselves from the political struggle for tribal and scheduled-caste equality or to jeopardize the partnership with the hospital on which our program was founded. We decided that our partnership with the hospital was so crucial to the functioning of our program that we would have to accept the attendant constraints. Thus ended our links to the tribal development group.

One morning, we traveled to a Dalit colony to visit Lalitha, a woman who was in need of our help. The colony was deserted because everyone was out working in the fields, but Lalitha was at home; she was lying on a straw mat in the corner of her one-room mud house. She had been unwell. Three years prior to our meeting she had started having health problems and had to stop working. She had two sons, who were 15 and 12 years old at the time. Both had been good students, but she had to take them out of school to work, to compensate for her lost wages.

Before her illness, Lalitha would go to the fields at about 6:30 in the morning and return home around 4 in the afternoon. Some of the landlords who are more generous give the workers some buttermilk and rice at lunchtime, but there are many that give absolutely no food at all. Therefore, many workers might eat something in the morning and then not eat again until 4 or 5 in the afternoon. The going wage in this area is 25 rupees a day (about 50 cents). The basic diet is rice and a watery curry with cucumbers, which has very little nutritional value. Lentils, which are part of the staple diet of the upper castes, are unaffordable for people like Lalitha. They cost about 15 to 20 rupees a kilo. The work was constant, and Lalitha and her husband were in the field every day, vowing to work so that their sons could finish school.

When her health problems led to economic hardship, Lalitha's relationship with her husband began to deteriorate. She had been experiencing burning, pain, and anger during sex. "I started to feel really tired. In the evenings he drinks. Then he calls me to sleep with him, and we fight because I do not want to. . . . My husband took me to see a doctor who gave me some tablets, saying that once my head was fixed, all my diseases would disappear."

It was difficult for me, as a nonphysician, to really make sense of Lalitha's symptoms. Much has been written in India about women's experience of fatigue, locally known as *susthu*. When we were presenting exercises to women in Vijaygiri, we would ask them—in groups and individually—to list the major health problems that women in their area experienced, and *susthu* was always mentioned. *Susthu* might be a result of anemia and the hard physical labor that most women engaged in, and may have been compounded by the other more psychosocial stresses (arising from poverty, marital discord, trouble with neighbors/landlords/bosses, raising children) that women, particularly poor, lower-caste women, coped with day in and day out.

The pills that Lalitha had been given were tranquilizers, meant to sedate rather than cure her. After several years of taking such drugs, trying to figure out what was wrong with her body, and receiving no answers, Lalitha was feeling weak and disinterested in life.

Although Lalitha and her husband spent whatever little money they had in visits to private physicians, the doctors could not diagnose her properly. They had gone to the full range of health-care providers: village healer, a man who used herbal remedies to treat illnesses, the local ayurvedic doctor, the registered medical practitioner, and allopathic/biomedical practitioners. They branded her neurotic, a "basket case" for whom little could be done. They did not see that when she left their office, she would return to the stresses of her everyday life—poverty, marital discord, and the burdens of raising two sons. These were invisible to the doctors. Caste segregation is so complete that the physicians could not know these things and so could not know of the despair that Lalitha felt about her life; in other words, they could never truly address her problems.

The Swasthya research teams found that Lalitha's case is not unique. Her story mirrors that of many women in Vijaygiri, who have no choice but to go to physicians with physical manifestations of problems related to stress and social and economic hardship. Although these women are in need of social and psychological support, physicians rarely recognized this.

I had accompanied our young physician interns on a weekly visit to one of our Swasthya health centers. We went in the Swasthya jeep, with the men—the two interns and the driver—in front and a Swasthya CHW, two nursing assistants from the hospital, and me (all women) in the back. The interns, young men in their early twenties studying at a nearby private medical school, were discussing the "regulars" they were expecting to find at the center.

"I hope that lady is not there," said one.

"Which one?" I asked from the back. I always tried to listen in on these conversations to get a sense of what was happening at the centers.

"You know, that crazy one. She comes every week, complaining of one thing or the other—headaches, stomachaches, exhaustion. There's nothing wrong with her. She looks totally healthy," was the reply.

Sure enough, when we reached the center, there she was.

These women, like Lalitha, typically walk away with a questionable set of tablets—vitamins and tranquilizers, for example. They walk away believing that these medicines will suffice to solve their problems. The fact that many of these problems arise from a combination of socioeconomic, cultural, and physical circumstances and call for more holistic interventions escaped both the physicians and the women themselves.

A Swasthya CHW visits Lalitha often, providing her with emotional support and encouraging her to participate in programs at the health center. The CHW also provides counseling to Lalitha's husband, attempting to make him more sensitive to the pressures Lalitha feels and to confront the violence in their relationship. The success of the CHW's efforts to support Lalitha is limited, however, by the sociopolitical and economic differences between them. The CHW is from an upper caste and is educated. Thus Lalitha and her husband, regardless of whether or not they wish to have her there, are obliged to allow the CHW in their home and to listen to her. They see her leave the colony every evening to return to her home in the more privileged section of the village. Although she is trained to be more sensitive than the physicians Lalitha has seen, she is also unable to truly understand what it is like to live as a Dalit in a colony. No matter how long she works there, the CHW will always be an outsider.

Gender, caste, class, and nationality create hierarchies of power and knowledge even within our own group. The authorities at our partner hospital and within the community tend to be men of the upper caste/class. The honorary secretary, the chief medical officer, the head of the laboratory, and even Jagan were all Brahmin men. Even among the nursing staff at the hospital, the matron and many nurses were either Brahmins, other upper castes, or Christians. The women who swept the hospital clean were Dalits. The CHWs, although relatively diverse in terms of caste and class, are privileged because of their training and employment. I, the program director, am a citizen of a globally dominant nation; in part, I have that citizenship because of the privileges that my family enjoyed based on our caste status in India. Given my own caste background and the fact that I was highly educated, to the level of a doctorate, gave me considerable voice. I was in a completely different category. And the struggle for me was to use this strategically—to protect and facilitate the interests of those who were not always heard, including the CHWs, within the prevailing power structures.

Community mobilization requires sustained community involvement and action. This was the weakest aspect of the student-driven model that we were pursuing. Given that students are students only for a short time, a model that is student-dependent is extremely difficult to sustain. In fact, it is likely to be unsustainable unless there is a stable core leadership. Our plan was to work with the CHWs until they could plan and carry out programs on their own. They would form the core group, with Jagan in a leadership position.

Over time, we grew concerned that Jagan was constantly torn between the needs and perspectives of the administration and the CHW/student group. We decided that the CHWs themselves should have greater leadership responsibility. In reality, we found that 3 years of working with the CHWs was not enough for them to reach this level of autonomy. They had not reached a point where they could continue to innovate and bring to fruition a vision on their own. Our trips to Vijaygiri over the fourth and fifth years revealed that, for the most part, the CHWs were carrying out activities that we had discussed and planned over the course of the first 3 years. Real innovation had not occurred.

According to one member of the student group who conducted an informal evaluation of Swasthya activities,

> When asked if they would like more education or would want any changes in the program, most community residents felt it was nice to have the CHWs come to their house and they would listen to whatever they said. However, these types of comments were made in a way suggesting that they did not really use the information—they just listened to it and were happy that someone was doing good work in their community. It did not seem that anyone was greatly dependent on these visits or that they would be greatly missed. However,

people did express that they had come in for certain tests and checkups to the hospital at Vijaygiri because the CHWs had encouraged them to do so. Most people seemed to feel that it was helping people in the community and good for the village, even if they themselves did not utilize the resources/information.[iii]

The project finally wound down 5 years after it began. The student group's involvement had come to a close after the first 3 years, but we continued to raise small amounts of money to keep the project going. However, we began to finish our degrees and move on with our lives. (I was 7 months pregnant with my second child and on the faculty of the University of California, San Francisco, by the time Swasthya closed.) In our occasional communications via e-mail, it became apparent that there was increasing unhappiness with Swasthya's governance, the lack of recognition and independence the CHWs had, and the evolution (or perhaps I should call it stagnation) of the program. A few members of the initial student group continued to visit Vijaygiri and found that the CHWs were still giving the same presentations, skits, and role plays that we had developed in the early years. The CHWs also voiced concerns during these visits: they wanted more stable employment.

At the end of a series of discussions with the hospital, we realized it was unlikely that we would be able to resolve these concerns to everyone's satisfaction. Finally in December 2002, we and the hospital decided to end the partnership.

Each of the CHWs has followed a unique trajectory. Each, I feel, has been touched deeply by the project. Swasthya did provide opportunities for self-expression and independent thought and action—opportunities that few young women, particularly those in rural areas, have access to even today. They opened and operated bank accounts—some with the support of their families and others clandestinely. Nearly all the CHWs continue to work and pursue careers today. Shantha and Anita are roommates and work as nurses in a large clinic run by a friend of Dr. Vasan's in a nearby district. Several others are in similar employment. One CHW became involved in village politics; another got married and stopped working.

Jagan remains at the hospital, continuing to run the "nurse aid" training program. The hospital has expanded since my time there. They now have a government-accredited undergraduate nursing college that has overshadowed Jagan's program. The nursing college is staffed by teachers with bachelor's and advanced degrees in nursing and follows a state-approved curriculum. However, the graduates of Jagan's program are still in demand; many small nursing homes continue to look for lower-paid nursing staff and do not care whether their employees have a recognized degree or not. Jagan continues to raise funds through local clubs and associations in order to run outreach clinics. In his desire to keep innovating and contributing to local health promotion, he became certified in counseling through a part-time program offered in a nearby city and received a degree in health administration through a distance learning program. He had hoped that this degree would help him move into a hospital management position. However, the power structure within the hospital has been so entrenched that his plans have not materialized.

Despite the loss in stature of his nursing program, his unrealized dreams of engaging in mass health education and outreach and his failed attempt to take on a greater administrative role at the hospital, Jagan remains cheerfully optimistic. He and his family visited me a few months ago. In response to my barrage of questions about everyone at the hospital and the goings on, he replied, laughing, "Everything is the same!"

ACKNOWLEDGMENTS

This chapter builds on a paper coauthored with Rajesh Vedanthan titled "Experiences of the Perils, Pitfalls and Inspirations of Public Health as Social Justice: The Swasthya Community Health Partnership, India." I am grateful to Raj and my other Swasthya colleagues for the enriching experiences and relationships that continue to inspire me.

NOTES

    i. Names of places and individuals have been changed.
    ii. Village government.
    iii. Tantri, A. Personal communication.

8 Applying Global Health Lessons to Syracuse, New York

Sandra D. Lane

She was 17 years old and 2 months pregnant; he was aged 19 when the police bat-tered down the door of her apartment to arrest him.[1] They were both from loving families who worked hard and attended church; they were well known in the community. Syracuse at the end of the 1990s had the twin tragedies of a collapsed legitimate economy combined with swelling illicit drug markets in which her boy-friend became entangled. She was attracted to his "thug" swagger, sporting dia-monds and the confidence that cash can provide. But he was also smart and caring; values that she knew her family would appreciate. She had become pregnant after his first arrest, in her adolescent denial not believing that either pregnancy or prison was a real possibility. When she told them about her pregnancy, her parents said they would support whatever decision she made, but in their clear-eyed assess-ment of the difficulties ahead, they offered to pay for an abortion. Her baby's fa-ther, via a collect call from the county jail, begged her, "Please don't terminate my baby." She continued with her pregnancy, beginning by making an appointment for prenatal care. For a 17-year-old, she was remarkably capable, working part time while attending high school and visiting her boyfriend every week, first in the county jail and then at the state correctional facility. Her mother attended the birth of her child, while her baby's father listened over the phone from prison, where he remains today. Her baby was full-term and healthy. Her baby's father never had his name entered on the birth certificate because, being unmarried, to enter his name would require his notarized signature or his presence. Neither he nor his family provided any financial help to her, but she accepted an average of $200 in collect phone calls from him during each month of his incarceration. She feels that the love and support he has given her in those telephone calls, and the frequent visits she makes with her child to him in prison, have kept him involved as a father for the past 7 years.

This is the story of an African-American woman in Syracuse, New York—a resourceful, intelligent woman whom I will call Mae. She currently works, attends college part time, and supports her child single-handedly. Mae's success in mothering her son—despite poverty and an incarcerated partner—is evidenced by the child's health, early reading ability, wide vocabulary, and self-confidence. Many of the young single mothers I have met, like Mae, struggle heroically to provide for their children's emotional, social, and financial needs. Despite the mothers' efforts, they often face insurmountable obstacles posed by high infant death rates, violent neighborhoods, dilapidated rental housing, failing schools, and missing fathers.

As one of his top five priorities, former Surgeon General Dr. David Satcher called for research and intervention to eliminate disparities in health and survival related to race and minority status. In response to Dr. Satcher's call, a landmark study entitled *Unequal Treatment*, from the Institute of Medicine, documented in a wealth of detail how people of color are treated differently by physicians, clinics, and hospitals in ways that are detrimental to their health.[2] Among the physicians, nurses, and other health professionals with whom I work in Syracuse, this study is receiving serious consideration, as it should. Access to and receipt of quality health care are critically important. But health is a bigger issue than health care. While access to quality health care cannot be overestimated, health care alone cannot make up for disease-inducing environments. Syracuse, a city of fewer than 150,000 residents, has five hospitals providing world-class medical care. Three of these hospitals have labor and delivery services and two feature neonatal intensive care units. Yet, within 2 miles of these sophisticated medical facilities are neighborhoods that have some of the highest rates of infant death in the United States. Clearly, we need to look beyond the clinic and hospital to the neighborhoods, schools, correctional facilities, and policies that create the context in which actual lives are lived. It is this crucible of disadvantage and discrimination that makes people of color sick.

Although this policy focus on health disparities only began at the turn of the millennium, unequal health of the poor, and most profoundly of people of color, has been recognized at least since public health's beginning in the nineteenth century. I became aware of the issue in 1972, as a first-year nurse on the pediatric ward at Boston City Hospital. There, I cared for children whose recurring admissions for lead poisoning resulted from their having been repeatedly returned to the same apartments in which they became ill, where lead-based paint crumbled into powder from doors and windowsills. Children were admitted with multiple fractures from being hit by cars while playing on city streets, and others who had been nearly killed by gunshots. Two Puerto Rican sisters, ages 3 and 5, could not escape a blaze in the tenement that was their home because the fire escape door had been nailed shut, blocking their escape. Third-degree burns—covering their faces, hands, and nearly three quarters of the skin on their bodies—healed into thick bands of scar that contrasted shockingly with the colorful ribbons tied in their tightly curled pigtails.

Most of the school-age children were barely literate, stumbling over simple words in the books we encouraged them to read. The Puerto Rican children were also unable to read the Spanish-language comic books we had obtained for them, as we thought that perhaps they were better educated in their native language. In an effort to coax their mastery of arithmetic, I taught the children blackjack during slow periods on the ward. At that point I realized that medicine, surgery, and advanced technology were often missing the point, coming too late, and patching up children damaged by their environments, only to send them back to those environments. I had grown up in what at that time was an all-white, largely working-class suburb of Boston, which was both less than 10 miles and a whole world away from the Roxbury, Mission Hill, Dorchester, and South Boston neighborhoods then served by Boston City Hospital.

Leaving Boston for California, I returned to school, earning a doctorate in medical anthropology and a master's degree in public health in epidemiology. I lived and worked in Egypt for 5 years, conducting research on gender and health, while serving as a Ford Foundation Program Officer for Child Survival and Reproductive Health for the Middle East. Since 1992, most of my work has been in the United States, with brief consultancies in the Middle East. I was part of a team that evaluated needle exchange programs for injection drug users in the United

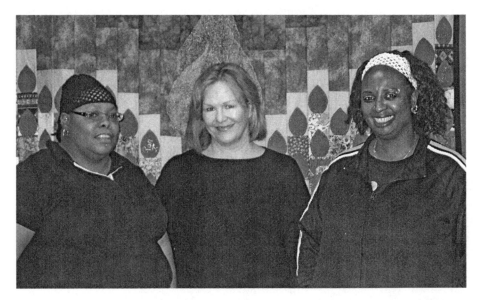

Sandra Lane with Tarah Tapley and Pam McKenzie of the Southwest Community Center FACES Program, which addresses HIV/AIDS among people of color in Syracuse. (Photo: Christina Pettinelli.)

States and Canada, spent 6 years as a behavioral scientist in a county health department, and conducted research and designed programs to eliminate the gap in health and survival facing people of color in Syracuse. I gradually realized that the differences in the causes of poor health between Egypt and Syracuse—between the so-called *developing world* and the *developed*—are overrated. The real differences are between those whose lives matter and those whose sickness and death are nearly invisible.

For example, I wrote the following field notes in 2000, while working as a short-term consultant on maternal mortality reduction in Ministry of Health Hospitals in Upper Egypt, the poorest part of Egypt, which is actually in the southern part of the country and is named after the south-to-north flow of the Nile:

> 1 A.M.: I was walking through the hospital's empty reception/emergency area, and came upon a group of people all yelling at once, half dragging a pregnant woman and being led by the hospital gatekeeper through the darkened first floor of the hospital to the elevator. The elevator doors remained shut, however, despite numerous pressings of buttons, banging and yelling for attention—the elevator operator, peacefully napping in a hidden corner, couldn't hear their clamor. We climbed the two flights to the delivery area, pulling and pushing the laboring woman who paused with each pain, arriving breathless, all calling at once to the lone first-year obstetrical resident, who was meanwhile massaging the fundus of yet another just-delivered woman in an effort to stanch her bleeding. The only other staff on duty—two nurses, inexperienced and under age 20, and an elderly cleaning woman—helped the newly arrived woman onto a delivery table, sternly admonishing her chaotic relatives to wait in the hall. The woman's lips stuck to her teeth, she was so dehydrated. The young female resident turned from the woman whose hemorrhaging had slowed to a trickle and proceeded to deliver the baby of the newly arrived woman. The resident urged the nurses and cleaning woman to push on the woman's abdomen to assist the baby's exit, a potentially dangerous maneuver for the mother, and all murmured *Al hamdu lellah* ("praises to God") when the baby emerged amid a gush of brown, meconium-stained amniotic fluid. The resident handed the baby to the nurses and cleaner, who shook and slapped the infant to bring on its first breath. Unaware of meconium's risk, the nurses did not suction the baby's mouth and trachea, so the infant's first breath drew the acid fluid deep into its lungs. When the swaddled babe was presented to the grateful kin, their ululations echoed in the hospital corridor.

Is there any doubt that if men got pregnant and delivered babies, the care and resources allocated would be greater? When the worldwide effort to prevent maternal mortality—the so-called Safe Motherhood Initiative—began in 1987, one of the key rationales for the focus on preventing the pregnancy-related death of women was stated as "If a mother dies giving birth, then her baby is more likely to die."[3] The death of the woman herself was viewed as an insufficient reason for action; her role as a mother was the redeeming factor in devoting resources to her health.

In fact, more women died from pregnancy and childbirth during the twentieth century in the United States than did military personnel during wars.[4] Yet to my knowledge, there is no monument for a woman who died bringing forth life, no scholarship in her name, no prayer or blessing or poem, no public recognition. In Europe, prior to the modern era, women who died in childbirth—and thus died in an impure state, according to the book of Leviticus—could be denied burial in sacred church grounds.[5] Clearly gender—the differential value, and socially prescribed roles of females and males—influences the quality and quantity of health care *and* the many other aspects of life that promote good health, such as food, education, housing, and employment.

Let us look now at race or, more fittingly, racism in New York State, by asking the question "If African Americans had the same death rates at each age as white residents of Onondaga County, where Syracuse is located, how many more would be alive?" Using data from the New York State Vital Records and the U.S. Census 2000, I calculated the answer to this question for the year 2000: 126 African Americans—75 males and 51 females—would still be alive on January 1, 2001, if blacks had the same death rates as their white neighbors. These lives lost are invisible to all but the family members and friends of the deceased. No governmental investigation sought the causes for their untimely deaths; no memorials remind us of their loss. And this was just 1 year in a pattern that likely repeats every year. In epidemiology, we call such deaths "excess mortality," meaning those fatalities that are over and above what would be expected, which is a way to distance ourselves from the implications of so many lives prematurely ended. Anyone who has lost a loved one knows that every death is a tragedy. The year 2000 was actually a pretty good year in terms of data for African-American infant deaths; fewer babies died that year than in the several previous years. Therefore the 126 African Americans who died in 2000 represent a smaller number than those recorded for many other years. These deaths involved African Americans of all ages, and their death certificates recorded a diverse set of causes, from premature birth among the infants to complications of diabetes among the elders. The one factor they shared was being African American, a category that is largely social and in the United States reflects a history of disadvantage. "Race" is a pre-nineteenth-century taxonomic construct, used by early European adventurers to explain differences in physical appearance to themselves and to justify the Europeans' colonial land grabs. The Human Genome Project failed to find a gene that mapped onto races as subgroups of our species.[6] The excess mortality of African Americans is not due to race as a biological difference but to rac*ism* as a source of inequality in the raw materials of health, including education, food, employment, safe housing, dignity, and health care. The thread that connects a poor rural Egyptian woman nearly dying during childbirth with urban African Americans' disproportionate mortality is that in both cases the lives of those at risk are devalued, resulting in insufficient effort to promote their health or save their lives.

SYRACUSE HEALTHY START

I arrived in Syracuse in the fall of 1996 and joined the Onondaga County Health Department to write grants for infant mortality reduction. Two weeks before I visited his office to seek employment, the commissioner of health had given a press conference in which he committed his administration to reducing infant mortality. Syracuse's infant mortality problem had been a source of shame for the city, since it was recognized in the late 1980s. In 1985–1987, infant mortality in Syracuse averaged 15 infant deaths per 1,000 live births, making it the fourth worst of 56 small U.S. cities surveyed by the Children's Defense Fund.[7] African-American infant mortality at that time, at 30.8 per 1,000 live births during 1985–1987, was the worst of 47 other U.S. comparably sized cities. Many intervention programs began or expanded in response to this crisis. The City of Syracuse Commission on Women was the first to publicly address these alarming rates and to call on health and human service leaders to work with them on this critical issue. The county health department conducted an Infant Mortality Review (1990–1993). A state-funded perinatal network—Family Ties Network, Inc.—and three case management agencies began serving impoverished pregnant women and families with infants. By 1997, African-American infant mortality in Syracuse had dropped to 22.7 per 1,000 live births, which, although a great improvement over the previous decade, was still higher than that in Tonga, Fiji, and Micronesia for that year, according to *The State of the World's Children 1997*. African-American infants died nearly three times as often as white infants, a disparity that was greater than that existing in any other upstate New York county and in the nation as a whole.

Syracuse, in Central New York State, has been characterized as a "typical . . . American midsized city" and is routinely used as a test market for consumer goods.[8] Casual visitors often remark on the lush green summer foliage, the parks, the beautifully preserved nineteenth-century architecture, and even the quality of the restaurants. Hidden from view, invisible even to many long-term residents, is the poverty and unequal mortality of people of color. Syracuse has spiraled down economically in recent decades, with the loss of industry and concomitant loss of jobs. These fiscal problems have hit worst the communities of color, which make up about one-third of the city. Because of urban renewal, African Americans and Latinos have been pushed out of their former homes and into decaying neighborhoods without grocery markets, with the highest levels of lead poisoning in the city, and with inadequate schools. Many residents of these impoverished areas see their only economic hope in the state-run lottery, on which they spend an inordinate part of their meager earnings. Some younger males find employment in the illicit drug markets, which draw customers from all parts of the city and the suburbs. Less than half of students get their high school diplomas in June after 4 years of education; some graduate high school later, some earn a general education diploma (GED), and some never finish.

Starting in the 1960s, urban renewal dramatically split the city into "haves" and "have nots." Following urban renewal and largely owing to housing discrimination, people of color who had been uprooted by eminent domain became concentrated in the south and southwest sides of the city. Numerous studies look at the impact of the built environment, such as houses and roads, on health outcomes. Broken windows, litter, and dilapidated housing characterize neighborhoods with high crime, poverty, and residents with inadequate health care.[9] Lead poisoning, for example, disproportionately affects impoverished Syracuse children, who account for 7.7% of all children with elevated blood lead (EBL) in New York State for the years 2000–2001.[10] Babies born to mothers living in devastated neighborhoods have higher rates of low birth weight and infant death. Beginning in the 1960s, supermarket chains moved away from the inner cities. This shift left smaller corner markets to serve as the primary food sources for many inner-city residents. By the late 1970s four of the major supermarkets in Syracuse had closed. The closing of these sources of healthy food makes it much more difficult for pregnant women and families with small children to eat healthily. Those without cars must take taxis, get rides from others, or take on average two buses each way to a full-service grocery, often accompanied by small children. The urban retail food sources remaining in Syracuse, mostly small corner groceries or convenience stores, not only feature very limited choices of healthy food but also charge more for such items than do the suburban supermarkets. The Syracuse Hunger Project documented the alarming number of city residents who require emergency food assistance from charitable food pantries run by faith communities and other nonprofit agencies, without which they would go hungry. In part owing to poor nutrition, the rates of obesity, heart disease, and diabetes are growing rapidly, particularly among African-American and other inner-city residents, often leading to disproportionate rates of premature death.

Increasing unemployment was coupled with a flourishing trade in illegal drugs. In response, in 1973 New York State implemented the "Rockefeller drug laws," mandating lengthy prison sentences for possession or sale of illicit substances.[11] Incarceration rates among African Americans tripled since that time, and female-headed households doubled.[12] Young males of color began experiencing arrest and jail time as a rite of passage to adulthood. Today's incarcerated adolescent males are the second and, in some families, the third generation whose children are brought to the correctional facility on visiting day to meet their fathers. Disproportionate incarceration may also be the key risk factor in the alarming rise of HIV and hepatitis B and C among African-American women and Latinas; all of the behavioral risks for transmission of these blood- and semen-born infections occur in prisons and jails, where the usual public health protections are illegal and where the rate of infection among inmates is many times that in the community.[13]

The per capita income in the 2000 census for Syracuse was $15,168, compared with the per capita income in the United States of $29,468. The 2000 Syracuse median family income was $33,026, compared with the median U.S. family income of $50,890. In Syracuse, whites are impoverished compared with their counterparts in other parts of the United States. On many indicators, African Americans fare about twice as badly as whites in Syracuse, and Latino rates of poverty and inadequate education are substantially worse than the African-American rates. White Syracuse residents, who see themselves as struggling, often find it difficult to perceive how much worse off are their neighbors of color. This poverty disproportionately affects children; Syracuse has New York State's third highest child poverty level, following Buffalo and Rochester, and the second highest Latino child poverty rate in the United States, according to the Children's Defense Fund.

With this level of poverty and despair, I realized that any intervention to reduce infant death would need to pull together all of the available resources. Immediately after being hired by the county health department, I began in the way that anthropologists have long initiated fieldwork in a new community. I started by meeting as many people as possible, including public health and elected officials, community leaders, minority agency staff, home visiting nurses, outreach workers, and adolescent group facilitators. I asked each person why he or she thought Syracuse had so many babies dying and then listened, took notes, and asked who else they thought I should speak with. I collected available statistics on many aspects of the city, trying to piece together a coherent picture. I requested and was given permission to go through the Medical Examiner's files on infant deaths for 1996, which were only in hard-copy paper archives at that time. The infant mortality review that the health department had conducted from 1991 to 1993 had been only partially analyzed and three boxes of the review's original files remained in storage. I requested these boxes and read through the medical charts of each of those deceased infants. With each new idea or hunch about what was going on, I searched through the medical literature, and made telephone calls to health researchers around the country in order to find out, as much as possible, what was known about the issue.

During this initial phase, I met with several community groups to discuss these preliminary findings and get feedback, which I have continued to do on a regular basis ever since. As a part of these community outreach efforts, we plotted the infant deaths from 1995 to 1997 on a 3-foot by 5-foot map of the city which had street names, enabling project area residents to locate their homes and neighborhoods. We placed a dot on the map for each dead baby. During 1995 to 1997, four census tracts on the south and southwest part of the city had the highest numbers of infant deaths. We held over 30 meetings in those four census tracts with clergy and congregants of faith communities, the Neighborhood Action Councils, Early Headstart mothers, the Syracuse chapter of the Association for Black Social Workers, and many others. At every meeting women would kneel before the map and gently stroke the areas where the dots clustered; we felt that the map was somewhat like the AIDS quilt; it made otherwise dehumanized statistics visible and easily understood.

At these meetings community members would ask, "Why are our babies dying?" They would sometimes speculate on esoteric causes, asking if there was something in the air or water that put them at risk. All of my subsequent work has been an effort to answer this question. Five months after being hired by the health department, I led a team that wrote a proposal for federal funding, bringing together many of the agencies and people with whom I had been meeting and from whom I had been learning. Through this work, Onondaga County was awarded a nearly $5 million Healthy Start grant (1997–2001) and a second Healthy Start grant (2001–2005) for $3.8 million. From 1997 to 2002, I served as Director of Syracuse Healthy Start (SHS), which continues to provide care to pregnant women and their families.

SHS brought together over 30 agencies to coordinate and enhance the care of pregnant women and families with infants throughout Syracuse. Rather than put in place a new and separate program, we sought to integrate and enhance the many existing but fragmented programs. These included four case management services and four obstetrical clinics serving the majority of lower-socioeconomic, teen, and minority clients. SHS staff and partners made links where there had been none; for example, between drug and alcohol treatment and obstetrical providers, who should have been coordinating their services all along. We revamped the literacy level, and the clarity, of health education materials across multiple agencies; introduced a co-ordinated risk screening and referral protocol, trained local hair stylists in infant mortality prevention and domestic violence recognition so that they could help their clients; and created five television commercials that aired during the *Jerry Springer* and *Judge Judy* programs.

As the work progressed, I began to see the following issues emerge. First, discrimination based on poverty and on gender, race, and ethnicity overlaps but it is not the same. Women and people of color with financial resources can afford better health care, food, and homes, but their resources cannot entirely protect them. Second, many health risks, such as childhood lead poisoning or asthma, have roots in infancy or the prenatal period. Some health risks grow cumulatively throughout life, in a manner that simple cross-sectional, "slice-in-time" analyses do not capture. A few social and health risks become intergenerational, making children suffer from the health inequalities of their parents' early development. Third, looking only at individual responsibility for health and disease is inadequate. A person's knowledge and ability to protect his or her health while reducing exposure to disease does not occur in isolation; unsafe, sickness-inducing environments are hard to overcome. History matters and place matters; the context in which people live— their neighborhoods as well as their culture and social institutions—shapes their health behavior. Finally, racial and ethnic health disparities emerge from unequal health care and from patterns of discrimination in housing, education, jobs, incarceration, and exposure to environmental toxins. Efforts to decrease health-care disparities are important. But even if all health-are disparities were eliminated, unequal health and survival rates would remain if we did not address the structural violence and embedded racism in environments, policies, and institutions.

THREE SUCCESSES: PREGNANT INMATES, TEEN MOTHERS, AND HEALTH LITERACY

By the year 2000, the network of SHS partner agencies was reaching half of all pregnant women in Syracuse with enhanced services. By 2000, infant mortality in Syracuse decreased by 25%, although, because SHS was not a controlled research study, we cannot say what part of the improvement was due to program efforts. By 2001, welfare reform had drastically reduced the proportion of pregnant women in Syracuse receiving public assistance. Later that year, the aftermath of the Twin Towers and Pentagon bombings diverted funding from traditional public health efforts to bioterrorism preparedness. Month by month in 2001, we frantically read the mounting death certificates of infants, and by the end of the year, we realized that infant deaths had again peaked. Although they would come down again in the subsequent 2 years, we realized with painful clarity that the prevention of infant death, like many public health achievements, is not a goal that can be reached once and for all. Our society tends to think of progress toward social objectives in terms of military campaigns or even holy crusades, like the "war on drugs" or the "war on poverty." But babies are conceived and born minute by minute, and programs developed and funded to enhance their survival must be guided by a different metaphor than war. Rather than a battle, with an initial confrontation leading sooner or later to a declaration of victory and medals to be displayed under glass, the prevention of infant death is more like housework. It will never finally be achieved, more will always remain to be done, and many of the people working hardest—the community health workers, the public health nurses, clinic social workers, and labor and delivery staff—will not receive medals.

Despite the challenges there are three areas in which we saw considerable success; these are each described below.

Pregnant Inmates

In the Onondaga County jail in 1996, a pregnant woman bled to death from a ruptured ectopic pregnancy.[14] The inmate, who did not realize she was pregnant, had complained of extreme cramps for several hours. According to news reports, a nurse practitioner made the inmate climb a down a flight of stairs to be examined and, when the woman stopped breathing, the physician merely watched on the television monitor rather than performing cardiopulmonary resuscitation.[15] A state inquiry into the death found that a physician, nurse practitioner, and three nurses had been negligent. Upon reading the state report, County Legislator Sid Oglesby said, "Her death certificate should not read that she bled to death. Based on this report, it should say she died from incompetence and indifference." The inmate was African American, the jail health staff were white.[16]

In response to this tragedy, and in part funded by Syracuse Healthy Start, the county health department overhauled the care of pregnant inmates. There are three correctional facilities in Onondaga County. In addition to the county jail, there is a state correctional facility and a juvenile detention center; all house women of reproductive age. As the director of Syracuse Healthy Start, I was occasionally very involved with helping individual women get the care they needed as they passed into and out of correctional facilities, chemical dependency treatment facilities, and back to the street. Almost all of the women were drug users, often of crack and other substances. They were such heavy smokers that their teeth and fingers were stained yellow. Some were infected with HIV, many were homeless and had long psychiatric histories with borderline personality disorder, depression, and other diagnoses. They often supported themselves by selling sex, usually oral sex, to men in cars. One day I was searching for a Healthy Start client who had stopped going to prenatal care. I was told that she had her lunch daily at St. Francis of Assumption, where the nuns provide free food to the homeless and destitute. The nuns said that she ate the lunch outside in fair weather, across the street on the steps of a boarded-up but once majestic church. As I waited on the corner where this homeless, pregnant, drug-using woman typically hung out, I noticed that cars with single male drivers swerved close to the sidewalk where I stood. I had, without realizing it, staked out a corner where sex workers ply their trade. As the first several men drove by, they looked expectantly at me and I looked back a bit sternly, but puzzled. I think that they must have taken me for a female police officer, because they drove quickly away after our mutual looks of inquiry. Finally the woman passed by and I was able to encourage her to return to prenatal care and to enter drug treatment.

Because most pregnant inmates in these facilities have problems with chemical dependency, SHS coordinates with local chemical dependency treatment agencies, the probation department, obstetrical providers, Correctional Health, and, at times, the Syracuse Community Policing Program. When a pregnant woman is arrested, staff from each of these agencies interact to help her get the clinical care and the social support needed for her to have a healthy baby. Usually the pregnant women are arrested for prostitution; about 150 women are arrested for prostitution each year in Syracuse; but since some women may have been arrested more than once, this may not be an unduplicated number. The chemical dependency agencies try immediately to open up treatment slots. Correctional Health ensures that the women see an obstetrician, according to the following protocol: Pregnant women in jail for at least 7 days receive (1) initial prenatal history, (2) physical exam, and (3) obstetrical ultrasound. All pregnant women in jail receive regular prenatal visits from an obstetrical physician on a schedule recommended by the American College of Obstetrics and Gynecologists. Public health nurses also begin "home visiting" the client while she is incarcerated in order to provide support, education, and coordination of services. SHS and Correctional Health staff evaluated this protocol from October 1, 2001, through September 30, 2002.[17] During that year, a total of 103 pregnant inmates were incarcerated in the local correctional facilities, most for only a couple of days but a some for up to several months. The speed with which the women come and go makes it very difficult to provide services to them, especially any services—such as tuberculosis testing—that require at least 2 days to assess. Often the women give false addresses upon release, which makes it difficult or impossible to provide ongoing services. Nevertheless, the evaluation demonstrated that over 80% of women incarcerated for 2 weeks or more received adequate prenatal care in the jail. The evaluation tracked the birth outcomes of all 60 inmates who delivered their babies in Onondaga County, most of whom had been released from the incarceration facility prior to their baby's birth. The inmates whose births were not included in the evaluation probably left the county before giving birth. Two of the 60 infants died, but the birth weights and gestational ages of the other infants were similar to those of babies of nonincarcerated Syracuse mothers. Of course we wished that all of the infants had survived, but given how difficult it was to provide care to women who were in and out of jail, often homeless, drug-using, and surviving on sex work, we were pleased that the large majority of infants appeared to have been born healthy.

Syracuse Healthy Start and Teen Birth Outcomes

When we conducted the analysis on the babies born to teen mothers in Syracuse, we were stunned and extremely pleased to see that the infants of teen mothers had *lower* rates of death than babies born to adult women. In most of the United States, the situation is exactly opposite. Nationwide, the babies of teen mothers die much more frequently than those of mothers age 20 and older. So, how did this result come about?

The network of partner agencies working together with Syracuse Healthy Start focused enormous attention on pregnant and parenting teens, including coordinated case management, outreach, and prenatal programs. Although our mandate was to care for pregnant women of all ages, we believed that teen parents were the most vulnerable and needed more attention than adult mothers. Case managers assisted teens with scheduling their prenatal and pediatric care, made sure that they attended their appointments, coordinated these preventive and clinical services with school health personnel to help the teens stay in school, and provided transportation as well as many other types of assistance. By 2000, about 90% of pregnant teens received at least some of our services and 79% received comprehensive care.

We focused a lot on making the services "teen friendly." For example, one of the prenatal clinics serving a majority of low-income women grouped the teen appointments on Thursday afternoons, when a nurse practitioner and physician who were particularly skilled at caring for pregnant teens were on duty. Sister Ida Gregoire, a Roman Catholic nun who is both a nurse and social worker, sat in a waiting room devoted specifically to the teens every Thursday afternoon, feeding the young clients granola bars and listening to them. Everyone who knows Sister Ida smiles when they speak of her. So tiny that she is often dwarfed by her teen patients, she exudes such compassion and acceptance that they open up with their life stories, bring their friends to the waiting room to meet her, and often come to the waiting room on Thursdays even when they do not have appointments. Sister Ida resisted well-meaning attempts to have her teach the teens in structured sessions, which I think would have turned them off. I once asked her what she talked about with the teens, and she replied that she mostly listened and that the teens themselves raised the issues with which they were struggling. I cannot quantify in an evaluation the magnitude of Sister Ida's contribution to the good outcomes of her teen patients, but my hunch is that it was considerable. Additional teen services include school-based early identification of pregnancy, risk assessment, and referral as well as case management and public health home visiting. The school-based program not only sought to promote the health of both mother and child but also to encourage and support the pregnant teens and new teen parents in academic progress.

Not only did our teens have fewer infant deaths than older mothers, but the racial gap in low birth weight, premature births, and infant death was eliminated among teens aged 13 to 17 years. African-American babies born to adult mothers, on the other hand, had higher rates of low birth weight, preterm delivery, and infant mortality than their European-American counterparts. Did the comprehensive case management, outreach, and teen-friendly prenatal services lead to lower infant mortality among teen mothers and the elimination of the racial gap in pregnancy outcomes? It seems quite likely that they did, but since SHS is not an experiment with a control group, I can only speculate that the case management and teen-friendly services were what worked. The projects' success in reaching so many teens in the city of Syracuse—with the various clinical, case management, and home visiting services—means that there is no comparison group of pregnant teens within the city that was not served. I would much rather reach the vast majority of teens with needed services than have a comparison group that lacked services.

Health Literacy

People with more education live longer, and mothers with more education have fewer infant deaths. Just completing high school confers greater longevity. Compared with high school graduates, the lives of those who dropped out before getting a diploma are almost 2 ½ times more likely to end before age 65.[18] Nationally in 2002, among mothers of all racial and ethnic groups, those who left high school between the 9th and 11th grades had the highest rates of infant death, followed by those who finished 12 years of education.[19] Mothers with at least some postsecondary education had the lowest rates of infant mortality. Educational inequality is a cornerstone of many disparities in pregnancy and infant health in Syracuse and elsewhere.

My colleagues and I in SHS developed a set of interventions directed toward parents with low education and low literacy. We began by reviewing local epidemiological data on maternal education and infant mortality from the New York State Vital Records. We compared mothers aged 20 and older who had completed high school with those the same age who had not gotten their diplomas. We limited the analysis to mothers above age 19 because we wanted to look specifically at the impact of finishing or not finishing high school. The death rate of babies born to dropout mothers was 50% higher. One cause of deaths—sudden infant death syndrome (SIDS)—stood out as much higher among the infants of non–graduating mothers. The chance of such a mother having a baby die of SIDS was nearly 9 times that among high school graduates.

But what was it about the failure to finish school that was causing these tragedies? One obvious root cause is low literacy. The reading comprehension of people who leave school early often lags about 4 years below their final completed grade, so that if a person quits school after the ninth grade, he or she probably reads at about the fifth-grade level. Local adult literacy specialists told us that only about half of Syracuse adults can read at or below the eighth-grade level, and a quarter can read only at or below the fifth-grade level. We wanted to make sure that the printed health advice for pregnant women was written at a level they could actually read. SHS staff, therefore, conducted an analysis of 28 health-education brochures and other documents given to pregnant women and families by local providers and by national agencies. This analysis was based on materials provided to pregnant women by a local prenatal care provider, consumer education brochures sent to SHS by local and national agencies, and an Internet search of the websites of organizations dedicated to disseminating health information focused on prenatal and postpartum care. These documents were evaluated according to three criteria: (1) The Fry Readability Index, which is a standardized method of determining reading level; (2) the "easy-to-read" criteria developed by Stableford,[20] which assess inclusion of white space, inclusion of culturally appropriate pictures, the type of material, and length of material ("white space" refers to short statements surrounded by ample space); and (3) cultural competence. Since it is difficult to analyze materials directed to a general audience in terms of cultural competence, we focused on the addition of graphics that represented a diverse audience. A panel of three individuals—a public health fellow, a medical student, and a graduate student in medical sociology—reviewed each of the documents. The panel had attended health literacy training where the Fry Readability Index and other measures used in this analysis were fully covered. The reviewers jointly discussed the document analysis to arrive at consensus.

We were stunned to realize that most of the printed health advice was only useful for kindling firewood. Over three quarters of the documents reviewed were above the 7th-grade reading level, and all of them were above the 6th-grade reading level. These often expensively produced educational materials for pregnant women and parents of infants were incomprehensible to half of the population.

Based on these findings, we revised our interventions so that we could better help mothers with low educational attainment to have healthy babies. First, we initiated a multiagency approach to changing how written health materials were prepared and what types of materials were purchased by training the staff of local health care, public health, human service, outreach, case management and community-based agencies in how to write materials that are "easy to read." We then conducted a follow-up assessment to determine whether the trained staff used these principles in their work. Of the approximately 21 agencies or programs whose staff attended one or more of the training sessions, 15 agencies/programs subsequently used the approach to prepare or purchase materials. In over three quarters of these agencies or programs, the staff reported that their approach to preparation or selection of health materials has been fundamentally revised.

Second, we put ads on television, trained hairstylists to impart our health messages, and increased the number of outreach staff who engaged community members in face-to-face communication. Third, we provided funding to 14 peer leadership/education programs to help adolescents complete their education. Fourth, we referred parents with low literacy to adult education programs. Fifth, we added a fatherhood component to the SHS program that included a paternal case manager to work with the fathers of the babies of adolescent mothers. The fathers were encouraged to read to their babies during two half-hour periods per week and were given culturally appropriate children's books such as *Guess How Much I Love You*, *Good Morning Baby*, and *Good Night Baby*.

So how did these low-literacy interventions work? We evaluated these efforts by looking at the pregnancy outcomes of adult women in Syracuse who had not graduated from high school. Among these births, we compared women who were or were not Healthy Start participants. Just as in our earlier analysis, SIDS and other causes of infant deaths that occurred after the babies reached 1 month of age—so called *postneonatal deaths*—were most common among mothers who had not graduated from high school. We were very pleased to find that Healthy Start participants were 75% less likely to have an infant die in the postneonatal period than nonparticipants.

Infants are the most vulnerable group in any society. Internationally, we use a country's infant mortality rate to assess its level of development. The shameful fact of Syracuse's history, of having among highest rates of infant death in the United States, indicates that the city's level of development—the access of its residents to health-promoting resources—is poor.

As a graduate student I learned about the ecosystem approach to understanding health and illness. My professors typically focused on the developing world, where, for instance, cutting down the rainforest in West Africa left clear pools of rainwater for mosquitoes to breed, thus creating the ideal conditions for malaria to proliferate. I remember discussions about how dam construction, in places such as Egypt or Tanzania, increased the spread of the schistosomiasis parasite. In these examples, alterations in the environment increased or decreased the risk of disease.

In the preceding discussion, I have used this ecosystem approach to understand the environmental and social conditions that lead to unequal infant death for the poor, primarily among African Americans and Latinos.

In Syracuse, the clearing of whole neighborhoods during urban renewal, coupled with an economic downturn due to the collapse of industry, brought unintended consequences. Dilapidated rental housing, abandoned houses, and empty lots provide the conditions for lead poisoning and illicit drug use to grow. White flight to the suburbs, the closure of small businesses, and expanding governmental offices and university facilities slash property tax revenues available to fund city public schools. Inadequate education, unemployment, the Rockefeller drug laws, and racially biased arrest and sentencing, underpin the epidemic of African-American male incarceration. Inmate fathers cannot provide financial support, and the emotional support they can offer during collect calls from jail or prison is limited. Neighborhood violence, likely a key reason that full-service supermarkets left the inner city, now clusters around corner stores that sell cigarettes, malt liquor, lottery tickets, and drug paraphernalia in place of healthy food. Residents' diets suffer when there are barriers of distance and expense to fresh produce, low-fat dairy products, and other good food. Fear of gunshots, assault, or being targeted by police keep residents indoors; children kept indoors lack vigorous exercise, with dramatically rising obesity being the result.

But the ecosystem model of health cannot completely account for the gap in infant death between people of color and their white neighbors in Syracuse. Hidden disadvantage and embedded racism form the crucible in which African Americans and Latinos die too soon of largely preventable or treatable causes. Since 1960, Syracuse's population has shrunk by one third, but the county jail was enlarged. Over 90% of loitering arrests are of young African-American males. Unemployment, incarceration, and poor health do not afflict all groups equally. Families of color in Syracuse have over twice the rate of poverty of white families. African-American males become inmates at over seven times the rate of white males. As mentioned earlier, if African Americans in Onondaga County had the same death rates as their white counterparts, about 125 fewer would die each year. Every 2 years, therefore, the equivalent of an airliner full of African-American residents of Onondaga County crashes; everyone dies and no one notices.

I imagine that some readers are thinking "What about individual responsibility?" Obviously individual efforts in health promotion are important. I struggle to eat the right foods to keep my cholesterol under control and I encourage my smoking friends to quit. I monitor my daughter's intake of junk food. I think a lot about how to be healthy and I often drive my family and friends to distraction with my suggestions. The analyses in this chapter, however, suggest that there are limits to how much individual will can accomplish. A baby cannot ensure that the house in which he or she learns to crawl is free of lead paint dust. A young mother cannot compel her baby's father to be involved with his child if he is incarcerated. Parents surviving on low-wage jobs cannot create a supermarket in their neighborhoods;

they cannot stop the gunshots or drug dealing surrounding their local corner stores.

Within this context of community stress, a worsening economy, welfare reform, and cuts in public health funding, Syracuse Healthy Start has been successful in three key areas. First, pregnant inmates receive high-quality prenatal services and integrated case management, helping many to give birth to healthy infants. Second, pregnant and parenting teens in Syracuse have generally good birth outcomes and lower rates of infant death than adult women. Because we designed such a comprehensive package of teen services, however, we cannot say what part of the care made the difference. Third, adult women who had not graduated from high school and were served by SHS were found to have significantly lower rates of postneonatal infant death than comparable women who were not SHS participants.

I believe our successes in these three areas are modest but important. We did not solve the problem of poverty in Syracuse, nor did we substantially reduce the many other social stresses that affect struggling parents. But infants who were served by our program, whose parents were among the most impoverished, were more likely to survive.

PART III

The Calculus of Health: Markets, Frontiers, Franchises

Daniel Perlman and Ananya Roy

As countries came together in 1978 in Alma-Ata to celebrate the concept of primary health care and commit to health equity for people of the developing world, a countervailing political and economic philosophy was brewing. Development strategies were about to undergo a transformation away from strengthening the state to enhancing the private sector and creating conditions for markets to flourish.

Starting in the 1990s, this new paradigm began to be called "neoliberalism" because it revives the model of nineteenth-century liberalism, which supported laissez faire policies. Despite the word *liberal* in its name, neoliberalism is associated with conservative politics in the United States and Great Britain, as exemplified by the U.S. Republican and British Conservative parties of Ronald Reagan and Margaret Thatcher, respectively. The rise of neoliberalism was furthered by the fall of the Soviet Union, which eroded the influence of Marxist theory on international politics. Neoliberalism has been aggressively promoted by the International Monetary Fund (IMF) and the World Bank as the underlying ideology of their development approach. A number of industrialized countries – including the United States, England, and Germany – began to apply neoliberal reforms in the 1980s by cutting taxes and reducing government social spending.

In developing countries, neoliberal policies were implemented in the context of heavy external debt. In order to ensure that governments would pay money back to private, often European and American, banks, the International Monetary Fund created structural adjustment programs in line with neoliberal philosophy to stabilize Third World economies. These programs were implemented broadly starting in the early 1980s. The key components of structural adjustment programs were trade liberalization; devaluation of currency; privatization; the removal of government subsidies for food, fuel, and other basic goods; increased interest rates; and the implementation of cost recovery for social services such as health and education.

These policies often had a devastating effect on the health of people in poor countries.[1] Governments reduced their spending in the health sector, limits were imposed on health workers' salaries and on the number of workers who could be hired, and fees were charged in public hospitals and health centers. As a result, health care providers were laid off, wages were frozen, and public sector expenditures declined. Public health became fragmented, with few resources to maintain the primary health care infrastructure established in earlier decades.

APPLYING THE MARKET MODEL TO HEALTH

The neoliberal mantra of the 1980s was "market failure is better than state failure." Whereas older theories of liberalism had sought to temper the market with concerns about public goods and social interest, the neoliberal revival inaugurated an unconditional celebration of markets. This is worth a closer look, because the market is a peculiar institution. Perhaps its greatest peculiarity is that while real markets are shot through with various forms of social and political power, its ideological rhetoric promotes ideas of freedom and fairness, ignoring structural barriers to participation that block access to poor people, the politically disenfranchised, and small businesses. But such issues were set aside in the neoliberal policies of the 1980s. Instead, the state came under great attack. International financial institutions emphasized governmental corruption and inefficiency as causes of underdevelopment and used these concerns to push for governmental downsizing and private-sector support. This approach ignored problems of corruption and inefficiency in business organizations as well as preexisting structural barriers to full participation by the disempowered.

Corruption is considered by many who work in the field of international development to be an inherent trait of developing country governments. In their case, Mbakwem and Smith point out that international health and development professionals are rarely able to reflect on their own contribution to corruption and how the overall structure of aid reinforces inequity. Similarly, the World Bank and the IMF have not recognized their historical role in promoting corruption by lending large quantities of money to unrepresentative governments that have used the money for personal wealth or to maintain power through war and repression.

One of the first global initiatives to promote the use of market incentives for health was the Bamako initiative launched in 1987 by the WHO and UNICEF. The idea behind the Bamako initiative was to ensure a constant supply of medicinal drugs at the local level by charging fees for pharmaceuticals in order to create a revolving fund. Under the initiative, a stock of essential generic drugs was provided to a dispensary management committee (composed of community representatives). The drugs were then sold at a profit to community members. This profit, in addition to payments by users for consultations (user fees), could be used to buy back the initial stock of drugs, and for improving access to care and quality of services.[2] According to the Bamako initiative, poor people in developing countries had proven their willingness to pay for pharmaceuticals, which would permit a shift away from dependence on central level financing.[3]

In the same year that the Bamako Initiative was launched, the World Bank released a document titled *Financing Health Services in Developing Countries: an Agenda for Reform*.[4] The World Bank argued that user fees would raise revenue for the health sector, reduce unnecessary utilization of services, and encourage people to use low-cost primary health care services instead of hospital services. Proponents claimed these policies would increase efficiency and improve equity. However, almost universally, the result of user fees has been a reduction in the use of health-care services and delay of care seeking until the problems became emergencies.[5] "Willingness to pay" proved not to be the same as "ability to pay," and in order to get access to pharmaceuticals and health-care services, poor families sacrifice food, school fees for children, domestic animals, and other basic needs. Furthermore, user fees have been found to raise very little additional revenue while also increasing administrative inefficiency.[6]

In parallel with the increasing reliance on fees, international agencies supporting health increasingly directed investments into a few cost-effective primary health care interventions. Walsh and Warren's 1979 analysis led UNICEF and USAID to redirect hundreds of millions of dollars through the 1980s into the child survival interventions: oral rehydration, vaccination, and breast feeding.[7]

In 1993 the World Bank published its annual development report *Investing in Health*, dedicated to the topic of health in developing countries. The report represented a major shift in global health policy making, with the World Bank taking front stage while the influence of the WHO and ministries of health in poor countries declined. *Investing in Health* proposes a four-pronged approach for improving the health of people in developing countries: (1) promoting economic growth to increase household incomes and expanding education, (2) redirecting government funds to a basic package of cost-effective interventions such as immunizations and infectious disease control, (3) promoting private-sector competition in health-care service delivery, and (4) diversifying health sector financing through user fees and private and social health insurance for services beyond the basic package of cost-effective interventions.[8]

Investing in Health recommends that five categories of cost-effective services be included in a countries' basic package of services: immunization and care for common childhood illnesses such as diarrhea and acute respiratory infections, pregnancy-related care, family planning, tuberculosis control, and control of sexually transmitted diseases.[9] These interventions are almost exclusively medical and do not include more systemic, nonmedical activities with multiple benefits. In fact, *Investing in Health* explicitly recommends that governments *not* broadly subsidize water and sanitation. The authors reason that households are willing to pay for such services and that the health benefits derived from water and sanitation are not sufficiently cost-effective to justify public subsidy.[10] While the authors of *Investing in Health* acknowledge the complications and limitations of using cost-effectiveness analysis, the logic outlined in the report continues to be the dominant trend in international health projects. As a result, in the name of "cost-effectiveness," treatment of diarrhea repeatedly with oral rehydration therapy is sanctioned but prevention of illness over the long term by providing communities with safe, potable water and reducing the hours of labor that women spend collecting water is not.[11] Critics point out that privatizing water systems furthers corporate aims by encouraging businesses to provide water services for fees instead of governments using tax moneys to improve the common good.[12]

Investing in Health lays out a blueprint for health-sector reform in developing countries, explaining how governments should go about changing their health-care financing and service delivery. These reforms were implemented throughout the developing world, generally with loan packages from the World Bank or from other partner agencies such as the Inter-American Development Bank. Each country has taken on its own version of the reform to make it palatable according to its political and social context: some have focused on health-care financing such as cost recovery through user fees, whereas others have emphasized private health-care service delivery by companies or nonprofit organizations. Alejandro Cerón and Meredith Fort discuss how Guatemala implemented health-sector reform in this section.

Reforms have been criticized for being top-down and externally imposed; in many countries they have been met with resistance.[13] Critics point to the failure of the reforms to address underlying social and economic problems and to engage local communities in the process. Following the recommendations of the World Bank, reforms are selective rather than comprehensive, emphasizing technical and primarily medical strategies without addressing the underlying social and economic determinants of health. Community involvement has essentially been nonexistent in bank-driven reforms with the exception of the utilization of community volunteers as free or low-cost labor.

A key component of the neoliberal model is the opening of markets to global trade. The policies of the IMF and World Bank are echoed in the World Trade Organization (WTO), created in 1995, which is the ultimate body on the setting of trade policy. In the WTO framework, trade agreements aim to reduce government restrictions on trade. However, trade liberalization and efforts to increase access to health care and services have come head to head. Jane Galvão describes how Brazil came into conflict with the WTO agreement on intellectual property (TRIPS) because of its efforts to make AIDS drugs widely available through a national program instead of allowing the right of multinational pharmaceutical companies to set the prices for antiretroviral treatments.

THE CURE: SOCIALIZING THE MARKET

By the early 1990s, even the institutions most enamored with the magic of the market, institutions such as the World Bank, were becoming acutely aware of the fallout from neoliberalism. In a surprising autocritique, the World Bank argued that its free-market policies had created a "lost development decade" in sub-Saharan Africa, exacerbating rather than mitigating poverty. This autocritique was reinforced by a new set of development ideas, such as the work of Nobel Laureate Joseph Stiglitz, which focused on market failures. In 1987 UNICEF published a critique of structural adjustment programs, titled *Adjustment with a Human Face*, which called for the protection of vulnerable populations.[14] Starting in the 1980s, "austerity riots" had exploded in various parts of the world, with the urban and rural poor protesting cuts in social spending and the rising prices of energy, food, education, and health care that accompanied privatization. Neoliberalism had undercut the "social contract" and there was now an overflowing of social energies and mobilizations. By the time the World Bank and International Monetary Fund marked the 50th anniversary of their establishment (1994), these mobilizations had crystallized into a set of global social movements calling for the shutdown of the apparatus of development. The World Bank was meant to cure underdevelopment; now it seemed, as Jane Galvão points out, that it was time for a "cure for the Bank."

The "cure" took many different forms. In countries hit hard by neoliberal policies, such as Bolivia and Egypt, the World Bank and IMF established "social funds" to soften the blow. These state-run institutions sought to find employment and establish enterprises for those rendered unemployed and otherwise affected by privatization. In other words, they tried to mitigate the harshest dimensions of the market and to create "safety valves" for the anger and frustration that had built up during the neoliberal years.

Perhaps the most significant "cure" that international organizations applied to themselves was the socialization of the market. In contrast to the idea of the "free" market, or even the idea of market "failures," a new paradigm asserted the "social market," a market embedded in society and subject to the moral calculus of social norms and social outcomes. The paradoxes of the twentieth-century market thus become the grand solution of twenty-first-century development. Janani's concept of "social franchising," described in this section, is emblematic of such a paradigm. It is worth exploring the paradigm and its icons.

Gopalakrishnan shows how Janani reconceptualized rural medical practitioners as entrepreneurs who own considerable assets in the form of "social" and "human" capital if not physical capital. The point is that such social assets (such as networks of trust or indigenous knowledge about medicinal plants) can be converted into capital and thus integrated into the global economic system. And through such a conversion the entrepreneur is not only set free to participate in markets but also enfranchised.

Janani works with commodities that are for sale. Its model reprises the approach of Section Two, asserting that reproduction is not simply biological or social reproduction but rather reproduction through the market—the buying and selling of condoms and pills as market commodities. But Janani reconciles such commodification with its social mission of access to contraception. Such a "double bottom line" is a central element of the "social market" paradigm, which imagines the poor as a viable market for innovative, low-priced, well-distributed products. Popularized by management guru C. K. Prahalad as the "fortune at the bottom of the pyramid," such a view also argues that the market can indeed deliver both commodities and social benefits.[15]

Janani is a franchise network that creates a market in reproductive health commodities and services. However, it is also a nongovernmental organization (NGO), seemingly autonomous of both market and state and yet closely affiliated with each. The turn of the century witnessed the proliferation of NGOs, community organizations, and other civil society groups. Hailed as "globalization from below," these associational forms were meant to provide a "third way," dominated by neither the market nor the state. But in many parts of the world, NGOs are extensions of state power or at least subject to state supervision and regulation. And with the rise of the "social market" paradigm, a new collaboration between NGOs and the market came into being; acting as partners of multinational or national corporations, NGOs began to facilitate the integration of the poor into markets, including credit markets, land markets, and the market for health products.

These three icons—entrepreneurship, the double bottom line, and civil society— are powerful and compelling. They can be interpreted in various ways. Are they "Band-Aid" reforms of free market capitalism, meant to ease and appease? Are they new frontiers of capital accumulation whereby the poor are reconstituted as consumers of new products? Are they a serious and successful effort to socialize and democratize markets? Are they a creative and innovative solution to the failures of top-down and top-heavy development? Tackling such questions requires coming to terms with the paradoxes of the market and particularly the paradoxes of the "social market." Is the "social market" an oxymoron, seeking to reconcile the irreconcilable logic of social justice and market profits? Or is it a novel hybrid, a way out of the dualisms of market efficiency and sociopolitical equality?

Social marketing has come into question by those who ask whether it fosters equity or reinforces social exclusion. For example, bed nets have been promoted throughout much of Africa by USAID's social marketing approach in an attempt to reduce malaria transmission. However, as has been seen in the Zambia and Mozambique, even when the nets are subsidized, the poorest families are not able to afford to buy bed nets and are more likely to go without them.[16,17] Social marketing efforts tend to be single interventions, implemented by NGOs that are divorced from the public-sector health system or only loosely linked to it. They have also been criticized for not addressing the broader determinants of health but instead focusing on individual and family behavior change.

As Janani and other experiments continue, two issues will emerge as a litmus test for the "social market": affordability and accountability. Can the calculus of entrepreneurship and social assets prove to be inclusive? Can all segments of the poor participate in the "social-market economy" as entrepreneurs or at the very least as consumers? Will such a calculus exclude the poorest of the poor, those with frayed social networks and few opportunities to invest in entrepreneurial opportunities? Will there be enough of an incentive in the calculus of the "double bottom line" to reach this frontier of dispossession? And who is accountable when the very poor are excluded from the "social market"? Does the market have accountability? To whom? Can the market be subject to the logic of democratic accountability? Is this the role that NGOs will play, by insisting on the right to participate for all? In the calculus of the "social market," can clients and consumers become *citizens*, or are such political and territorial notions of accountability now outdated and irrelevant?

A GLOBAL CALL FOR CHANGE: REFORM OR REVOLUTION?

The end of the last century and the turn of the new one came to be marked by global campaigns of generosity: global funds, global initiatives, global goals—all meant to direct attention and spending on the travesty of disease and death in a prosperous modern world. The Millennium Development Goals, ratified by the United Nations, are bold: the reduction of hunger and extreme poverty; the reduction of maternal and child mortality; a dramatic response to the killer diseases of AIDS, tuberculosis, and malaria; the empowerment of women; and universal primary education for children. Together they articulate a new global social contract for human development. It is this contract that is evident in the Gates Neonatal Initiative and its commitment to the global eradication of neonatal deaths. It is this contract that animates Jeffrey Sachs's claim that the "end of poverty" is one of the possibilities of our times.[18]

Despite the multitude of such seemingly generous campaigns, donor governments have fallen far below their commitment to address the global burden of disease. In 1969, industrialized countries committed to contributing 0.7% of their gross national income (GNI) to the developing world in overseas development assistance, but few donor countries have met that goal almost 40 years later, and the United States lags behind almost all the other industrialized nations, spending only 0.22% of GNI on foreign assistance. The Global Fund for AIDS, Malaria, and Tuberculosis had the goal of distributing $8 billion annually to governments to respond to these three major killers, but the fund has yet to reach its goal.

And although there have been numerous international meetings and forums where Third World debt has been discussed and analyzed and where agreements have been made to cancel or reduce debt, African countries have not been able to free themselves from its stronghold and health indicators on the continent are devastating. Almost 3 years after the Gleneagles G-8 meeting, in which the year 2005 was proclaimed "The Year for Africa" and leaders agreed to write off the debts of 18 of the poorest countries, Africa's debt crisis is far from over. Despite the growing crisis and after the Gleneagles debt cancellation, African countries still spend about $14 billion in debt service payments each year – money that otherwise could be spent on health-care services and other social protections, such as nutrition, sanitation, education, and housing. Furthermore, those countries that have qualified for debt reduction through the Heavily Indebted Poor Countries (HIPC) initiative have had to undergo economic reforms such as the privatization of public companies and the implementation of trade regulations, which can have negative consequences for their citizens.[19]

Global philanthropists have directed their attention to the problems of global disease and death. The Bill and Melinda Gates Foundation has received continual praise for its contributions to global health, including an astounding $31 billion donation from Warren Buffett. The Gates Foundation emphasizes breakthrough technologies and cost-effective interventions instead of investing in health-system strengthening and in addressing the underlying causes of disease. The foundation generally operates through grants that partially fund projects, and other international agencies complement the remaining portion; the scale of the foundation and its approach to lending have given the Gates Foundation tremendous agenda-setting power in global health policy.[20]

But an alternative has been brewing. As the century turned, so did Latin America. Battered by the market prescriptions of the World Bank and the IMF, confronted by social mobilizations that insist on justice and equity, and shaped by a long history of populism, South America entered the new millennium and turned left. From Venezuela to Brazil, leftist parties were voted into power. In Bolivia and Peru, leaders of indigenous origin were hailed and celebrated. While the majority of Third World countries remain under the dominant international health and development paradigm, South America is leading a retreat from neoliberalism.

The promises are immense: of a twenty-first-century socialism, of development owned by the people, of social redistribution before market profits. But the pathways are many. In May 2007, Venezuela, Argentina, Brazil, Bolivia, Ecuador, and Paraguay began discussions to launch a Banco y Fondo del Sur in order to no longer have to depend on the Bretton Woods institutions. Since 1999, Latin American countries have been borrowing one-fourth to one-half less from the World Bank in order to increase their autonomy.[21] President Rafael Correa of Ecuador has paid off the country's debt to the IMF and in April of 2007 ordered the expulsion of the World Bank representative from his country.[22] In Bolivia, Evo Morales, once a coca farmer and now president, has nationalized the gas industry and managed to maintain international relations with countries whose multinational corporations have taken a big cut.

In Brazil, a long history of "insurgent citizenship" has created the conditions for better access to health care, housing, food, and education for the country's poor.[23] Prompted by Brazil, which in turn had been prompted by its insurgent citizens, the world was compelled to debate the ethics of the market and decide whether it was fair to maintain the logic of market profits in the face of pandemics. Although access to treatment has not been guaranteed for most of the world's people living with AIDS, the unfettered right to profits is no longer considered acceptable, and pharmaceutical companies have come under scrutiny the world over.

Though not revolutionary, changes at the World Health Organization and the Pan American Health Organization show a commitment to promoting health equity and social justice. A recent document from the Pan American Health Organization (PAHO) on the renewal of primary health care returns to the fundamental ideals of Alma-Ata and critically analyzes the policies that were implemented over the last quarter-century.[24]

But have all Latin American governments presented a set of real alternatives to both neoliberalism and its legacy, the "social market"? This is the important and provocative question posed by Cerón and Fort in their analysis of reform in Guatemala. After the Peace Accords were signed, ending a brutal civil war that lasted more than 30 years, the Guatemalan government implemented a health-sector reform in line with the social-market paradigm which took the form of a system of community health aimed at reducing maternal and child mortality and was implemented through a network of village volunteers. Funded by the InterAmerican Development Bank, the program has all the hallmark features of the social market—entrepreneurial communities with entrepreneurial volunteers, the mobilization of social capital by NGOs, and the ambitions of a "double bottom line." The alternative has come in the form of the Instancia Nacional de Salud, a grassroots effort to create an inclusive and comprehensive primary health care infrastructure. The Instancia seeks to create a health system characterized not by limited, low-cost interventions but rather by comprehensive care based on communities' needs, a health system where health knowledge is not simply packaged into specialties and products for efficient distribution but rather where ways of knowing are rooted in the long history of indigenous peoples and their communities. In doing so, it has made an effort to address the issues of affordability and accountability that seem to confound the social-market paradigm.

The way forward seems obvious, but is it? As some Latin American countries offer possibility for improved health, Africa sinks deeper into the AIDS crisis. Can the ambitious promises of redistribution be met in the face of economic globalization and its pressures? How can the right to health be ensured and who is responsible for assessing whether we are getting closer or further away from the goal of health? It will be for future generations to decide whether we are on the pathway toward improved heath or if there is a new bend in the road just ahead that we cannot yet see.

9 A Collective Response to the Health Sector Reform in Guatemala

Alejandro Cerón and Meredith Fort

More than a decade has passed since internal conflict officially ended in Guatemala, but the state terror that plagued the country is not easily forgotten. The complete toll is unknown, but it is estimated that more than 200,000 people were killed and disappeared and that 1.5 million people were displaced during the war.

After a socially just, democratically elected government was cut short by a CIA-sponsored coup in 1954, a rebel group took up arms against the government. The government, in turn, worked to wipe out the rebels over a period of more than 30 years. The country's majority Mayan population living in rural communities was most affected by the violence, especially during the "scorched earth" campaign in the early 1980s. The war officially came to an end when the Peace Accords were signed in December of 1996, providing the country with hope for a peaceful future.

A year after the accords were signed, the government launched a health-sector reform at the primary care level that changed the way health care services were provided to communities. This chapter describes our individual experiences during the initial years of the health-sector reform and our collective participation in a coalition of grassroots organizations called the Instancia Nacional de Salud, which was formed in response to the reform.

ALEJANDRO

I was born and raised in Guatemala in a working-class neighborhood where parents tried to ensure better futures for their children. My parents gave my siblings and me the best education and example that they could. Although there was not much discussion of politics in my family, we grew up with the values of responsibility and solidarity and strove to be good, upright people.

My family lived quite sheltered from the turmoil that was going on in the country. Even so, I have memories of the war. When I was 6 years old, the government projected counterinsurgency images and messages in the papers and on television of soldiers, people captured with blindfolds, and cadavers. I did not understand the message, but it made me scared. I remember asking my parents and my teacher what it meant, and, as one might expect, they tried to calm my fears. About the same time, a neighbor of mine who studied at the university was killed; I never knew exactly what happened, but I did know that his death was linked to the violent counterinsurgency, which was often directed at the civilian population. When I was 9 years old, the father of a school friend was "disappeared" for being a union leader.

I remember seeing messages spray-painted on the walls of buildings in favor of the guerrillas or against the government. Soldiers were everywhere, as was news of bridges or electrical stations having been destroyed by the guerrillas, massacres committed by the army, kidnappings by both sides, and a number of coups. I was surrounded by the war, but we did not talk much about it and always only halfway. It was dangerous to speak and better not to know too much.

In my first years in medical school I participated in medical *jornadas* to different rural parts of the country. The medical *jornadas* are common in Guatemala, both in rural and marginal urban areas. Generally community leaders or political candidates appeal to different organizations and institutions—those having access to medicines and employing technically trained health workers capable of diagnosing illness and prescribing treatment—asking them to go to certain villages to provide health services. The *jornadas* sometimes last an entire day, and any villager who has time shows up in order to get medicine for their health problems.

Many of the people attending do not have acute illnesses but rather suffer from chronic problems that are often impossible for health care workers to diagnose adequately with the resources available during a *jornada*. Also, many people who are not actually sick say that they have a fever or cold or pain in order to get medicine to have on hand. The *jornadas* are so common because of the population's poverty and their limited access to health-care services on a day-to-day basis.

I was confronted with a dilemma during the *jornadas*: I knew that they did not resolve the people's health problems (the majority of patients had chronic illnesses or recurring acute illnesses directly related to their living conditions), but our *jornadas* were among the few opportunities that people had to receive medical care. For 2 more years I participated in the *jornadas*, which were personally satisfying but also raised many new questions for me. Why did the Guatemalan health system not reach these people in need? What was our role as medical students in trying to promote change in the national health system?

One of the aspects of this work that was most disconcerting to me was the graphic, emotional, and eloquent way in which many people described their ailments and the logic behind their comprehension of the human body and the causes of illness.

I remember one *jornada* vividly:

It was almost noon in the village on a sunny and dry Sunday. The wind blew garbage and dust along the road. On the patio of the school, there was a long line of people of all ages but mostly children accompanied by their mothers. A vendor selling *granizadas* yelled out to the crowd to buy his icy treat. A group of thin dogs roamed around. The women talked, the older children played, and the younger ones cried with boredom. The people who had woken up at the crack of dawn had already been seen by the university doctors, but those who had arrived by 8 A.M. were still in line, waiting. In the classrooms, 10 medical students attended to the villagers, using school chairs and tables, stethoscopes, blood pressure cuffs, thermometers, an emergency medical kit, basic medicines donated to the university, and samples from pharmaceutical companies. By noon, each pair had seen about 40 patients. One student went outside to the patio and called the next patient: "¡Doña Adriana Chávez!"[i] A black-haired, smiling 40-year-old woman who was moderately obese and eating green *jocotes* with salt stepped forward. The fourth-year medical student said, "Come on in and please have a seat. What can I help you with Doña Adriana?"

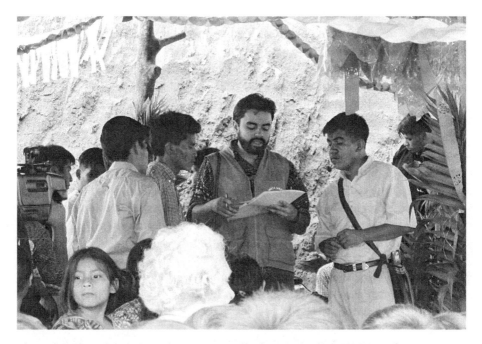

Alejandro Cerón meeting with community leaders at the inauguration of the community health house in the village of Tzamabaj in 2004. (Photo: Andrew Bryant.)

"Ay doctor." Her smile turned into a worried look. "I have a headache. It is very painful." She emphasized the word "pain" as she leant her head to the right and put her hand on her forehead.

The medical student wrote *cefalea*. He read the next question: "How long have you had the pain?"

"It began yesterday but it is worse today."

"So does it hurt you right now?"

"Yes."

The medical student wrote "one day of evolution" on the form in order to finish what he had filled in as the patient's complaint. "Please, show me with your fingers—where does it hurt the most?"

"Right here," she touched with her two hands the back of her head, "and then it comes through here. . . ." She leaned her body to the left and passed her hand slowly from the right side of the neck to the shoulder and then the elbow. "And sometimes I feel it in my knees . . . but what affects me the most is the fever." She looked more worried now, "And it hurts when I urinate." She leaned forward holding her lower back with both hands. "It is like a hot ball that suddenly attacks me and then changes places."

"Okay," the young student said gently, "but right now where does your head hurt?" He was required to write down an adequate description.

"Actually, right now my head doesn't hurt. I just feel feverish."

"Well, let me examine you." Using the schoolteacher's desk as an examining table, the doctor took her temperature, blood pressure, and pulse. He looked at the color of her skin; her eyes, nails, and the palms of her hands; tried touching the spots that Doña Adriana said were painful in order to see if she had a muscle spasm or something more; listened to her heart and lungs.

"Right there, right there hurts me," said Doña Adriana, "and my vision, Doctor, I see dark." The doctor finished his physical exam and went over to where the medicines were to select what he would give to her.

"Okay Doña Adriana, please take these medicines." He explained in detail how each one should be taken and wrote the directions down so that one of her children or a neighbor could remind her of the dosage. "In addition, you have to watch what you eat." He explained the importance of a balanced diet, thinking of what would be within her socioeconomic reach. "And drink a lot of water. And please, if you continue to feel bad, please go to the health center."

"Doctor, you wouldn't happen to have an injection?" She now looked almost disappointed. "I think that an injection would help get rid of my pain."

"No Doña Adriana, you do not need an injection. It is better for you to take these pills." He tried to give his best explanation about how the medications work.

I did not understand exactly what the problem was that Doña Adriana had and certainly did not know how the doctor had diagnosed her illness. After she left, I asked him, "What do you think she has?"

"Well, it is possible that she has a urinary tract infection and anemia, which could explain her pains, so I gave her an antibiotic and vitamins and medicines to reduce fever. I would have liked to run some tests, but that is not possible on a *jornada*." The doctor tried to give me the best possible explanation that he could about her case. I was appreciative of his insight and advice, but I was left with the sensation that Doña Adriana was not going to be cured and that she would not have an opportunity for follow-up.

While patients spoke about *calambres* (cramps) that passed from their legs to their heads to their chests and abdomens and then returned back to their legs and had something to do with cold air, work in the fields, or washing clothes with cold water, doctors understood the patients to be talking about muscle spasms and might prescribe a muscle relaxant. Patients expressed their problem of *nervios* (nerves) and doctors prescribed pain relievers or vitamins. I, as a new medical student participating in the *jornadas* mostly to learn and support the effort, could see clearly that the patients said one thing and the doctors understood another. At the end of the consultation, the patients left satisfied with their medicines, the doctors were satisfied because they had treated another patient and were ready to move on to the next; I asked myself if either of them had noticed that they were talking about different things. Following up on my interest in what I had seen led me to learn about medical anthropology, some of its pioneers in Guatemala, and leaders in alternative medicine, all of whom were outside of the medical school. I asked myself, "Why had such an important topic been omitted from my medical training?"

At the university I learned that the government had undertaken a health sector reform that would bring health-care services to the same excluded populations I had visited during the *jornadas*. I still have the documents that we had to read about the reform, along with my handwritten notes: "How are they going to do this?" "How will it play out?" and "Who will do this work?" These documents were very general and we were taught about the reform in a nonanalytical way. I think that at the time I wanted to believe that the reform would be the answer to the problem's of Guatemala's health system, even though I knew that the state carrying out the reform was the same one that, during the recent civil war, had been responsible for assassinating and "disappearing" people living in some of the same rural communities to which they now wanted to extend health care.

During my early years in medical school, the Peace Accords officially ending the armed conflict were being negotiated and were at last signed in December of 1996. As a public university student who had experienced a certain level of political participation both in and outside of the university, these times generated contradictions for me. Previously, the government was considered to be the enemy. and now we were to work within the government in order to strengthen the state. Our instruments for change would be the Peace Accords and the new political party that we would create. For me, a young man from the capital city who had heard a lot about the history of the war—the massacres, fear, pain, atrocities—this new scenario of peace and a progressive political party was encouraging, an opportunity

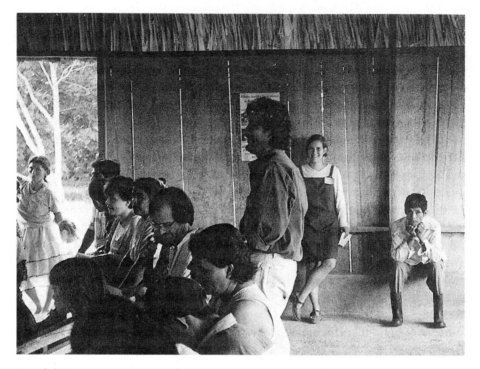

Meredith Fort at a meeting to form the Association of Health Promoters and Midwives of the Petén in 1998. (Photo: Liza Grandia.)

to build a more just society. I still remember when a classmate gave me a copy of the Peace Accords agreement on the "socioeconomic and agrarian situation," about which she was very hopeful and which included a section on health. I read it avidly but felt that something was missing.

The section about health in the agreement included only a few goals that were not very different from what the Ministry of Health proposed, and although there was mention of universal access to services and of "reclaiming" Mayan medicine, the agreement did not seem very revolutionary to me. People with more "political clarity" told me that I had to understand it as an agreement in which not all of the details could be explained and that it had been negotiated, but that at any rate it was a beginning from which a just health system could be built. As the new political party began to take shape, I had some opportunities to ask its leaders about the kind of health system they thought Guatemala needed, and I realized that, in general, they had no concrete ideas; some mentioned the Cuban example while others said that the reform currently under way in Guatemala was on the right track. And these were the leaders of the revolutionary party!

In 1996, as I listened to a talk by Juan Carlos Verdugo, who had studied social medicine in Mexico, I felt that I was making connections between health and policy on a different level than I had before. Never before had I learned about international financial institutions such as the International Monetary Fund and the World Bank, and I had not known how they influenced the social and economic policies implemented in Guatemala. Juan Carlos explained to us that through his research, he had found that the Inter-American Development Bank was driving the reform process in Guatemala through a loan and that this was based on guidelines set forth in a 1993 World Bank document titled *Investing in Health*.

I had not known that the health goals in the Peace Accords coincided with the goals that these institutions were promoting in all of Latin America. That day, I felt that the blinders I had had on were removed, and since then, the way I perceive reality has never been the same. That day I learned about the political, social, and economic factors that condition health, and I realized that improving people's health would require a lot more than my personal commitment to being a good, technically trained doctor.

I was impressed that Juan Carlos treated us with respect and that he listened closely to our questions and concerns. At the end of the talk, he asked us, "Should we be guided by human values or economic rationality?" But overall I remember his enthusiasm, the hope in his eyes, and his positive attitude. He finished his talk with a phrase inspired by the writer Ernesto Sábato: "I believe that out of desperation comes hope; I try to search for what is positive and instill optimism in young people. One must struggle for hope in everything."

From that day until my graduation I carried with me a copy of the document that Juan Carlos gave us, and from time to time today I still use it as a reference. I saw him again several times in the following years. In 2001, I was invited to participate in a course on health policy analysis with Juan Carlos, and a year later I was invited to join him to work with the Instancia Nacional de Salud in working toward a healthier, more just Guatemala.

MEREDITH

I first started hearing about the country of Guatemala as a high school student in Seattle, Washington. The idea of Guatemala stuck in my mind after watching a movie called *El Norte*; it starts off with a scene of a brother and sister who have to flee their town as the military move in to search out rebel sympathizers and take out anyone in their path, including their father, who was murdered, and their mother, who was "disappeared." As flames ravage their home and amid screams and shots, the brother and sister flee for safety in the middle of the night and begin a treacherous journey north to the United States.

Later, in college, I learned about the ancient Mayan civilization and the tremendous archeological sites throughout Central America and Mexico; I wondered how such an advanced civilization had collapsed. With concerns about environmental conservation, increasing people's access to basic services, and understanding more about the recent political history in the country, I was granted a fellowship to work in Guatemala upon graduating from college in 1997.

I moved to the Petén, the northernmost department in Guatemala, to assist in developing a new health component to a nongovernmental organization (NGO) called ProPetén, which had a focus on conservation and community development. The Petén is one of the most remote departments in the country and is the least densely populated. I had grown up in an urban setting; therefore the pigs walking in front of my house, the roosters crowing, and the unpaved roads that we traveled to reach villages took just about as much getting used to as the language and cultural differences. I arrived to Guatemala in the hope of being able to help improve access to health-care services for the rural poor, but I had only a limited knowledge of how I would most effectively be able to contribute. I entered on to the scene just as a new debate was heating up.

I was invited to participate in a series of meetings facilitated by the Association of Community Health Services (ASECSA), which had just recently opened an office in the Petén. ASECSA was founded in 1978 and is based in Chimaltenango, Guatemala. It has worked with NGOs throughout the country to provide rural communities with trainings for health promoters. The organizations participating in ASECSA had begun to train health promoters because of the government's limited involvement in community care and because they felt that government institutions could not be trusted, especially during the late 1970s and 1980s, the worst years of repression and genocide. In much of the countryside, communities lived in resistance to or hiding from the military and did not have access to services; rural villages were assisted only occasionally by nurses and doctors, mostly from NGOs and primarily by health promoters trained to use the village health-care handbook *Where There Is No Doctor*. Health promoters played the role of being "community doctors," treating patients for just about every illness imaginable.

The health sector reform in Guatemala has been at the primary care level. The state's role was reduced to low-cost interventions organized in a basic package of services. The government signed agreements with preexisting NGOs to provide health-care services and many new NGOs were created in order to obtain government funds for service delivery. Social investment funds were temporarily set up to provide funding to a limited number of communities not included in the health-care system, for infrastructure such as clinics and water systems; these funds were not sufficient to provide this infrastructure to everybody, but they effectively removed this responsibility from the Ministry of Health. Communities were obliged to select nonsalaried community health workers in order to receive health-care services. The 5% to 10% of health-care workers who received salaries were given annual contracts rather than long-term jobs in health-service delivery, and many did not receive benefits.

ASECSA and its member organizations were concerned about what the new health sector reform would mean for the health promoters who had been trained and the communities they served. In response, ASECSA began to hold meetings in order to understand and analyze what the reform would entail. The organizations were particularly concerned about the new government program called Sistema Integral de Atención en Salud (SIAS), an example of the larger reform that was happening across Latin America. While the consultants designing the technical aspects of SIAS were Guatemalans, the overall plan for the reform was guided by the loan package defined by the Inter-American Development Bank in Washington, DC. The problems with Guatemala's health-care system, as SIAS defined them, were that 40% of the people had no access to health care and that the public facilities had limited equipment, were poorly maintained, and were staffed by personnel who received little pay and were therefore unmotivated.

Unfamiliar with the details of how the health-care system worked prior to this new service delivery approach and without a thorough understanding of the pros and cons of the reform, I participated in the meetings, mostly as an observer, in order to familiarize myself with the debate.

In one of the first meetings, held in a room of CARITAS, a Catholic relief agency, the health area director for the Ministry of Health was invited to present the SIAS model for health-service delivery, which the organizations had begun to analyze with great concern. An NGO working just south of the Petén in the department of Alta Verapaz had also been invited to the meeting in order to explain its experience working with the new model. There were about 30 people at the meeting, 6 were in decision-making positions in their community-based organizations and the others were health promoters and traditional birth attendants who volunteered their time to serve their communities.

Even before the health area director began to present SIAS, I could feel the tension in the room. The health promoters and the directors of the community-based health organizations were not accustomed to having to work with the Ministry of Health and were, for the most part, critical and suspicious of government services.

The health area director knew what he was up against but hoped that the organizations would be impressed by the presentation and would consider working with the Ministry of Health. He was sweating in the warm, poorly ventilated room, and he looked around, quickly trying to size up the group. After the ASECSA representative nodded his head that it was time to begin, he spoke as follows:

> I know that you have probably all heard something about the new government program called SIAS, and some of you have expressed concerns to me about it. Today we want to take the opportunity to explain the model in detail so that you understand it, and we have a representative here from an NGO in Alta Verapaz who will tell us about its experience implementing SIAS. He has traveled 5 hours to be here with us today, so let's give him a warm welcome.

The representative from the NGO in Alta Verapaz stood up, wiped the sweat off his brow, and handed out an informational packet with a diagram of SIAS to the participants. He did not have enough copies and asked if people could share. He had been forewarned that the group in the Petén had organized the meeting to learn about SIAS not because they wanted to be SIAS providers but rather because they were concerned about the role of health promoters and community organizations. He began his explanation:

> Thank you for inviting me here today. The Ministry of Health approached us last year to see if we wanted to provide health-care services to rural communities in Alta Verapaz that had very limited access to care. We agreed to do so, which meant a big change for our organization, since we had focused on girls' education and medicinal plants.
>
> You may be asking yourselves, what exactly is SIAS? SIAS is a health-service delivery package offered by NGOs that receive government funding to provide care to one or more jurisdictions, in which each jurisdiction is approximately 10,000 people. Currently we have seven jurisdictions. We receive a budget based on an average per capita amount of Q30, [ii] or $5. With the money we receive we hire a team of health workers to provide a basic package of services in four intervention areas: maternal care, infant care, emergencies and common illness, and environmental sanitation. The money is used to pay for staff, medicines, and other operating costs and includes a percentage of overhead for the organization.
>
> Who are the health-care workers? According to the model that the Ministry of Health has designed, for every 10,000 person jurisdiction, there should be one ambulatory doctor, one institutional facilitator (generally an auxiliary nurse or a rural health technician), 4 to 6 community facilitators (who receive an incentive for their time), 84 *guardianes* [volunteer health agents], and a handful of birth attendants. Each *guardian* is responsible for 20 families, and they are supposed to dedicate 5 hours per week to SIAS and receive Q50 [$8] per month. The community facilitators are supposed to dedicate 20 hours per week and receive Q500 [$80] per month.

He showed some slides with photos of the work that the organization was doing, and then the health area director stepped in front of the group again to wind up the presentation.

> You all know that up until now health-care access has been very limited. Forty percent of the population is not covered by government care through health centers and health posts; here in the Petén that number is probably higher. We see SIAS as a way to provide care to those communities that do not have services. SIAS is a way to put the Peace Accords in practice. As you know, the Peace Accords call for a 50% reduction in maternal and child mortality between 1995 and 2000. If we work together, we can make a difference. I want you all to consider the option of becoming a SIAS provider for the communities that you work with, because SIAS is the new model that will be implemented in all of Guatemala.

The participants in the meeting had read an analysis about SIAS prepared by Juan Carlos Verdugo, who was working in ASECSA. In his analysis, Dr. Verdugo argued that the SIAS model was unjust because it depended on volunteer labor. He stated in the document that only the doctor and the institutional facilitator worked full time and received salaries, whereas the remaining health-care workers (more than 90% of the work force in the model) were volunteers. His analysis explained that a system dependent on volunteers is not dependable, because farmers cannot be expected to give up unlimited time each week, even if they genuinely care about the health-care problems in their communities. He questioned why the urban and middle-class families were not told to volunteer their time in order to receive health-care services while the rural poor were expected to do so. He also stated that the reform was top-down; communities had not been involved in its formulation.

I looked around the room to see the reactions on the faces of the people at the meeting. It appeared to me that the health promoters and midwives had only captured bits and pieces of this technical presentation, and they looked to the directors of their organizations to ask questions.

A doctor working with a health-promoter training program through the Catholic Church was the first to ask a question: "Where there are already health promoters who have been working for decades, how will they coordinate with the new *guardianes?* Will it be divisive for the community? Will the Ministry of Health respect where we are already working if we decide not to be SIAS providers?"

A nurse working to cocoordinate a health promoter and midwife training program asked the next question: "What about the quality of care? It seems that SIAS is focused just on producing numbers."

Then a health promoter asked about the reform itself: "Isn't SIAS a move toward privatization of health-care services, considering that the government is giving over responsibilities to NGOs? I think that it is the government's responsibility to provide care for our communities even though they have always neglected us. If the government only gives us Q50 a month, we are not going to be able to spend time working with the communities; we are going to have to be in the fields harvesting corn."

The meeting ended much as it had begun. The Ministry of Health representative and the invited speaker left before the modest lunch that ASECSA had ordered arrived. The rest of the participants stayed to talk over their discontent with SIAS and to begin planning for another meeting.

The community-based organizations, led by ASECSA, continued to meet on a regular basis to analyze and monitor what was happening with SIAS.

Seeing that there was no hope of convincing the community-based organizations connected with ASECSA to become SIAS providers, the health area director eventually approached ProPetén to see if the organization was interested in becoming a SIAS provider. The attempt seemed almost desperate to me; the health areas were receiving a lot of pressure from the central government to put SIAS into practice. I was surprised that the Ministry of Health would approach us, considering that ProPetén had no previous experience in health-care service delivery. Both because of the concerns that the organizations presented in the meetings and our lack of experience, we declined the offer. Instead, we began a program to train traditional birth attendants in communities that had none and to focus on reproductive health.

ALEJANDRO

I was interested in learning more about the government's SIAS program firsthand so that I could compare it with what I had heard and read. In 2001, therefore, I began my first job after medical school as an ambulatory doctor with one of the better-respected NGO service providers in the jurisdiction of Cahabón, Alta Verapaz.

Alta Verapaz was one of three departments in which the SIAS program was initiated. Ninety-five percent of the people in the department are of Q'eqchi' origin. This department rates as one of the lowest on the human development index; it has some of the highest rates of poverty and extreme poverty as well as some of the worst health indicators in the country. The department is characterized by large plantations from which coffee and cardamom are exported and by the largest number of land conflicts between peasants and plantation owners. Cahabón, a municipality with about 40,000 inhabitants, primarily Q'eqchi,' is located 98 kilometers to the east of Cobán, the capital city of the department of Alta Verapaz. On a road that was then unpaved, it took about 4 hours to travel the distance. About one-fifth of the municipality's population lived in the town center, where the government buildings, the Catholic Church, and the market were located. The rest of the population was dispersed among villages of fewer than 1,500 people or lived as *mozos colonos*, working on plantations in exchange for permission to live on the *finca* owners' property and cultivate a small part of it for subsistence. Generally they receive no pay; because their living situations are so fragile, they do not organize for better conditions.

At the time I worked in Cahabón, a Ministry of Health medical director (who often left for Guatemala City or Cobán for administrative functions) was stationed at the town's health center along with a professional nurse, four auxiliary nurses, an environmental sanitation inspector, a rural health technician, and an ambulance driver. Of all the staff, only the ambulance driver was Q'eqchi.' Everybody else was *Ladino* and did not speak the language, although the auxiliary nurses, rural health technician, and environmental sanitation inspector could get by with Q'eqchi,' as they were natives of the town. They were all good workers who made an effort to do their jobs well, but many times they were limited by few material resources, their limited training, and their social prejudices. In the town there were also four pharmacies and an undetermined number of traditional healers.

My time in Cahabón with SIAS was full of unforgettable and enriching experiences, although many were sad. I was exposed to life in rural communities, which has many satisfying aspects: solidarity, positive ancestral knowledge, reciprocity, a will to improve the family and the community, the disposition to share resources and knowledge, etc., and also many that are frustrating: community conflicts, envy, apathy in the face of other people's suffering, leaders taking advantage of villagers, etc.

The population of about 10,000 with whom I directly worked lived in some 30 communities. There was a dirt road to the largest community, Tuhilá, a community formed by the repatriated population in which people of *Q'eqchi,' Q'anjob'al, Mam,* and *Ixil* origin lived together. From Cahabón to Tuhilá it was a little more than a half an hour on a motorcycle. From Tuhilá, it took between a half hour and 5 hours to get to the other communities, usually on foot.

I wondered how the jurisdiction for the government's SIAS program was assigned to these communities. Although it is clear that they suffered poor living conditions and were in need of health care, the communities to the northeast of the municipality were in much greater need. In the northeast, the majority of people were *mozos colonos*. They had no organized legal structure and no government development projects; for that reason their living conditions were more precarious. This was something that authorities in Cahabón agreed on, and they asked the same question that I did. Some speculated that the communities were chosen so that it would be easier for the EC/SIAS program to achieve better results. Others thought that Tuhilá had been chosen for political reasons because it was a repatriated population, or that the rural health technician had interests in a political party and it was helpful for his campaign to offer health-care services to these communities.

The people were told that there would be a new health program, but in order to receive services they had to choose community members to volunteer as health *guardianes*. If the communities were not able to come up with these volunteers, they would not receive services. The selection process caused conflicts and the rural health technician selected volunteers strategically, paying debts for political favors and buying support from the community leaders. Sadly, the small monthly 50 quetzales that the volunteers would receive was sufficient political enticement.

For the most part, people who had been health promoters prior to the SIAS program did not become *guardianes* because it was time-consuming and reduced their community status. For trained, experienced, respected health promoters, it was demeaning to be subordinated to a translator or a lackey for the doctor or nurse. Instead, health promoters continued to work as they had prior to the SIAS program. One time, when I arrived at a community to offer care to patients, nobody was waiting for me. Later I found out that the people who had needed care had gone to the health promoter in a neighboring community despite the fact that the medicines I offered were free and that the health promoter charged a fee. Evidently health promoters offered a service that was more culturally acceptable and appropriate, in a more comfortable setting, during hours more convenient to community members.

To compensate for the lack of birth services in the SIAS package, community birth attendants were to have a close working relationship with the institutional health workers. The birth attendants were instructed to take part in a monthly training, for which they would be reimbursed with Q50 for their time and travel costs. In addition, once a year they received a kit for attending births. In the jurisdiction where I worked, SIAS only had funding for 35 traditional birth attendants, although there were close to 50 actively attending births in the communities. Some of the birth attendants took part in the monthly meetings, even though they were not reimbursed, but others simply could not afford to.

Although in theory SIAS is based on continual care by *guardianes*, community facilitators, and the visits by the ambulatory doctor, in practice the *guardianes* and community facilitators where I worked in Cahabón did not have the training, resources, or incentive to carry out this task. In the logic of SIAS, *guardianes* were to work at least an hour every day, in addition to working several hours or even full days during the medical *jornadas* and when it was time to update the census. They did not receive any pay for this work; the 50 quetzales was only to cover the costs of making it to the monthly trainings. Because the volunteer *guardianes* were typically people who did not have the time, interest, or capacity to do the work expected of them, the tendency was for the community facilitator and the *guardianes* to only notify the communities which days I would arrive for a *jornada*, and the people would show up. On the day of the *jornada*, the *guardianes* would organize the people and translate between Q'eqchi' and Spanish during the consultation. I carried out these *jornadas* in buildings based in one community that served a total of three to five others. Often, patients had to travel 1 to 2 hours and sometimes as many as 4 hours in order to attend.

This way of working provoked a variety of problems. First, I could travel to these convergence centers only once or twice a month. This meant that when people became sick and needed care, I was generally not nearby or easy to locate. For that reason, on the days that I did travel to a convergence center, people would arrive for a consultation with me, some of whom were not even sick but would feign a fever or cough in the hope that I would give them medicine that they could have on reserve for a day when they would need it and I might not be there.

It was not possible to provide quality care to all of the people who showed up to be seen. Twice I "gave consultations" to more than 110 people. My option on those days was to provide more thorough care to 30 to 35 people and leave 70 people without care (asking them to return in a month), or attend all 110 people poorly; I chose the latter option. Another difficulty was that in the SIAS program, I had goals of providing prenatal care and checkups for healthy children. These goals of preventive care were relegated to a secondary place owing to the scores of people with common illnesses who were waiting to be seen and the fact that many pregnant women, particularly from the most remote communities, would not travel to the convergence centers for prenatal care, as they considered it to be too far away.

Something that was very moving to me was that people in the most remote communities of my jurisdiction assumed that I was from another country, because they had never before been visited by a Guatemalan doctor. Those that had seen doctors had seen only Spanish doctors, who were present when the repatriated population was settled. In one community, members wrote in a notebook recording important community events that, for the first time, a doctor had arrived to their community.

During my time working in the communities of Cahabón, I had a number of experiences illustrating what the Guatemalan health system means for the indigenous population in rural areas and for the health personnel that connect this population to the institutional system. Here I share one of them.

There was a family with whom I became friendly. It was a couple, about 35 years old, with two adolescent girls and three younger children aged 6, 3, and 1. They were very active in the community and had been open and helpful to me. The husband knew how to read and had achieved a relatively high economic level in the community; he even had a pickup truck. One afternoon, when I was leaving the community after having seen patients, I passed by the house to say hello to the family. When I entered the house, I realized that the youngest son appeared to be undernourished; his parents told me that he had had pneumonia the week before. I asked what they were giving him to eat and recommended Incaparina, a nutritional drink that would help him gain weight. I wrote down how to prepare it and in what quantities they should administer it.

The following week I returned and saw that their son was worse. He was sick with a new episode of pneumonia. I gave the family medicine, explained what was happening, and told them that their best option was to bring their son to the hospital in Cobán. They told me that if their son got worse, they would. Together we prepared the Incaparina drink and I showed them what amount to use and how to give it to their son. I asked that they notify me right away if he was not consuming enough Incaparina. When I returned 3 days later he was even worse. I insisted that they should not wait any longer; that they should bring him to the hospital immediately. The father's words were candid and unnerving: "Children that go to the hospital go there to die, and the official procedures make it very hard to bury them here in the village. If it is God's will that he die, I prefer that he die here." I gave the child his treatment for pneumonia, but by the time I returned the next night, he had died.

A feeling of frustration and sadness invaded me. I have reflected a lot and analyzed this case, including what I could have done differently. Why had this child died in spite of the fact that his family cared for him with love and tried to help him recuperate? Why is it that what I had done was not enough? And why did families consider government hospitals to be their worst option?

The SIAS program encountered many difficulties. Since the funding for the high- and mid-level technical work of SIAS comes from the Inter-American Development Bank, SIAS was developed as a structure parallel to the Ministry of

Health. However, the technical–administrative workers in SIAS have much higher salaries than those with similar responsibilities in the Ministry of Health; those working under SIAS have to report separately to the Ministry of Health's information system and to one set up by the project administering the Inter-American Development Bank's loan. Often the priorities of these two entities are different, and the employees of the Ministry of Health have stated that the priorities of the Inter-American Development Bank usually prevail. For example, in some cases the NGOs that are SIAS providers have been well rated by the Inter-American Development Bank (with indicators that focus primarily on the quantity of services produced), while they are poorly rated by Ministry of Health employees (using indicators of maternal and infant mortality or the referral or lack thereof of patients with complications).

At an operational level, the problems are multiplied. The SIAS health-care workers are evaluated by a central SIAS technical team, but their day-to-day work depends on the coordination with local health district directors. Although in the discourse SIAS is considered to be an integral part of the Ministry of Health, in practice sentiments are different. And although employees in both SIAS and the Ministry of Health district levels try to do their jobs well, they are frequently caught in the middle of conflicts and contradictions owing to structural problems.

After I had spent a little more than a year working with the SIAS program, the Instancia Nacional de Salud offered me a position. I accepted and spent a year working to analyze the health sector reform. During this period, I reflected on the many operational and structural difficulties that I had seen in the SIAS program. I also witnessed directly the large disconnect between what the government offers and what the population is looking for, which I had also seen when I took part in *jornadas* in medical school. By attempting to provide care to communities that had never before received health-care services, the government was taking an important step, but I was convinced that rural communities deserved more than what the SIAS program had to offer.

MEREDITH

While I was attending meetings to analyze the reform in the Petén, similar meetings were taking place in different parts of the country, and groups had come together as a coalition called the Instancia Nacional de Salud. In 2001, I learned about the Instancia Nacional de Salud initiative while reading a Pan American Health Organization document describing their efforts. I immediately called ASECSA to find out more about this new initiative. Since that first phone call and meeting with the co-founder of the Instancia Nacional de Salud, I have worked to support the efforts of the coalition and the team working to implement its alternative health-care proposal.

I first met with Juan Carlos Verdugo, who was the coordinator of the technical–operational team of the Instancia Nacional de Salud, in a bookstore in Guatemala

City. I was impressed to meet such a tall, dignified-looking man working to start this new social movement. We met for coffee just briefly, as he had to teach a public health course in the evening to master's degree students at the Rafael Landivar University.

Juan Carlos asked, "Remind me how you heard about the Instancia Nacional de Salud and why you are interested in what we are doing."

I felt the need to demonstrate that I would support their efforts and try to do whatever I could to help. After listening to my explanation, Juan Carlos was convinced and agreed that I could carry out my public health practicum with the Instancia Nacional de Salud for the master's degree in public health that I was pursuing.

Years later, in a conversation about the founding of the Instancia Nacional de Salud, Hugo Icú, the director of ASECSA, told me how it began:

> In 1998, the Ministry of Health invited ASECSA to take part in a meeting about SIAS, with the hope that they could be convinced to sign an agreement with the government to be a SIAS administrator or provider. When I received the invitation, I decided that instead of going alone to the meeting, it would be more effective to have other organizations take part in the meeting to show the Ministry of Health the widespread discontent. I also invited the Public Health Workers' Union and an Association of Rural Health Technicians.

The first meeting with the Ministry of Health turned into a series of meetings that continued over a 6-month period. Finally, after many months of disagreeing, the Ministry of Health decided to call an end to the meetings. While ASECSA had made many attempts to convince the Ministry of Health that SIAS was not the appropriate model, it appeared that they had made little headway.

During the 6 months of meetings with the Ministry of Health, the coalition of organizations learned some important lessons. The Instancia Nacional de Salud recognized the need to strengthen its advocacy capacity since they felt unprepared in the meetings. The Instancia also learned that the Ministry of Health is limited as an advocacy target because, after all, the funding and specifications for the reform came from an Inter-American Development Bank loan. The coalition learned that it was not enough to solely resist; in order to influence the government, the Instancia would also have to work proactively to create a viable alternative proposal to serve as something concrete around which to lobby. During the years prior to the creation of the Instancia, the member organizations had not worked on alternative proposals or lobbying the government as they had been responding to the immediate needs of the communities.

The coalition decided to base a technical–operational team centrally, just outside of the capital, to work full time on advocacy efforts and proposal development. The member organizations would come together several times a year for national and regional assemblies and would elect a small group of representatives as a coordinating council to meet on a more regular basis.

In the summer of 2001, I began helping out the technical–operational team of the Instancia Nacional de Salud in the area of health sector monitoring at the central government level. I interviewed officials in the Ministry of Health, the Guatemalan Social Security Institute, the Inter-American Development Bank, the Congress, and other government offices about the health sector reform. As I carried out interviews with government officials, I was struck by how easy it was to gather information. I remember feeling that as a North American, I was probably being treated differently than my Guatemalan colleagues would be if they entered the same offices requesting the same information. On some level, I was pleased to see how easily I could access information because I knew that I was helping the Instancia Nacional de Salud understand the reform, but I also felt almost ashamed for receiving special treatment.

After a number of people recommended that I contact the office that administered the loan, I scheduled a meeting with a high-level official there. The first time I met with him his office was not on the premises of the Ministry of Health building but in a residential part of Guatemala City. During our first meeting, I sensed that he was quite distressed and needed to talk with somebody about what he was seeing. He closed the door and, after a few questions about my background, began to talk almost incessantly for 2 hours.

> The main achievement of SIAS has been that health-service coverage is now available in rural areas that previously had no care. However, there are important problems with the coverage. During the first 4 years, there was essentially no evaluation of the NGOs. When an internal evaluation was finally done, 70% of the NGOs did not meet the requirements. When SIAS began, NGOs, many of which did not even have any health experience, saw it as an easy way to get a hold of funds. Since the government needed to have counterparts to carry out SIAS, there was no real selection process.

When he stopped for a moment to take a breath, I took the opportunity to slip in a question: "I understand that the money for the reform comes from a loan from the Inter-American Development Bank. What does that mean for the sustainability of the SIAS program?" I was concerned about what an increasing foreign debt and dependency on foreign agencies would mean for the Guatemalan government.

He looked at me with a smile and I realized that I had touched precisely on a topic that he was very interested in.

> Sustainability, that is a very important topic. The money from the first portion of the loan was used mostly to pay consultants to design SIAS, whereas the Guatemalan government paid for the direct service delivery. The concern is whether the government will be able to pay for SIAS in the future. I am concerned about the $55 million loan that the government will receive for the second phase of the reform and what that money will really go for.

During the summer I conducted more than 15 interviews with key informants and reviewed numerous government documents. What became clear to me was that there were a slew of different decentralization initiatives and concepts of health reform in the different offices. And the people who were responsible for implementing the reforms had doubts themselves about what should be done. The one constant that appeared to receive the most emphasis in the reform was SIAS, which was now being referred to as the "program to extend coverage."

During my first few months with the Instancia Nacional de Salud, I sat in on a health policy course. There, I met Alejandro Cerón in a session analyzing the role of health workers in health sector reform. I was impressed that he had made the decision not just to criticize the reform from the outside but rather to understand the reform by taking part in it directly as a rural ambulatory doctor in SIAS. I visited Alejandro in Cahabón and saw for myself what SIAS was like.

ALEJANDRO AND MEREDITH

At the same time that our separate paths led us to the Instancia Nacional de Salud, the technical–operational team was finishing an alternative proposal for the primary care level in Guatemala. The proposal, now called *Hacia un Primer Nivel de Atención en Salud Incluyente: Bases y Lineamientos* ("Working toward an Inclusive Primary Care Level: Foundation and Guidelines), was presented publicly in 2002. The coalition had recognized the need for an alternative proposal in the initial meetings with the Ministry of Health but took on the task of developing one that would not only respond to the present health sector reform but also counter the historical exclusion of Mayan people and women.

The Mayan people have suffered discrimination and exclusion for 500 years, starting with the Spanish conquest and followed by a liberal reform in the 1870s, which forced Mayans to work as laborers on European-owned plantations, followed by the horror of the internal conflict, which was particularly bloody in the 1980s, during the rule of the dictator Rios Montt. And women, as is true in most societies, have been treated as second class citizens, with limited opportunities to study, work, or even make decisions to improve the health and well-being of themselves and their families.

From 2003 to 2006, we worked together in the implementation of the Instancia Nacional de Salud's inclusive primary health care proposal. The alternative proposal calls for a comprehensive approach to health, including promotion, prevention, curative care, and rehabilitation. Through a balance of interventions in three programs (individual, family, and community programs) paid, full-time health workers—*agentes de salud comunitaria*—provide care to the whole assigned population. The proposal has three guiding principles: the right to health, gender equity, and interculturality.

The right to health takes into account that health care is not a gift communities should feel thankful for when they receive it but rather a service they can and should demand. The principle of gender equity recognizes that women and men should be provided care in an equitable manner and should have equal opportunities to participate and take part in the decision-making process. The principle of interculturality recognizes the cultural diversity of Guatemalan society and promotes horizontal and respectful relations between the different ethnic groups to combat the prevailing discrimination. One example is to establish "parallel coordination" between community healers, including those of the Mayan medical model, and the institutional system. In addition, the proposal requires health workers to consider the patient's diagnosis and understanding of health–illness. The proposal also states that the community plays a critical role in working to influence the determinants and conditioning factors that cause people to be healthy or unhealthy.

The experience of implementing the proposal has taught us many lessons about the challenges of providing primary health care. Because the program is an "alternative" to the SIAS model, we have felt that it is important to design our own technical instruments and protocols. However, during the process, we have always used what the Ministry of Health has designed as a reference. We recognize that within the Ministry of Health, during the years of the SIAS model, many useful ideas have been developed (for example: a guide for carrying out health-situation analysis), but they had not been implemented because of limited resources.

There are a number of major differences between SIAS and the Instancia's proposal. From a policy perspective, the concept of the state underlying the SIAS model is to intervene minimally and only where the market fails to do so. As a part of the health sector reform process, the Congress approved a new health code and the Ministry of Health's bylaws were modified; these changes redefined the state's role with respect to health care, allowing for the participation of private entities in the delivery of government health-care services and leaving open the option of the demonopolization of the Social Security Institute. The aim of the state in the Instancia proposal is to guarantee the individual, social, and economic rights of the population, including the right to health. The Instancia model is being implemented in close coordination with health district directors and is strengthening the Ministry of Health by moving toward a universal health-care system.

Health–disease in SIAS is conceptualized exclusively as a biological phenomenon. In the Instancia proposal, health–disease is conceptualized in a comprehensive way, acknowledging its social origins. During the family visits, health workers consider and assess the social and cultural factors that influence family members' health. Families are then classified according to risk level in order to define interventions specific to their needs.

SIAS, based on classic epidemiology, does not take into account other models of health. Differently, the Instancia proposal is designing a sociocultural epidemiology framework that takes into account other models of health, such as the Mayan model. In practice, health workers implementing the Instancia proposal ask patients about how they understand their health problems, sociocultural illnesses are registered and reported, and a referral and counterreferral system is being developed with community therapists.

Gender in SIAS is limited to providing maternal health care. The Instancia proposal aims to promote gender equity by offering health care according to the specific needs and health risks of men and women. Based on the primary motives for women's consultations, clinical guidelines were developed by the Instancia team for a range of women's health problems, which go beyond their roles as mothers and include menstrual anomalies, stress, back pain, menopause, and female-specific sociocultural illnesses. The health workers have also made an effort to offer consultations at hours that men can attend. Domestic violence and alcohol abuse are addressed in the family and community programs as important risks that affect men and women differently.

The basis for the programmatic design of SIAS is vertical, cost-effective, and disease-specific interventions; whereas in the Instancia proposal, programs are comprehensive and geared toward individuals, families, and communities. The Instancia programs are for the entire population, using comprehensive primary health care as a model for service delivery rather than limited, select interventions.

SIAS has a top-down management structure in which planning is done at the central level without community or operational level input. While abiding by national health standards, the Instancia proposal emphasizes teamwork and local input and encourages community involvement. In the Instancia proposal, the community is expected to participate in the planning and evaluation of health efforts; participation is a process that is limited initially and increases with time. Health workers implementing the Instancia proposal have helped communities obtain resources for needs that they have defined, understanding health in a broad sense (e. g., the repair of roads after Hurricane Stan in 2005).

Health care in SIAS is provided periodically, whereas in the Instancia model, health care is ongoing. In the SIAS program, health-care providers arrive in villages once or twice a month to offer physician consultations and vaccinations. In the Instancia proposal, health-care workers provide care on a permanent basis from community health houses equipped with medicines and medical supplies.

More than 90% of the SIAS workforce are volunteers, whereas in the Instancia proposal, trained community health agents are paid full salaries and have a professional support team for referrals, ongoing training, and supervision. The SIAS model has changed very little from how it was described earlier in this chapter. In the Instancia proposal, the number of health-care providers is determined according to local needs, depending on topographical and geographic characteristics and distances between communities in order to ensure that populations receive equitable care. In practice, this has translated to there being 14 community health workers per approximately 10,000 people and a support team including a doctor, nurse, family and community program animators, an accountant, data-entry staff, and a team coordinator.

The first of the three programs that we launched was the individual program. We visited the *agentes de salud comunitaria* (ASC) regularly in the community health houses where they work, to provide them with ongoing training and support. On one visit to the community health house in Patzité just months after its inauguration, we realized that community members would immediately put their trust in the ASC and that we would quickly need to define responses to not only simple health problems but also to more complex social and cultural problems, such as the ones illustrated here.

Diego, an *agente de salud comunitaria* in his early thirties, said to the next woman in line, who was studying the posters on the walls of the community health house, that he was ready to see her. The woman, who was at most 20 years old and had a small baby slung on her back, slowly walked through the door to the examination room, and Diego motioned to her to be seated on the padded table. She sat down with an expectant look and—after writing down her background information, including her family's geographic code, her age, and her sex—Diego asked, "Please, tell me why you have come in for a consultation today."

She looked down at the floor and said, "I think that I am pregnant again and I am scared."

"Why are you scared?"

"Because my husband hits me and I am afraid that he may harm my baby." Diego did not appear to be fazed by her comment; he has seen domestic violence many times in his own village just 5 kilometers from Patzité. Although he knew that he could not respond to the larger problem that this woman faced in the consultation, he could offer her compassion and care during her visit and explain that it was not right for her to be suffering such violence. Also, working through the family and community programs, he was able to address domestic violence by counseling with family members, leading community meetings, and sending referrals to organizations that help families suffering domestic violence.

In the family program, which we started a year after the individual program was under way, the ASC made home visits to every household in the catchment area of their community health house—between 1,000 and 2,000 people—in order to screen for possible risks and illnesses such as malnutrition; promote the use of vaccines, pap smears, prenatal care, micronutrients, and other services offered by the program; as well as to encourage the use of the community health house. On the first round of family visits, we realized that we were going to have to make some changes in how we organized the services.

Juana, an ASC with two children of her own and with years of experience treating patients in her community before she started working for a salary as an ASC, asked during a monthly planning and evaluation meeting, "What do we do about the six other children who we found are malnourished in Pacanal? Now we have more than 20 in our catchment area, and I am worried about what will happen to them. When we were just providing care with the individual program, not all of the malnourished children showed up to the community health house, so we did not see the problem. But now that we know that they are here, what can we do?" After we saw just how many malnourished children we were finding, we began to provide families with a nutritional supplement.

In our minds, the community program was to be the last of the three programs implemented. In reality, we were not able to wait, and the ASC became involved in community organizing almost from the beginning. In November 2005, as Hurricane Stan swept through the communities in which we were providing care, the ASC helped communities in the search for shelter, food supplies, and tubing for community water systems.

The implementation of the Instancia Nacional de Salud's alternative primary health-care proposal is the closest that we have come to feeling that we are responding in an appropriate way to villagers' health needs. But we feel that there is a lot more work to be done. In years to come, we will continue striving to improve primary health care in Guatemala. We know that through the balance of direct service delivery and health-care policy, we can contribute to a genuine implementation of the Peace Accords and to the three guiding principles of the Instancia proposal.

NOTES

i. Dona Adriana Chavez' name has been changed to protect her identity.
ii. The exchange rate was around Q6/USD at the time of the presentation. Currently it is approximately Q8/USD.

10 Social Marketing and Franchising for Reproductive Health in India

Gopi Gopalakrishnan and Paromita Ukil

The two pregnant women walked up to the metal road and stopped. Once they had confirmed that our car had halted, they made their way across the road. Sitting inside the car, we could make out their swollen bellies even through the thick December fog.

"Rajkishore Bhaiyya [brother], open the door, we have come for the checkup." The two women were now banging the door of a shop on this highway outside Patna city. The signboard hanging outside said "Dr Rajkishore Kumar, General Physician"; at the bottom right corner was written in tiny letters, "Ayurveda." Beside it hung another sign, bright yellow, with a colorful butterfly. At the bottom of this board was written, "Titli Center." A weatherbeaten roof of earthenware tiles sloped down to rest on eucalyptus poles on the verandah, where the two women stood. To the right of the verandah was a cow shed where a big brown cow was dipping into a trough full of hay, its stomach wrapped in a thick sheet to protect it from the biting cold.

We got out of our car and joined the women on the verandah, just as Rajkishore opened the door and stepped out, a blanket wrapped around his shoulders like a giant shawl. The women smiled and said, "We have come for the second checkup," and they handed him their pregnancy registration card.

By this time Shanti, Rajkishore's wife, had stepped out and greeted the two pregnant women. Rajkishore then turned to us. He brought out chairs for us to sit on in the open space between the road and his shop-cum-residence. He said he would be with us shortly and went to attend to his clients. We looked on from a distance.

Shanti had made the two women comfortable on a bench standing on the verandah; it had an armrest on each side and a back, resembling a rugged couch. She brought out weighing scales and a small stool on which she placed the blood pressure apparatus. Rajkishore sat on a plastic chair and measured each woman's blood pressure. Then he asked each of them to stand on the scales while he noted their weights and pressures on the pregnancy registration card.

A look of worry appeared on Rajkishore's face each time he examined the frailer of the two women. He told her that her blood pressure was high and that she weighed very little. He checked her pregnancy card, issued by the government health center, and said: "It's good that you have taken two tetanus shots. And make sure that you take all of the 100 tablets you got from the health center." He asked Shanti to take her inside and have her lie her down on their bed. He then went in and, as he later told us, he and his wife palpated the woman's fetus. They both felt it was too small for 6 months of pregnancy.

There were definite indications of a complicated pregnancy, and Rajkishore would have to try to persuade the family to consult a gynecologist. He asked the woman when her husband would be home, because he would have to go over and discuss the matter with him and her in-laws. The best course for her, he told her, would be to register with the Surya Clinic, which was only 2 kilometers from his shop. The village the two women came from was across the metal road, just a few meters on the other side.

He told the other woman also that it was always advisable to go to a hospital for delivery. The other woman, the one with the healthier fetus, then asked Rajkishore to drop in at her house too and speak to her in-laws. Rajkishore said that he would, and his patients went in with Shanti to make the nominal payments.

Rajkishore dragged his plastic chair to join us outside his verandah. Answering our many queries, he explained that although these women had registered their pregnancies at a government health center, they came to him for their antenatal checkup because it was more convenient. The health center was 5 kilometers from their village, and it was not certain that the auxiliary nurse midwife would be available when they went there. So they preferred to get the checkup from Rajkishore and his wife, even though they had to pay for it.

By now piping hot tea, so welcome in the biting cold, arrived, and we concentrated on balancing our cups. As we silently sipped, Rajkishore reclined on his chair, stretching his bare feet in rubber slippers. A shy smile spread across his face, which seemed to say, quite humbly, that he was proud of what he had made of his life.

When I came to Bihar from Delhi in the 1990s, I was not at all sure how things would turn out. Bihar, one of the most populous states in India, was frequently making national headlines for all the wrong reasons—no law or order, no governance, rampant corruption. The list was endless, and much of it was true. Even people I knew in Delhi, whose parental or ancestral homes were in Bihar, warned, "Don't go. Nothing works out there."

Yet my boss, Phil Harvey, felt that something should be done to meet the needs of Bihar's poor.

"Why Bihar?" I had asked over the phone when he first mentioned it.

"There's much that needs to be done there. No one wants to go to Bihar," he said.

I had telephoned Phil to tell him I was leaving. He was not my boss yet, as I was still working for Population Services International (PSI). Phil Harvey was a PSI board member, with whom I got along well, although we were continents apart. I worked with the program in India and he was at the head office of another social marketing organization, DKT International, as president.

During our phone conversation it became clear to Phil that I had not taken a new job, and he brought up the urgency of meeting some of Bihar's unmet family planning needs. The population at the time was close to 96 million and the 10-year growth rate 28.4% (against the national average of 21.3%); 42% of the people were extremely poor. It was estimated that 40% of the couples did not want to have another child or that they wanted a gap between children but were not using

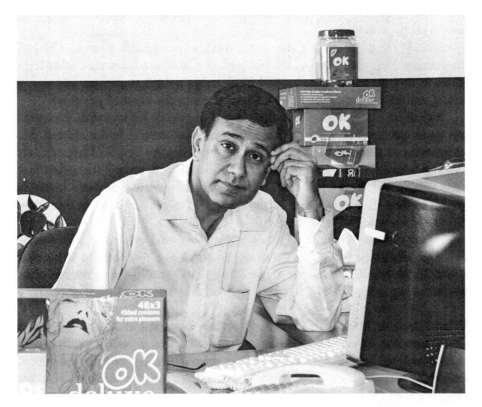

Gopi Gopalakrishnan at work surrounded (as usual) by boxes of condoms.

contraception because they had no access to it. There was a huge need for family planning services, which remained unmet by government and private providers.

It was evident that Phil was dropping not-so-subtle hints. I told him I would go—it would be easier for an Indian than for an expatriate to set up something up there.

Later that day, Phil called me again and asked, "Were you serious when you said you would go to Bihar?"

"Of course I was serious," I replied.

Talking to Phil had made me realize the enormous potential to do something worthwhile in Bihar. I was confident that the 8 years of social marketing experience I had gained at PSI had given me the experience I needed to be successful there. Like any social marketing outfit, PSI marketed family planning products using a network of distributors and retailers. I had no doubt that we would be able to successfully market condoms and oral contraceptive pills even in Bihar. But Phil had greater ideas for the program. Bihar's needs were far greater than what conventional social marketing offered.

I went to Bihar soon after. I made it a point to understand the ground reality before developing a plan. I wanted to take time to conceptualize so that we could get it right.

I arrived in Patna on June 3, 1995. I had a theoretical knowledge of the need for family planning products in Bihar. But that's all it was—theoretical knowledge. It was only after I traveled through the towns and villages of Bihar that my eyes opened to the acute demand and the lax supply. It was not, as many city folks wrongly believed, that the Indian villager is averse to family planning and does not want to limit the size of his family because he believes it is God's gift. A large number of people I met did not want any more children because they had enough—they could not deal with another newborn every 2 or 3 years. Still, babies were being born all the time because many of the villagers did not know how to stop having children.

I traveled through the interior of Bihar to get a feel of the land and its socioeconomic constraints. One winter I and a woman manager of our team journeyed to the village of Lalpur. When we arrived, we found the women of the village enjoying the warmth of the sun as they kept a watchful eye on the goats, cows, and buffaloes grazing the fields. We approached them and soon got to talking. As we sat by the lush green wheat field, some men also joined in. When my colleague raised the issue of unwanted pregnancies and contraception, three women in the group burst forth in an urgent plea.

"Please do something, Didiji, do something for us, dear sister."

All three women were quite evidently pregnant. For each of them it was their fourth or fifth pregnancy, which they did not want. Because there would be so much work in the fields at the time of delivery, they knew it would be very tough for them and their families to cope. They could not afford to hire an extra hand—it would mean paying with wheat, which they would need for the family's food security.

The men too joined in: "Yes sir, do something. You say you are in this business."

They wanted us to take them to a clinic for female sterilization. "Take us to a good place," said one of the women. The other women also joined in, until they were almost pleading. Then all of them, men and women, told us about the two instances in the village where the women had ligation done in a government-sponsored camp, only to conceive within a few months.

"We don't mind paying even 1,000 rupees," they said, "but it has to be a good and reliable place."

After meeting with the men and women of Lalpur, I worked out a one-page concept note and sent it to Phil. The note said if the program was to be relevant to Bihar's needs, it would have to go beyond urban areas and nonclinical products such as contraceptives—it would have to extend to the villages, and it would need to establish clinics that offered high-quality yet affordable services.

The clinics could not be located in a village because there would not be a large enough clientele for them to become viable. And further—which doctor, having studied medicine for a minimum of 5 years, would want to practice in a place where there was no electricity, no running water, and no trace of any of the usual modern conveniences?

The clinics would have to be located in the smaller district towns. Every village was connected to some such town by a public road. The resource was therefore available for the program, but we would need to remodel it to meet people's needs. Although every town had mushrooming clinics practicing curative medicine, very few offered family planning services, and those that did were of doubtful quality.

The question was how to link the target clientele with these clinics. Who would, for example, tell the women of Lalpur that what they are looking for is available at this clinic in this town, under 15 kilometers from their village? Immediately, I thought of the informal medics known as rural medical practitioners (RMPs).

In poor states like Bihar, where health indicators are far below the national average, the government health delivery system is almost nonfunctioning, even more so in rural areas. Unlicensed medical practitioners such as the RMPs are virtually the only medical service providers in the vast rural areas of India. Rajkishore was an RMP when I came to Bihar to set up the Janani program as its country director.

As a general rule, in northern India, in states like Bihar and adjoining Jharkhand and Uttar Pradesh, RMPs are men. There are a few women RMPs in the central state of Madhya Pradesh, but they are an exception.

Villagers have deep faith and trust in their RMPs. Although government and private doctors call them quacks, villagers address them as doctors. They come on their bicycle once every second or third day to the village, carrying large cloth bags full of medicines for common ailments, injection syringes, bandages, scissors, and various other things they may need. The RMP parks in a central location in the village and people gather around him with their complaints. He listens to each one patiently, and to each he hands almost a fistful of yellow, pink, green, and brown pills that can supposedly cure anything, from malaria to diarrhea to simple fever. The pills work most of the time, so the RMPs are what village folk look for. They cannot afford transportation to the nearest town or a visit to a city doctor. They cannot afford to lose the work and wages that this would involve. Here, "quality cure" means quick cure. Injections are preferred over pills because they are known to work faster, so the first thing an RMP learns to do is to give injections.

In Bihar, I learned, RMPs provide virtually all the health-care treatment and advice to 80 million rural people. They offer diagnosis and treatment and make much of their money from the sale of drugs. They are present in every village. Some villages have more than one RMP. They are the only regular link with the outside world because they have to go to a nearby market town to get their supply of medicines.

The Janani program saw the RMP as a resource. We would not have to identify, train, and then relocate a person in a village when all he wanted was to get away from there. There would be nothing to hold that person to life in the village. An RMP, on the other hand, was part of the social fabric. He was also a link between the village and the market. If the program took him as a component, the connection could be established at little extra cost and made sustainable.

The program was now all chalked out: RMPs. Shops. Clinics. These were the three components, the three interlinking networks of a composite social marketing program in family planning services.

TITLI CENTERS

My concept now focused on the RMP. Our Janani program would elevate him to the status of a man you first turned to for all your family planning needs. But I knew that village women would not feel free to discuss their family planning needs and problems with a man. A solution was to incorporate the RMPs' wives into the program. The wife would help to make the RMP acceptable to female patients and would serve as the first point of contact. If the RMP's wife knew enough to recommend appropriate methods of contraception and to do pregnancy tests, the two together would be perceived as a team. Gradually, as the ice was broken, the women would slowly open up to seek the RMP's advice on more complicated clinical issues. Then, it would only be a matter of logistics to get the women to the Janani clinics in nearby district towns.

We decided to start with the RMPs because we did not know how things would go in the rural sector. This is when we met Rajkishore and learned his story.

By the time Janani came into contact with Rajkishore, he was a full-fledged RMP, it is true, but a chain of events in his early life had led him to become a nonformal medical practitioner. After completing high school, when Rajkishore was at loose ends wondering what to do next, he would spend a lot of time with his friends in Patna, the state's capital city. One of them was studying for a degree in Ayurveda, a system of traditional medicine. On his recommendation, Rajkishore completed a 2-year correspondence course in Ayurvedic medicine. Not long after he received his diploma, Rajkishore fractured a leg and thus came in contact with a doctor, who was to define the course his life would take. This doctor ran a clinic on the main road in a town not far from his village. As he was taking off the plaster cast, he made Rajkishore an offer to work as his assistant at the clinic. Rajkishore's family encouraged him to accept the offer.

"Go ahead, son, take the job. At least there will be a regular source of income in the family," his father told him. He assured Rajkishore that he himself was still strong enough and could manage the farm work with a few hired help.

Rajkishore therefore accepted the doctor's offer. In the beginning, all Rajkishore did was clean the floors, the examination tables, and the instruments and equipment. The clinic was rather small, with just two tiny rooms; there was not much cleaning to do. Rajkishore therefore spent much of his time observing the doctor and doing errands for him in the clinic, like fetching bottles of medicine, sterilizing instruments, and other odd jobs. In time and with the doctor's encouragement, Rajkishore acquired the skills of a compounder. He began by sterilizing bandages and dressing wounds and later graduated to giving injections. He remembers even now how nervous he was when he gave an injection for the first time. He was afraid the needle would touch the patient's bone. He recalls that he even asked the patient, "I hope it didn't hurt too much?"

Rajkishore now went into villages in the vicinity to give injections to regular patients. For each injection he got paid 2 rupees by his patient. He also administered glucose and saline to patients in their homes for 25 rupees per bottle. This expanded the doctor's practice and also helped Rajkishore earn a few extra rupees. At the end of 5 years, Rajkishore felt confident enough to branch off on his own. There was a growing demand for his services in the villages he visited, and by now he knew enough about curing common ailments like fever, diarrhea, and vomiting. He had acquired some knowledge of antibiotics during the time he spent with the doctor. He knew that he would be able to make more money on his own.

That is how Rajkishore came to be a halfway doctor, offering quick cures for ailments that commonly occurred in his village.

Experience gave exposure to Rajkishore; education gave him the ability to negotiate. He knew many doctors and hospitals by now, some in Patna. This placed Rajkishore far ahead of many in his village. They came to depend on him for his street smarts. Those who were uneducated in his village, those who could not read or write, were reluctant to venture into uncharted territory. They lived their lives more or less confined to the village. They felt intimidated in a world demarcated by numbers and letters, where at every step you had to fill out forms or sign papers. How would they read the number of the destination written on the bus? How does one know which is the bus to one's village? City people are so rude, they don't tell you everything. And how do I know they are giving me the right directions?

Unlettered villagers were also wary of being taken for a ride, of being duped for money.

The illiterate villagers depend on savvy people like Rajkishore. He, in response, began helping out relatives and friends. When someone was seriously ill and Rajkishore's antibiotics were no longer working, he would take the patient to the doctor with whom he had apprenticed. Sometimes, after his wife had had repeated miscarriages, a friend would come to him for help. Rajkishore would take him and his wife to a "lady doctor." Soon it became a trend. The clinics to which he brought patients would sometimes reward him with a commission. There was no system in the payment of commission; it was solely discretionary.

With time, more and more women wanted to be taken to a doctor for their "female" problems. Sometimes this doctor did procedures like hysterectomies, abortions, or ligation of the fallopian tubes. Since, most of the time the "lady doctor" in such a district town was actually not a medical graduate but simply the doctor's wife, who picked up things on the job, there would often be mishaps and botched operations. Poor and uneducated, patients had no other recourse but to blame it on "kismet." In such situations, Rajkishore would be compensated handsomely if he managed public opinion in the village and made sure that blame did not fall on the doctor.

Rajkishore's small business as go-between for his women patients picked up between November and April, between sowing and harvesting of the winter crop. During this period, his women clients would be relatively free from their farm duties and be willing to undergo invasive surgical procedures, such as those already mentioned. Since these procedures required patients to rest after their surgery, they also found these months opportune.

When we, at Janani, came into contact with Rajkishore, he was looking for a way to improve his service package to his women clients. By now there were four other RMPs practicing in his area. Competition was stiff.

When we approached Rajkishore to ask if he would be interested in doing training on reproductive health and afterward run his own rural center for family planning products and other basic services, he showed immediate interest. Yes, he said, he and his wife, Shanti, would like to do the training we suggested. The couple filled out a form and together attended the training with Janani. It was conducted in a big hospital in Patna and lasted for 3 days. There Rajkishore learned how to detect complications of pregnancy or a prolapsed uterus and how to predict an obstetric emergency, so that he could refer such patients to a clinic. With each case he referred to a clinic of the Janani network, he would earn a commission.

Rajkishore and Shanti were also trained in dip-stick pregnancy tests and blood pressure measurement. They learned of the different kinds of contraception available, so that they could offer counseling to couples seeking protection and offer the method most suited to their needs.

Rajkishore came back a different man after the training. Now he had a professional partner—his wife. After the training, Janani helped him set up a shop he could run from his house—a shop that sold condoms, pills, and services like pregnancy tests, blood pressure measurements, and referral services in family planning. In addition, Rajkishore continued to cure patients of common ailments. He hung bright yellow board outside his shop, adjacent to the board that normally hung on his door, announcing as the services of a general physician. This new board had the picture of a very colorful butterfly; it said Titli (Butterfly) Center.

When Rajkishore set up the bright yellow board of the Titli Center, men and women from the village came crowding by to see what this new object was. Over the next few months, Rajkishore and Shanti did a lot of explaining to curious villagers about their training and all the services that were available at the Titli Center. At times women came in groups of three or four to their house-cum-shop, wanting to speak to Shanti in private. On these occasions they wanted to learn in detail about contraceptive pills and their possible side effects. Shanti would explain to each group about the number of pills to be taken, when to take them, and how they offered protection from unwanted pregnancies. Most importantly, she explained that the nausea that women often complained of regarding contraceptive pills lasted only a few days while the body became adjusted to the new regimen.

The efforts paid off—women began to buy the pills. The younger women who came to Shanti bought the pills for themselves, the older women bought them for their daughters-in-law. Now women could also have pregnancies confirmed in the village the first time they skipped a period. It cost them only 40 rupees (about a dollar).

Shanti also spoke to the women of the importance of prenatal checkups to avoid complications during childbirth. She told them of the benefits of trained assistance at the time of giving birth and how a doctor's presence could prevent many a mishap.

When they learned that the Titli Center also checked blood pressure, the elderly among the villagers came as well; they had learned of implications of high blood pressure from the health programs on the government-run All India Radio.

The rural Titli Center sold nonclinical family planning products and advised villagers on clinical remedies when required. If a patient was interested, the Titli Center arranged for clinical procedures like female sterilization, hysterectomy, or abortion. When Rajkishore detected complications in a pregnancy, he encouraged the family to have the delivery at a clinic, and he made all arrangements for that at the nearest clinic of the Janani network. Once they were set up, these clinics came to be called Surya Clinics.

Seeing Rajkishore in action that winter morning, in his little shop that sold condoms, oral contraceptives, and oral rehydration salts, and noting all the services it offered, I felt that it had been worth it all—staying away from my family and missing out on watching our daughter grow. The program I came to set up almost 9 years ago has been able to achieve what it set out to do. Rajkishore too was overwhelmed, talking to my colleagues and me about his life after Janani. Joining the program gave him stability and status, he said. It opened up a whole new dimension by enabling him to learn about reproductive health and offer these new services.

He was no longer insecure about competition from fellow RMPs, as he was doing much more than peddling cures for common ailments.

Rajkishore and Shanti belonged to the first batch of RMP couples we trained under the Janani program. In the beginning, we were apprehensive about being able to recruit RMPs. When we got 20 couples together for the first group to be trained, we had a tremendous sense of achievement. We bused them to the capital, fed them full meals for free, and even gave each couple a small stipend for participating in the training. We had thought that we would have to lure them; only some time later, we learned that the training itself was what attracted RMPs to the program. In fact, it turned out that couples were even willing to pay for it.

With each camp we got bolder and bolder. First we phased out the food. It was quite a task, setting up an open-air kitchen to cook food for all participants, including small children, because both parents were called to these training sessions. We now asked people to bring their own food because the training sessions were no longer residential; the RMPs went home in the evenings.

When we saw that this approach did not lead to a drop in numbers, we introduced a small fee, first 10 then 15 rupees. Now, after so many years, Janani charges 250 rupees for training an RMP couple. There is also an annual membership fee of 300 rupees for every Titli Center. Rajkishore and his fellow RMPs have been renewing their memberships quite regularly so far.

The training was our winning strategy both with RMPs and, as we found out a few years later, also with doctors, who wanted their clinics to be part of the Janani network. At the camps for RMPs we taught very basic facts: a little about physiology as well as about menstruation, reproductive health, reproductive tract infections, and sexually transmitted infections. Some of the training was devoted to an explanation of antibiotics. That was important because RMPs had a high degree of comfort with medications; they had been prescribing trimethoprim/sulfamethoxazole (Septran) and other broad-spectrum antibiotics to their rural patients. The problem with most RMPs is that they do not have a clue about different types of antibiotics. So they give the broadest-spectrum antibiotics for the simplest ailments. We taught them how antibiotics worked and what could go wrong.

At the end of the training, there was a small celebration and both the RMPs and their wives received a certificate. At this ceremony they took an oath with their hands raised, the way doctors do when they receive their medical degrees. Here, they represented a team.

Right from the beginning we had the woman with the man; she was an integral part of the rural center that we envisaged. That was why we trained them in couples. The woman was there for a strategic reason. She would take us to the vast clientele of women in need of social marketing products and services. We were not sure, at this stage, how appealing family planning services would be as a business venture to RMPs. But of we were more certain of reproductive tract infections (RTIs) and sexually transmitted diseases (STDs), because various studies showed that up to 80% of rural women in India suffered from some form of gynecological disorder.

We thought that if RMPs were trained to RTIs and STDs, it would bring the clients to the service providers. The woman would be the bridge. Without her, we would make no progress; rural Indian women would hesitate to discuss gynecological matters with a man, especially someone from their own village community. Now that the Titli Center has been around for some time, things have progressed a great deal. Women feel comfortable buying condoms. I am happy we got that right from the very start.

SHOPS

The major reason condoms and oral contraceptives did not penetrate into rural areas before Janani was not the scarcity of shops—it was the inherent disinterest among shop owners in stocking such low-cost, low-volume, and hence low-profit products. Consider a village whose population is 2,000. Even if all eligible couples in the village, under current levels of protection, bought condoms and oral contraceptives from one shop, the profit in a month would not be more than 2 rupees. This does not even buy a cup of tea.

Rural shops, particularly small village shops, do not have supplies brought to them by company salesmen, again for reasons of low volume. So village shopkeepers have to go and get their own supplies, usually from the nearest town with a wholesale market, two or three times a month. During my travels through rural areas, I would often see a man off-loading two huge bags from the bus and walking to his village with a heavy bag in each hand; periodically he would stop under a shady tree to catch his breath or share a smoke with a farmer. Women who run shops in villages have to do the same; they prefer to carry the loads on their heads. And for this reason goods cost a little more in village shops, to compensate for the transportation and effort put in by the shopkeeper. It is a service charge for bringing the commodity within reach of villagers. And villagers do not mind paying a rupee extra for, say, a packet of biscuits that is available right in their village.

One of the reasons why Janani chose RMPs as a vital component of the program was that they were linked with the market. An RMP would regularly visit the nearest town and procure his supply of antibiotics, injections, and sundry other things that he needed in order to dispense his medical practice from atop his bicycle in the village square. So the RMPs could easily buy contraceptive commodities during these visits. A traditional birth attendant was also another medical service provider who could be found in every village, but she would not have been as useful a member in the program because she did not have any link with the market.

Urban shops, on the other hand, functioned on entirely different principles. Here, salesmen of various companies came to the shopkeeper, took a list of the needed supplies, and later returned to deliver these. Manufacturers of high-cost, high-volume products did not bother to send their salesmen as they knew it was in the shopkeeper's interest to seek out their goods.

In the urban shops, low-cost nonclinical family planning products circulated within the trading system. Salesmen placed jars of condoms and oral pills on the shop shelves. Shopkeepers did not mind because, however little it might be, the profit came home without effort. The profits were not significant, but shopkeepers did not have to lift a finger to move these products.

Janani had the marketing organization up and going within about 4 months of getting permission from government of India. We established a network of distributors who bought the products in bulk. Janani sent specially appointed salespersons to the distributors who placed the products with retailers. This is the model in conventional social marketing all over the world. The government supplies the products to NGOs like ours. We then store them in our warehouses and appoint distributors in the area. Currently we have about 120 distributors who buy the products in bulk. The minimum shipment to them is 1 case containing about 5,000 condoms in jars. Distributors place their orders with us. From the distributors the products move to the retailers. We use the field force for that; the main job of the salesmen is to move the products from the distributors to the retailers. And the retailer is the one who sells to the consumers. The NGO publicizes this service so that the consumers become aware of it and patronize the retail shops.

When we started out, we created a brand called Apsara Oral Contraceptives. The pills were supplied by the government. We designed the packet and got the material manufactured and the packaging done at our end. We could not start with condoms because at that time there was a shortage and the government could not supply them to us. However, it was well that we started with oral contraceptives.

To let people know about Apsara, we had what is called a "teaser" campaign. We put posters all over Bihar with a picture of a woman and a caption that read *Itni khush kyun hai sajni* ("Why is my wife so happy?"). The brand name, Apsara, was announced at the bottom of the poster, but the ad did not say what the product was. We let the suspense build up. We pasted these posters on walls in villages. Because there was little clutter on the message platforms used for advertising, our poster drew a lot of attention. Visibility was high. Speculation grew as to what the poster meant.

Then, when we launched Apsara, we had the same photograph of the woman on the packet. When Apsara became available in the shops, the posters again had the same photograph of the woman with the same caption, but they now spoke of the product and answered the question of why the wife was so happy: she was happy because she could control her fertility. The campaign must have been quite effective, as there were brisk sales of our brand from the very beginning. We were quickly able to gain the trust of distributors, who had to invest in our products up front. Sales zoomed.

After the teaser campaign was over and Apsara products were in distribution, we had to think of other ways to let people know about our products. Advertising channels were very few for the target client we wanted reach in rural and semiurban areas. But I remembered that when I was traveling through the interiors of Bihar,

I noticed there were only two kinds of posters up—film posters and political posters. There was not much else. That gave us the idea to tie up with the film distributors.

The movie theater owners in the district towns would come to Patna 15 days before a screening and book the film they wanted to exhibit with the distributor, who then sent him the print. We printed posters for the film and asked the distributor to send them along with the film. The poster had the name of the film, the name of the theater, and the show times. At the bottom of this poster, we advertised our products. One third of the space was taken by our products and two thirds went into advertising the film. The theater owners were only too happy with the posters because we saved them the cost and trouble of printing.

We tried the same strategy at village fairs, printing posters for daredevil motorcycle and magic shows. It took us a while to understand the rural world and explore the avenues it offered. In the beginning, I lost some time because I was looking for the urban channels and felt frustrated at not finding them. This did not mean that no channels existed; I just had to open my eyes to the world around me.

Our condoms too did well from the very beginning, and the reason was quite interesting. We started marketing condoms once the government resumed supplies. We designed a packet, gave it a brand name, and launched it. Our condoms were way ahead of others because, unlike all other brands, whose packets showed provocative photographs of scantily clad women, we had an illustration of a charging bull, the symbol of male virility. Our packaging proved to be a good decision, because most shops could keep the transparent jars full of condoms on full public display; they were not embarrassed to do so, as in the case of other brands. Most of these shops in small district towns also have sons dropping in to give the shopkeeper a break for his midday meal. Having photographs of nude women on publicity material and products puts the father in a tricky situation. Mithun, Janani's brand of condoms, with a picture of a bull instead of nudity, did not compromise anyone.

These condoms and the pills were placed not just in chemist's shops. They were to be found at all the tiny kiosks that sold cigarettes, betel leaves, and tobacco and became popular among men. The salespersons also placed them in cosmetics shops. Standing amid glass bangles, creams, lotions, vermilion, and *bindis* (the intricate dots Indian women wear on their foreheads) would be jars of condoms or strips of pills dangling in prominent display. This prominence made it easier for people who felt hesitant, as most did, to buy them. They preferred to point to the condoms or pills rather than ask for them by name. Placing them in shops frequented by women not only gave those women greater access but also pushed sales. Today, Apsara and Mithun lead the market.

With shops, as with RMPs, our strategy was the same: to use whatever resources were available on the ground. We did not create any, nor did we "motivate" anyone to do something. *Motivation* is a word that is very popular with NGOs, but it is not practicable to go on motivating people to carry out their work-related responsibilities. How long can you sustain a repetitive activity on motivation alone? A person will do something because he or she stands to gain from it. In our case we are talking about monetary gain. We determined what would appeal to the self-interest of the people we identified as resources, the RMPs, and those involved in the marketing network, and made them stakeholders. Later, when we established the network of clinics all across the district towns of Bihar, we appealed to the self-interest of the doctors who were already running those clinics.

CLINICS

It was not difficult to find doctors with private clinics—the small towns of Bihar were teeming with them. We found that there were about 35,000 private doctors in Bihar, yet their contribution to family planning was negligible. Preventive services did not interest them because they were not lucrative enough. There was far more money to be made in curative services.

To get the doctors on board, Janani had to convince them that family planning procedures would become lucrative once there was a sizable patient load. We told them of the network of Titli Centers that would refer people to them and ensure a jump in the number of patients seeking family planning procedures.

In the end, what drew doctors to Janani was not so much the program as the 15-day training we offered in reproductive health—in female and male sterilization, abortion, the insertion of intrauterine devices (IUDs), and hysterectomy. It helped the doctors to acquire a new range of skills and new channels of income. Much more than any other component, it was the training in abortion and the certificate the doctors received for it that was the greatest attraction. Abortion is legal in India, but only a qualified doctor with government-approved training in abortion can do a medical termination of pregnancy (MTP). We trained them in clinical family planning procedures and linked them with a network of rural RMPs who brought in more patients and thus increased the doctors' incomes.

Here, as with the RMPs and our products, we created a brand image for the network of clinics. We called them Surya ("Sun") Clinics and customized them by painting the walls a uniform white and blue with an emblem of the sun on the signboard. And, as in the case of the Titli Centers, we charged Surya Clinics an annual fee as a franchise.

The Janani network of clinics was thus run by private qualified doctors who paid a fee to be part of the franchise called Surya Clinics. Once they became franchisees, they had to conform to Janani's standard of hygiene and cleanliness, which was strictly monitored. These clinics, as part of the Surya brand, offered standardized reproductive health services and charged rates prescribed and widely publicized by Janani. The Surya Clinic came to be perceived as a place where one could receive quality medical treatment at an affordable price. But we had to go through some rough and tumble before that happened.

We made a mistake early on: we were apprehensive that we would not have enough doctors with us, so we took in anyone who showed interest. We ended up establishing a total of 505 Surya Clinics. Sometimes there would be several Surya Clinics in a single town, often as many as seven. This became counterproductive, because the referral patients brought in by Titli Center RMPs were thus divided among these several clinics, which, of course, also reduced their income.

After 4 years, Janani has learned from its mistakes. We are restructuring the network to bring down the total number of clinics to 360, which are much better spread out. Now we intend to have only one Surya Clinic per town, which works out to an average of six clinics per district.

A typical Surya Clinic has anywhere from 80 to 150 RMPs attached to it, bringing in patients from their villages. Rajkishore regularly brings women from his village and its surrounding areas to the Surya Clinic located 2 kilometers from his own Titli Center. The patients he brings are mostly interested in sterilization, IUD insertion, or abortion. On occasion he also brings in women whose families have been persuaded of the advantages of trained assistance at the time of delivery, which they can find at the clinic.

In order for a rural family to take advantage of any of the Surya Clinic services, it is important that the price of these services be kept low. The doctor, on the other hand, has to see his clinic make a profit after paying for maintenance and staff salaries. The balance can be attained only if there is a large enough caseload. The increase in volume that the RMPs bring makes the clinic viable even with low prices.

There can be no comparison between a Surya Clinic and the doctors' clinics in district towns as far as quality of service is concerned. The latter do not even adhere to accepted standards of treatment and hygiene. Often, it takes time to persuade poor villagers that it is worthwhile to go to a qualified doctor, but once such patients visit one of the clinics in our network, they will come back again and again and also bring members of their families. A clinic coordinator, appointed by and accountable to Janani, is placed with each franchisee Surya Clinic to enforce standards of cleanliness and hygiene, monitor infection control, do promotional work in the catchment area, and troubleshoot for the doctor. He also makes sure the RMPs are paid their commission each time they bring in a patient.

The cleanliness and the efficiency of the treatment are the winning factors.

In addition to the franchisee clinics, Janani has established its own Surya Clinics in key towns and cities. These clinics set the standards of hygiene and treatment for the entire network. They serve as a benchmark.

As soon as a patient enters a Janani-owned Surya Clinic, he or she is given a slip to hold that notes the presenting ailment and other details. When the person's name is called, the doctor examines him or her, writes down the tests needed, and directs the patient to the lab. The tests are done there and then. With the results, the patient goes back to the doctor for proper consultation.

A very large percentage of Surya Clinics' patients are poor. Not all of them are educated, as they often work as domestic help, as mechanics or mechanics' helpers, rickshaw pullers, vegetable vendors, and the like. Janani made sure that even as it went for quality, it did not make the ambience intimidating for patients of modest background, who feel comfortable at the clinics and have access to quality treatment there. Surya Clinics are popular because they are one-stop shops. It is often difficult to ask a poor patient to go elsewhere to get tests done. That is one of the main reasons why qualified doctors lose patients to unlicensed medical practitioners, who do not bother with tests at all in order to retain the patients. They are even known to write prescriptions for malaria or tuberculosis without pathological confirmation.

Whether it is a Janani-owned or a franchisee Surya Clinic, publicity is as important here as it was for our branded condoms and contraceptive pills. It lets people know that what they need or are looking for is to be found at these clinics. Surya Clinics are well advertised on the government-owned All India Radio, which has a near total listenership in rural areas. The district towns are also dotted with billboards and posters prominently advertising the clinical procedures people can undergo at Surya Clinics and at what cost.

Advertising the services with their costs not only informs people but also empowers them. Their knowledge of the costs serves as a monitoring tool. Franchisee clinics must think twice before overcharging patients, so as not to lose their trust. Patients are well informed as a result of widespread advertising; they can easily inquire why they are being charged more than the advertised rate.

When a new Surya Clinic is set up, Janani organizes a female sterilization camp, which runs for 3 or 4 days. This creates tremendous publicity in the whole catchment area. RMPs go from house to house to tell families about the sterilization camp. Cycle rickshaws are commissioned, with an announcer whose job is to inform people over a loudspeaker about the sterilization camp. The main draw at these camps is the extremely low cost of 20 rupees (50 cents) for a tubal ligation, requiring only a small incision. Outside of a camp, the procedure would cost 499 rupees in a Surya Clinic.

From a distance such a camp could be mistaken for a wedding. Colorful tents are put up on the terrace of the building; hired mattresses are lined up in rows, and here the women are brought to recover after surgery. They spend the night there; a female relative also remains to nurse them back to consciousness and help them through the night. In the morning the team of doctors, who have been brought in by Janani to handle such a large number of patients, examine the patients before releasing them. The stitches dissolve in a week.

After every sterilization camp there is steady increase in the number of patients visiting the clinic.

I devised these sterilization camps with the women of Lalpur in mind. I remember how they wanted me to help them gain access to quality clinical procedures. They were even willing to pay up to 1,000 rupees for such a service. It is not easy for humble farmers or their spouses to pay such a large sum, and these camps answered their needs.

The demand for family planning procedures is so high in Bihar that our periodic exercise in female sterilization camps is mere tokenism. The Surya Clinics cater to the middle segment of a semiurban and rural population that can afford to pay. But beyond that there is a huge cross-section of the population that remains underserved. They have almost no access to quality treatment, as the government's health delivery system in Bihar is in complete disarray. It is not able to serve the poorest of the poor, who need the nearly free service that the government system is supposed to provide.

Janani could make these clinical services available to this segment, but only when the government looks at Janani as an opportunity that can be utilized. We do not have the resources to absorb the cost, especially if we have to get this done through franchise. Using devices like coupons and vouchers, Janani could meet the needs of the poorest, even the very poor women in remote villages. If such a woman had a coupon that permitted her to access service from any Surya Clinic, the doctor could treat her without cost and later be compensated by the government.

People in families that are below the poverty line already have ration cards for buying wheat, rice, and sugar at subsidized rates. I am quite optimistic that one of these days the government will agree to a partnership with Janani to bring quality services deeper into the poorest rural areas of Bihar and its neighboring state of Jharkhand.

In the past 9 years Janani has made condoms and contraceptives widely available in these two states. It is now among the largest public/private networks delivering family planning and reproductive health care in India. Janani has, in nine years of programming, had averted 5.52 million unwanted births. In 2005 alone, the program protected 1.68 million couples in reproductive union, averting 962,000 births.

Now when I look back, I ask myself how we survived the challenges of operating in Bihar. Many of the warnings we received in the beginning were accurate. Bihar's main problem was corruption. Not a single file moved without lining pockets. Corruption was rampant particularly at the time when we were starting out. In response, we made our norms all the more stringent. We made it a rule that every single payment would be made by cheque. We also made sure we never paid any bribe to get our work done. We knew that once you start on that road, there is no end. If we started paying bribes, the amount would have to be falsified on our books. And that becomes a chink in the armor, it makes you vulnerable. Our fundamentals, we made sure, were strong.

If Janani was able to reach out to a large percentage of the people who needed its services, if Janani was able to build a program relevant to the vast underserved sections, it was because we were good listeners. Every so often there is a mismatch between what people want and what development agencies offer them. We made it our priority to understand what it was the people were asking for. I never did go back to Lalpur, I admit, to find out if the three pregnant women we met that day had been able to access sterilization in one of the camps we organized. But Janani owes much of the structure of its program to the impassioned articulation of their need. And if we succeeded in doing what we set out to do, it is because we listened to what those women were saying. We made sure that we understood the problem well before we attempted to offer a solution.

11   "Returned to Sender": Corruption in International Health in Nigeria

Benjamin C. Mbakwem and Daniel Jordan Smith

Almost everyone who works in international health has experienced the problem of corruption. Yet remarkably few firsthand accounts have studied the contexts and complex dynamics that facilitate it. Rarely do reports honestly address the shared complicity of public health practitioners—including expatriates, host government officials, and civil society actors—in perpetuating these practices. We believe that people who pursue international health as a vocation and a career would benefit by confronting more openly how well-intentioned people and organizations both wittingly and unwittingly participate in corruption and find innovative ways to navigate around it in order to achieve their more noble objectives.

In this chapter we offer an up-close account of these issues through the story of public health work in Nigeria and in particular of our experiences with international and local nongovernmental organizations (NGOs). Our perspective is that corruption is a real problem for the successful implementation of public health programs but that it is also widely misunderstood. The obsession with the "problem" of corruption obscures the extent to which western donor organizations and the expatriates who work for them in places like Nigeria are among the primary beneficiaries of these international health programs. The large dollar salaries, air-conditioned project vehicles, and posh capital city residences of many foreign aid workers are authorized and legitimized in official program budgets, but the local project fieldworker who hires some of his kin to carry out a survey and an administrative officer who steers a contract for office supplies to a friend who says "thank you" with a gift are branded as corrupt. We are, of course, aware of tremendous venality on the part of local elites, many of whom avail themselves of the budgets of internationally funded health programs as if they were their personal funds. This fact is part of the story, but so too are the pressures that well-meaning people feel to participate in "corruption" in health programs.

Ours is a story of friendship, collaboration, and a shared commitment to combating Nigeria's multiple health crises. We intend this to be a humble story. Neither of us has changed the face of public health in Nigeria or elsewhere. We have not led an effort that eradicated an entire disease from a continent; we did not single-handedly change a country's laws and approach to women's reproductive health. Unlike many of the authors in this volume, we cannot be labeled as heroes in the fight for global health. Our sense of humility is also the outcome of our experience that we have often been, mostly unwittingly, agents in perpetuating some of the very practices that sustain the inequalities we find so troubling. Part of the story we want to tell is about the problem of translating good intentions into good outcomes, and we view that problem through the complexity and conundrums of corruption.

Although the story we share here is both troubling and humbling, we also intend this to be a hopeful account. We have enjoyed immensely our work together and we believe that we have made some difference in the lives of the people we work with. Despite the fact that each of us has experienced great frustrations—as well as some painful soul-searching—in trying to reduce the suffering created by Nigeria's health inequities and facilitate measurably better outcomes, we have experienced tremendous satisfaction as well. We tell our story through the lens of corruption, even though we could tell it in many other ways, because it is instructive with regard to the issues we think are most important for people envisioning or training for a career in international public health or reevaluating such a career. In particular, a focus on corruption highlights the inequalities between donors and recipients, the role of culture in both obscuring and enabling the structures and behaviors that perpetuate inequality, and perhaps most important, some ways in which we have managed to navigate this complex terrain both successfully and unsuccessfully.

We first met in the mid-1990s in Lagos, Nigeria's largest city, while Benjamin was a program assistant working for the U.S.-based nongovernmental organization Africare and Dan was conducting dissertation research in southeastern Nigeria for a doctorate in anthropology. Dan had worked for Africare from 1989 to 1992, advising a child survival project in Imo State. Benjamin is a native of Imo State. Because of our common experiences with Africare and in the region, we had much to talk about. Below, we each narrate a version our work in Nigeria, focused on our encounters with and understandings of corruption and the lessons we feel we have learned, which speak, we think, to both the pitfalls in international collaboration and its possibilities.

EXPATRIATES, INEQUALITY AND CORRUPTION (DANIEL)

After 3½ years as a Peace Corps volunteer in Sierra Leone working in a primary health care program, I received a master of public health degree from Johns Hopkins

University. Upon graduating from Johns Hopkins, I got my first "real job" as the project advisor for Africare's child survival project in Nigeria in 1989. It was during the 3 years working for Africare that I became much more attuned to the problem of corruption but also to the ways in which prevalent views of corruption in the donor community tended to blame the victim and elide the role of expatriates and international organizations in a phenomenon we so easily condemned.

The Africare child survival project was funded by the United States Agency for International Development (USAID). I was based in the Imo State capital of Owerri, a small city that had few foreigners and no expatriate development community. But during the several trips a year I made to Lagos to meet with my supervisor and with officials from USAID and other development agencies, I recall having numerous conversations with expatriates, where the favorite topic was Nigerian corruption. Ironically, little is said about corruption in official development settings and in program documents. Indeed, most development agency documents paint a remarkably rosy picture of their projects and portray relationships between donors and recipients as equal and successful partnerships. But in more informal settings, both the problems with internationally funded projects and the true perceptions that expatriates have of their partners are often revealed. At parties and over drinks and dinner at the expensive restaurants in Ikoyi and Victoria Island, the upscale areas in Lagos where the development and diplomatic communities entertained themselves in the early 1990s, expatriates told seemingly endless stories of Nigerian corruption.

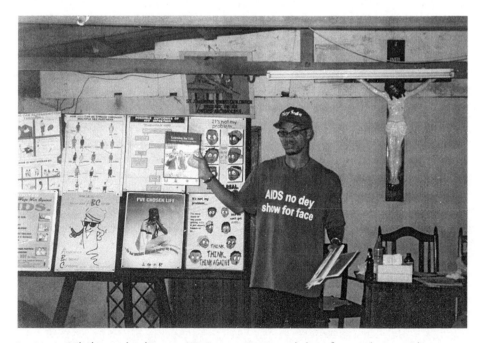

Benjamin Mbakwem leading an AIDS prevention workshop for youth in southeastern Nigeria.

These stories included cases where Nigerians working in internationally funded development organizations secretly hired relatives, steered agency contracts to friends, created ghost workers, submitted fake receipts, or just plain stole project money. For example, over dinner at an expensive Indian restaurant in Lagos, an American official at USAID told a story of how a very senior Nigerian staff member in his office hired her son in a midlevel position. The son managed to work at USAID for almost 2 years during which no Americans discovered this relationship, in part because mother and son had different surnames. In telling the story, the American official emphasized that other Nigerians in the office had known about the situation and had colluded to hide what the American regarded as nepotism. The tenor of the story and the laughter it produced in the all-American audience reinforced an "us" against "them" mentality that frequently surfaces in expatriate discourse about corruption.

I feel obliged to emphasize that in many expatriate circles, the kinds of issues I am raising here, such as the misplaced perceptions of foreigners or the failures of development projects to benefit the neediest populations, were common topics of concern and conversation. But it is the manner in which even the most seemingly culturally sensitive expatriates could be sucked into prevalent assumptions about the dynamics of corruption that is most insidious and most revealing about the powerful ways in which prevailing patterns of inequality are reproduced and tightly intertwined with corruption.

A few examples of the kinds of things that worried me when I worked as a project advisor suffice to illustrate how presumptions about Nigerians' corruption infused my thinking and my actions. I report them because I have come to believe that my experience was not unique. Many expatriates who work for development organizations in Nigeria and in other developing country contexts embark on their work full of good intentions but frequently end up participating in discourses and practices that contribute to the maintenance of inequality and the reproduction of stereotypes about the corruption of Third World partners.

The primary strategy of our project was to improve child survival. We would do this by raising mothers' knowledge and promoting health-protective behaviors through the training of village health workers, who would work directly with mothers in their communities. This strategy meant that our staff spent a lot of time in the intervention communities, organizing the training of village health workers and supervising their work. When our program officers would go to the intervention communities to train the village health workers, I wondered whether they always paid the trainees the full amount of the per diems allocated. They often came back late in the evening, and I sometimes suspected they had used the project vehicles for personal purposes. Occasionally, I would later ask a village health worker how much she had been paid for the training or ask a driver whether the team had come back directly from the field site.

The project had a number of vendors who regularly provided us with services—for example, the mechanics who repaired our cars, the printer who produced many of the materials used in project training and monitoring activities, the technician who serviced our photocopiers, and the vendor who provided our office supplies. I sometimes suspected that these vendors had reciprocal relationships with the senior staff. On a couple occasions I checked prices on things on my own to try to make sure that we were getting a fair deal. The reality was that my Nigerian colleagues could almost certainly negotiate better prices than I could, but I wondered whether they also got small kickbacks or favors from our biggest vendors. In truth, I never discovered any significant corruption on the part of our staff, and I am not sure exactly how I would have handled it if I had.

In hindsight, it is now much easier to see that I was not, in fact, a watchdog against corruption but a culpable and complicit actor in the whole enterprise of development-related corruption. By any conventional western standard I could not be reasonably accused of involvement in corruption. But if I examine my life as an expatriate working for a development project critically, it becomes clear that my vigilance regarding corruption among my Nigerian counterparts involved significant hypocrisy. My assumptions, my privileges, and my lifestyle were at least as morally problematic as anything I feared my Nigerian colleagues might have done with project resources.

It is not my intention to make a confession. I relate these personal stories because I believe that they represent common patterns of inequality and self-justifying perceptions of appropriate behavior on the part of many expatriate development workers. First and foremost, the hypocrisy of expatriates who criticize Nigerian corruption is evident in the inequality that characterizes the differences in economic position between expatriate staff and even the most senior local staff. For example, when I started as the Africare's expatriate project advisor in 1989, I was paid a salary of $23,000 per annum. Even in 1989, that was a very modest salary by American standards. Indeed, Africare had a reputation in the development community of being stingy about salaries. But consider the following: the Nigerian project manager, who was supposed to be my counterpart and whose job description gave her authority at least equal to if not superior to mine, was paid less than $400 per month. In other words, she made less than a fifth of what I did, although by "Nigerian standards," her salary was very good. The project's other personnel were paid much less, with the watchmen making as little as $50 a month. Further, I was provided free housing by the project, and because my project-provided house was inside the NGO compound, the office generator supplied my fully furnished house with electricity when there was no town power supply. The project's watchmen looked after my house at night, and the project's compound supervisor doubled as my steward, helping me with shopping and cooking, cleaning my house, and washing my laundry.

Compared with the palatial quarters of expatriates working for bigger agencies like USAID or UNICEF, my house in Owerri was relatively humble. Many expatriates' houses are far more luxurious than anything they could afford in their own countries. Further, no expatriates working in public health earned salaries that could, in their home countries, support the drivers, stewards, cooks, and watchmen that were routine benefits of working in developing countries. I remember feeling particularly empowered controlling a fleet of vehicles. Before I left Nigeria, our project had acquired four cars for our work, and at the end of each day all of the keys were handed over to me. In off hours I used those vehicles for my personal purposes, and I was especially fond of our white Toyota Landcruiser—a vehicle that has become the mobile symbol of international aid worldwide. I can remember times when I would argue with our Nigerian project manager about whether the Ministry of Health should be allowed to commandeer our vehicles for their purposes—suspecting that the commissioner for health was more interested in a nice ride than actually supporting an immunization exercise, for example. But I somehow managed to ignore the hypocrisy of my own all too happy use of the vehicles to meet my Nigerian friends for an evening of tennis.

Of course very few westerners would take a job in Nigeria for less than $400 a month and with accommodations equivalent to those of local counterparts. Maybe as a Peace Corps volunteer, but not as a development "professional." Further, it would be impossible for organizations like Africare to implement programs in places like Nigeria if local staff were paid salaries at American levels. But what is rarely discussed are the cultural assumptions and mental blinders necessary to sustain a system of inequality wherein my time is worth at least 5 times as much as that of a more senior Nigerian colleague and more than 25 times as much as the night watchman who has 10 children to feed. Part of the context of understanding western culpability, and in this case my own complicity, in sustaining Nigeria's notorious corruption is recognizing the peculiarity of a system that legitimizes my privilege but is on the lookout for a local staff person who awards a contract to provide office stationery to an in-law to help a struggling business or might terminate a driver who carries passengers for a fee in the office vehicle on his way back from an assignment in order to raise some extra cash for his children's school fees. These actions are viewed by westerners as forms of corruption. But the larger system of inequality is taken for granted, at least by most of us who are its principal beneficiaries.

I went back to school for a doctorate in anthropology partly in reaction to my growing frustrations with the realities of working in international public health. But by the time I had finished my doctorate and embarked on a career as a professor, I was hungering for opportunities to make some kind of practical difference. Enter Benjamin.

Benjamin and I had shared many discussions about the challenges of public health and development in Nigeria. I knew that he wanted to take his growing skills and use them to address more directly the burgeoning HIV/AIDS epidemic in his native Imo State. We had talked about Benjamin's dream of starting an NGO through which he could assist young people at risk of HIV infection, especially urban youths who had dropped out of school and were struggling to survive through various forms of employment and trade apprenticeships or participation in the informal economy. When I learned from a friend that the Ashoka Foundation—a unique organization that makes 3-year grants to "social entrepreneurs" to help them put their innovative ideas into practice—was restarting its program in Nigeria, I encouraged Benjamin to apply. Benjamin was awarded an Ashoka fellowship and founded a local NGO, Community and Youth Development Initiatives (CYDI), in 2001.

Benjamin and CYDI have, for the past 7 years, been engaged in numerous excellent projects in Imo State, including working with a large number of youths in the marketplace and in the informal economy by taking advantage of the guild-like associations run by the businessmen and women who hire these young people. CYDI also established the first and most popular HIV/AIDS counseling and resource center in Owerri, and they helped form the first support group for people living with HIV/AIDS, working directly with the only antiretroviral treatment program in the region. Benjamin and CYDI are widely respected by state and local health officials. He or his organization has been regularly hired by government and by agencies like UNICEF to run educational and training programs. By many measures, CYDI is a tremendous success.

Yet CYDI has never received a grant larger than $30,000—indeed, its $30,000 project has been by far the organization's largest. I have no doubt that Benjamin and his staff could do more excellent work if they had access to greater resources. The story of CYDI's struggle for funds is partly a story of corruption—both in the mechanisms of Nigerian government and in the ways that donors contribute to and are complicit in keeping money flowing in directions that benefit the "haves" more than the "have nots." Benjamin can tell this story much better than I can.

FACING UP TO CORRUPTION IN PUBLIC HEALTH PROJECTS (BENJAMIN)

Early in 2007, CYDI was hired by one of the state ministries in Nigeria to provide HIV/AIDS training to the ministry's community extension workers. We signed a contract for about half a million naira (approximately $4,000) to carry out the training activities. When we were paid for our work, we received a check from the government for only 300,000 naira. When we inquired about the outstanding balance, we were told that the remaining funds had been "returned to sender," local slang for a kickback on a contract that went to the official(s) who awarded it. We lamented the loss of funds but realized that any effort to contest the arrangement would jeopardize future contracts from the government. Such realities are part of what my countrymen commonly call "the Nigerian factor," a euphemism for corruption. It has been one of the challenges of working to address a major public health crisis in Nigeria.

Since 2001 I have spent most of my waking hours focused on the HIV/AIDS epidemic in Imo State, where I and my ancestors were born. In Owerri, the state capital where I live and where CYDI has its headquarters, many people know me as the man who works with AIDS. Indeed, I have become so associated with the disease that when my friends and clients who are HIV-positive invite me to a wedding or a funeral, I caution them that my presence might signal that someone involved is living with (or has died from) HIV/AIDS. Because the stigma associated with AIDS continues to be strong, I often demur and decline such invitations in order to protect people's privacy. Fighting HIV/AIDS has opened my eyes to many realities in Nigeria. The story of our national battle against this disease is a window onto many dimensions of the problems that plague efforts to raise the quality of life for ordinary citizens.

When I meet my friends from secondary school and university days, they wonder how I got to where I am now. In those days I had a reputation as a bit of a ruffian, an image I suppose I cultivated by keeping a collection of live reptiles in my dormitory room. In Nigeria, reptiles—particularly snakes—are generally feared, and the idea that someone would purposely keep them, much less handle them comfortably, evokes a combination of revulsion and respect. In some ways I suppose my affinity for snakes prepared me for my current work, because my work with people living with HIV requires confronting and overcoming popular misconceptions and prejudices about the disease and its victims.

As Dan has already explained, I worked for several years for Africare in Lagos. In my various capacities as a program and administrative officer, I learned a great deal about the business of development. I certainly feel that I owe many people a great debt for the skills and perspectives they shared with me. But in time, I came to feel that I needed to work more directly with my people. Although I respect the motives and am grateful for the help provided by many of the expatriates and organizations that work to provide public health and other developmental assistance to Nigeria, I also found that reliance on foreign aid can promote a climate in which we do not take responsibility for our own problems. This certainly seemed to be the case with HIV/AIDS. When I would visit my home region, AIDS was often spoken of as a foreign disease—even to the point where some people thought foreigners either made it up or deliberately infected African people. But the reality of people getting sick and dying and the failure of donor-supported interventions to stem the tide contradicted the belief that this was not really a Nigerian problem.

One of my own relatives died of AIDS, and I learned of other people I knew who were sick and dying. I became convinced that any effective effort to address HIV/AIDS would require a truly local response. Much as we may need the assistance of other governments, international NGOs, and so on, until we adopt HIV/AIDS as our responsibility, I do not think we will make real progress. It was this conclusion that led to the excitement I felt when Dan showed me the information about the Ashoka Foundation and encouraged me to apply. I very much wanted to return to southeastern Nigeria to start dealing with the growing epidemic. But it was no simple matter; if I quit Africare, I would have no income. Although my family is not as poor as many in my country, my father died some years ago and there would be no money without work. I kept my job at Africare while the Ashoka Foundation application process unfolded, and when I was fortunate enough to win a fellowship—after spending many hours in interviews explaining my vision for CYDI—I quit and returned to Owerri to start the work.

Together with my girlfriend, Oby, who would later become my wife, we launched CYDI from a small cubicle we rented in the upstairs offices of a local bookshop. Using just the funds from Ashoka, which were really meant as a stipend to the fellow and not for carrying our programs, we started with a project designed to reach young men who were apprenticed to automobile mechanics. In Nigeria, young men and women are commonly apprenticed to "masters" and "madams" to learn artisanal or commercial trades. These young people are typically school dropouts who have not completed a secondary school education. In Owerri, as in much of Nigeria, mechanic workshops are located in a "mechanics' village," where hundreds of mechanics have their small sheds. The young men who work as apprentices frequently sleep in their masters' workshops at night. We know from our work with them that they constitute a powerful peer group for each other and that they frequently spend their small wages on commercial sex. Our aim was to educate them about HIV/AIDS while also providing them with business skills that would enhance their value to their masters and enable them to be more successful when they launched their own workshops.

Our initial effort was plagued by many problems that I think are best explained by the pervasive culture of corruption that characterizes aid efforts in Nigeria. The first obstacle we faced was that the masters did not believe that we could be implementing our project purely for the benefit of them and their apprentices. We were not promising them any significant resources. Therefore, they doubted our legitimacy and suspected that we might be using our project with them to enrich ourselves—a common reality in Nigeria. When Dan brought two American students to Nigeria that summer, I thought that having him and his students visit the leaders of the mechanics' village might confer some legitimacy on our project and convince the masters to be more cooperative. In this strategy I was playing on the common perception in Nigeria that "real" aid programs are supported by expatriates—an idea that is related to both the imagined amounts of money involved and a somewhat common belief that foreigners are more likely to provide aid that will reach the intended beneficiaries. This latter perception is fueled by the extent of corruption in Nigeria but is complicated in reality by the kinds of issues Dan has described about the ways in which donors and expatriates are rewarded unequally via legitimized structures.

I invited Dan and his students to visit mechanics' village, and Dan spoke to the leaders. At one level, the strategy worked. The mechanics and their apprentices viewed our project with new respect—or, perhaps more accurately, with a new appetite. But this new desire to participate in our activities led to further problems. The mechanics' village is divided into two different unions, a fact that did not much inhibit our work when we had trouble stimulating interest. But after we were associated with foreigners—and therefore dollars—our little project became entangled in competition between these two groups. We managed to run some successful workshops for the apprentices and, perhaps most important, many of the apprentices learned of our work and our office, enabling them to come for individual counseling when they became concerned about their HIV status. But we learned a lot about the pitfalls of running even a small-scale health education project in the context of the tremendous problems and presumptions of corruption that permeate public health programs and other development initiatives in Nigeria.

As already mentioned, at first most of our activities were supported through my Ashoka Fellowship and through consultancies I would get to do training workshops for UNICEF and other agencies working on HIV/AIDS in Nigeria. We had yet to find a source of money to wean us off dependence on my small Ashoka stipend. In 2001, the World Bank loaned Nigeria approximately $90 million to fight HIV/AIDS. The money was targeted to benefit 18 states, including Imo State. The Imo State Action Committee on AIDS (SACA) used part of its multimillion-dollar portion of the loan to support the work of NGOs working to combat HIV/AIDS. In 2004, the Imo SACA issued a request for proposals through which local NGOs could compete for grants of up to $30,000 to finance their activities. At best, no more than a handful of NGOs in Imo State had been doing any serious work on HIV/AIDS in the previous decade. But the SACA competition attracted 79 applications, including many from organizations created purely in order to apply for the World Bank/SACA grants. The SACA grant-awarding process highlights how the corruption endemic in the aid apparatus in Nigeria affects even those with the best of intentions.

At CYDI we conceived and wrote a strong proposal for the SACA grant competition, building on our experiences with the mechanics to work with adult male traders and their young apprentices in the timber, building materials, and related trade sectors in Owerri's markets. If we won a $30,000 grant, it would be the largest amount of money CYDI had ever had to work with. The Imo State AIDS coordinator, who frequently consulted me for advice, indirectly assured us that funding CYDI would be one of SACA's highest priorities. The 79 applications would be reviewed by a technical committee appointed by the Ministry of Health, but the state coordinator said he was sure that our proposal would rank at or near the top. I joked with Dan that because of all the help I gave the state coordinator, I might not even be expected to subtract the typical "returned to sender" portion from the grant.

In the weeks leading up to the proposal deadline in October, I was deluged with requests from other local NGOs wanting help with their proposals. Even though they would be my competitors, I provided help to all that I believed were engaged in legitimate efforts. I was also bombarded with appeals from people who wanted to start NGOs in order to compete for the money. In those cases I simply referred them to the SACA office, where the proposal application was available. The proposal's guidelines stated that to be eligible for the World Bank money, competing NGOs had to have been registered with an appropriate federal or state bureaucracy for at least 3 years. A colleague informed me that all the newly formed

NGOs were getting backdated registration certificates from an official in one of the state ministries, who seized an opportunity to address the new demand for 3-year-old registration certificates.

I provided help on two proposals where I felt I had no choice but to assist if we wanted CYDI's project to be funded. The state coordinator came to me requesting help with a proposal for his own NGO; he also pleaded that I assist him with a proposal on behalf of the Imo State governor's wife. She wanted to use the $30,000 to support AIDS orphans, a seemingly noble gesture, except that actually identifying such orphans conclusively has proved notoriously difficult in Nigeria, where continuing stigma means that few families will openly admit that one of their own has died from AIDS. The governor's wife asked the state coordinator to write her proposal, and he passed the task to me. The state coordinator practically begged for my help, saying, "I don't want to lose my job." Who could blame him? He was doing very well for himself as the state's AIDS coordinator. I helped craft these proposals and ensured that, at the very least, they met the criteria of the proposal guidelines, but I was skeptical about the efficacy and sustainability of the governor's wife's plan to aid orphans.

The proposals were reviewed in November 2004 by a technical committee, a group made up mostly of academics from the local universities. After a week at a resort hotel and with consultant payments of approximately $100 a day (a sizable sum in Nigeria, even for the relatively well off), the technical committee presented its ranking. The first lady's project ranked first and was praised by the technical committee's chairman in a press release. The state coordinator's NGO was also among the 10 slated for funding. Our CYDI proposal did not rank in the top 10. It fell in the second 10, and by the original SACA criteria, it would not be funded. I was crestfallen. I knew that some of the NGOs that were going to get the money existed only on paper.

The state coordinator seemed genuinely shocked and embarrassed that CYDI was not ranked in the fundable category. He had just assumed that our proposal would rank at or near the top, and he had not really monitored the review process. In the end, he initiated a course of action to get the second tier of high-ranking proposals funded, and CYDI eventually received a portion of the World Bank money. But so did 15 other NGOs, and some of them appeared not to be the least bit credible or capable (and perhaps had no intention) of carrying out effective HIV/AIDS-related projects. Our experience illustrates a common pattern in Nigeria, where aid dollars flow in ways that further corruption as much as (or more than) they promote their ostensible public health and development objectives.

While there is little doubt that foreign donors and the governments of developing countries manage aid in ways that enable and perpetuate corruption in public health, I would be remiss if I did not acknowledge and try to explain something about how recipients—in our case ordinary Nigerians—also contribute to the dynamics that sustain corruption. One example from our work at CYDI is particularly revealing.

Not long after we started CYDI in Imo State, the Federal Medical Center in Owerri became one of the pilot sites for the implementation of Nigeria's initial program to deliver antiretroviral therapy to people living with HIV/AIDS. As we had experience in counseling, we worked closely with doctors running the clinical program to try to organize social support systems for people on therapy. In this effort I helped a number of people in the treatment program start the first support group for people living with HIV in Imo State. The group, called the Association for Positive Care (AsPoCa), met once a month on one of the main clinic days when people came to the hospital to collect their antiretroviral drugs.

In many respects, helping to form AsPoCa was one of the most gratifying achievements of our first years of work at CYDI. In Nigeria, the vast majority of people who know they are HIV-positive learn of their status because they are sick and are tested by a doctor on the basis of their symptoms. The testing of people who are not obviously sick is uncommon. As a result, most people receiving antiretroviral therapy have learned of their status only fairly recently. In the context of the stigma still associated with the disease, it is difficult for people who are HIV-positive to decide whether and whom to tell about their status, to manage their treatment when many people in their lives do not know they have HIV/AIDS, and to adjust to the reality of their illness; these are extremely challenging propositions. It was obvious to any observer that the gatherings with fellow sufferers offered welcome opportunities to share anxieties, relate common experiences, seek advice, and benefit from collective support.

Over time, however, it became clear that AsPoCa would encounter many problems. Significant conflicts emerged within the group over leadership. Gender inequalities similar to those in the wider society created problems for women in the group, both with regard to adequate representation in leadership and in terms of sexual harassment. The conflicts in the group were the result not only of interpersonal and gendered dynamics but of the emerging awareness that the group might be able to attract resources from the government or international donors. These issues came to a head during the competition for World Bank/SACA money described above.

CYDI had helped AsPoCa to register as an NGO precisely so that the association could become viable and independent. With our help, AsPoCa crafted and submitted a proposal for the $30,000 grants. In the process, significant rifts occurred in the group, and some members left to form their own support group, driven largely by competition to control possible government and donor resources. AsPoCa was funded under the World Bank/SACA mechanism, and since it received its grant, I have heard numerous complaints about how the leadership spent the money. In Nigeria, it is always hard to judge the veracity of accusations of corruption. On the one hand, experience demonstrates that corruption is extremely common, so that one is predisposed to believe such accusations—based as much on the presumption that corruption is ubiquitous as on the merits of the evidence. On the other hand, allegations of corruption are the common currency of complaint and are just as likely to be made by those who want greater control to facilitate their own malfeasance. Regardless of the relative integrity or culpability of the accusers and the leaders, it has been striking how deeply embroiled AsPoCa has become in the machinations of corruption.

None of these stories is reason to cease our work, or even, I think, to conclude that external aid for public health and development is a failure. I would argue that, in various ways, each of the programs, projects, and activities described here has contributed positively to addressing the HIV/AIDS epidemic in Nigeria. Our work with the mechanics' apprentices, and since then with young men and women in other trades in Owerri, has introduced knowledge, spurred dialogue, and created access to counseling, testing, and services that were unknown to these populations previous to our projects. Despite the fact that the World Bank/SACA grant competition awarded money to questionable organizations and projects, they also funded many worthy groups and activities. Although the internal politics at AsPoCa have become more strained with its formal establishment as a registered NGO and the consequent access to resources, the support group continues to provide an invaluable and irreplaceable forum for people who might otherwise feel alone in their misfortune. Our experiences at CYDI do not amount to failure, but they do suggest that people committed to careers in international health must be realistic about the obstacles that exist.

CONCLUSION: SOME SHARED THOUGHTS (BENJAMIN AND DANIEL)

From both an expatriate and a local point of view, we have experienced the realities of corruption in the implementation of public health programs in Nigeria. These problems are not unique to Nigeria, nor are they peculiar to public health programs. Far from casting any particular aspersions on Nigeria, we think that our experiences reflect much broader realities and that the lessons are applicable across a wide range of contexts. The primary lesson, in our view, is that the dominant structures and taken-for-granted practices in international health often play a role in facilitating and perpetuating corruption to the detriment of public health. While donors and their international expatriate (mostly western) implementing partners are often quick to locate corruption in the culture and practices of recipient countries and local people, in our experience forms of inequality that are legitimized in the current system can be just as pernicious as the practices that are more commonly labeled as corrupt. But we also recognize that corruption exists at multiple levels, including in the world of local NGOs. Ordinary Nigerians—like people elsewhere—participate in activities that reproduce the very patterns of corruption that operate to their overall detriment.

We cannot offer any magic solutions to these difficult problems, but we can say that we have found our collaboration extremely fruitful. Partly, we each feel that the perspective of the other keeps us more honest, so to speak. We both agree that there is more than enough blame to go around when it comes to the responsibility for corruption in public health and developmental activities. We are both sensitive to the fact that we can too easily become complicit in the very processes that we recognize to be harmful to the people most in need of better public health services and outcomes. We have also learned from our work that we—and we think others—can do better work when we confront these issues openly and realistically, asking ourselves regularly whether we are really doing the right thing.

12   Betinho: Celebration of a Life in Brazil

Jane Galvão

I am part of a group of people in Brazil who for many years have combined the world of academia with political activism and which have refused to accept HIV and AIDS as givens for marginalized groups. Together, through the creation of health policies, we confronted the disease, and we never accepted that a virus could have sexual preference, confine itself within borders, respect socio-economic status, or religion orientation.

But I am getting ahead of myself; I believe it is impossible to speak about the struggle for prevention and treatment of HIV and AIDS in Brazil without paying homage to the work of Herbert de Souza, known to most simply as "Betinho." The fight for adequate and equal health care, and Betinho's life and death, are two stories deeply intertwined.

In the 1960s and 1970s, for nearly two decades of Betinho's life, Brazil was governed by a repressive military regime. Like many others, Betinho became active in the student movement, fighting against the military rule. He was a part of the nucleus that formed the political organization Ação Popular (Popular Action), a primarily Catholic group that focused on social justice issues within the country. Betinho fought for basic reforms in the public health and education systems; he also worked with the Ministry of Culture and Education.

As the 1960s drew to a close, the level of repression from the government increased in intensity. In 1971, Betinho, along with many other activists and artists, went into exile. He first went to Chile, where he served as an advisor to President Salvador Allende, who was deposed by the military in 1973. Betinho escaped the bloody coup by seeking asylum in the Panamanian embassy; he then lived in Panama for 5 months. In 1974 he went to Canada, where he pursued his doctorate in political science, and in 1978 to Mexico. During this period, Betinho, together with other Brazilians living in exile, continued fighting to bring democracy back to Brazil. By the late 1970s, the pressure for change had intensified in Brazil. Betinho's name, which was well known because of his earlier activist work, became a symbol in the campaign calling for the return of those in exile. A popular song of the time, O *Bêbado e a Equilibrista* ("The Drunk and the Tightrope Walker"), mentions Betinho specifically as it dreams of the day of the exiles' return. Betinho returned to Brazil in 1979. As the dismantling of the regime was taking place in the early and mid-1980s, many of the former exiles, including Betinho, began to form organizations to address the socioeconomic inequalities affecting the country. A new agenda for issues such as education and health began to take shape, and the prodemocracy movement was, therefore, from the beginning, inextricably linked with activism surrounding health and social issues.

In 1981, shortly after his return to Brazil, Betinho helped to found the Brazilian Institute of Social and Economic Analyses (IBASE) in Rio de Janeiro. IBASE was where Betinho's office was located and where he thought through his ideas and actions. His office at IBASE was perfectly representative of his passions and of the work to which he devoted his life. The walls were covered with photographs, cut from magazines and newspapers, relating to various social movements, and caricatures of him drawn by local artists. In the caricatures, Betinho's nose and ears are enormous, the bags under his eyes in prominent shadow, the eyes themselves full of kindness and light. There were also colorful posters, each representing one of the many campaigns in which he was involved. Betinho conveyed an informal leadership style, and he treated everyone he came across equally, from cleaners and factory workers to CEOs and influential politicians. He was also a model "executive" in meetings, tending to avoid excessively long discussions and quick to make decisions. He had, in general, a very positive demeanor, with an occasionally biting sense of humor, and was often self-deprecating. He had a small refrigerator in one office and would often invite his colleagues to share a beer during meetings, which lightened the mood and made the gatherings more enjoyable even when dealing with difficult subject matter.

In 1986, Betinho learned that he had been infected with HIV from a blood transfusion, which, along with his two brothers, Chico Mario and Henfil, he received periodically for hemophilia. All three men had acquired the virus. In 1986 Betinho founded the Brazilian Interdisciplinary AIDS Association (ABIA), a nongovernmental, nonprofit organization, and was its president until his death in 1997. It was with ABIA, as its executive director from 1993 to 1999, that I worked most closely with Betinho. The organization was intended to take action against the spread of the epidemic by creating awareness of the disease and mobilizing Brazilian society as well as by advocating for the rights of people living with AIDS. ABIA's first headquarters were located on a quiet street in the middle-class Botafogo neighborhood of Rio de Janeiro; they were in a building so modest that the name of the organization seemed bigger than its office space. Although ABIA was small initially, there was always a flurry of activity inside the tiny headquarters. Later, in August 1992, ABIA moved to downtown Rio de Janeiro to be closer to the target populations of the various interventions and outreach projects that ABIA was developing and executing. The center of Rio is a meeting zone between the richer southern district and the northern and western regions of the city, which are traditionally poorer. It houses a collection of establishments patronized by gay community members, female and male sex workers, and the Afro-Brazilian community, which increases accessibility of the ABIA to these populations, and vice versa.

At the time of the ABIA's beginnings, the federal and state response to AIDS in Brazil was characterized by denial of the epidemic's severity. The Brazilian media, as in other countries including the United States, were complicit in this reaction, and mentions of the disease in newspapers treated it as if it were something affecting only homosexuals. As a hemophiliac, Betinho had a different understanding and used the newly created ABIA to promote public awareness of the disease.

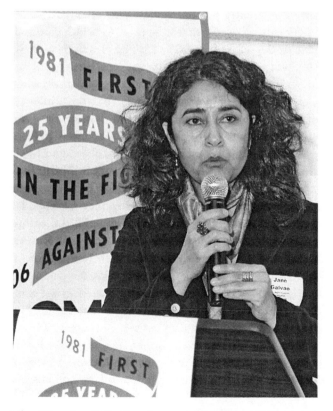

Jane Galvão at the "Drawing It Out" cartoon exhibit. The exhibition opened at the United Nations in New York City on World AIDS Day, December 1, 2006. (Photo credit: Donna Aceto.)

The label of "risk groups" was very popular at the time and served only to further marginalize people such as sex workers, gay men, and injecting drug users; an important part of ABIA's agenda was to increase access to information on AIDS and HIV for the general public. It was difficult for the public sector to connect with the health-care movement surrounding AIDS; the media portrayed the disease as connected to particular population groups and therefore as not a public health problem.

To highlight the HIV infection among hemophiliacs as an indicator of a problem facing the public health system, in 1988 Betinho, through ABIA, launched a massive campaign called Save the Blood of the Brazilian People. In order to rally Brazilian citizens to this cause and dispel the myth that those in certain "risk groups" were the only people susceptible to HIV, Brazil needed a human face of HIV/AIDS. Betinho knew which face to use– his own. He spoke in public about acquiring HIV and talked openly to the media about the disease and the difficulties of living with HIV/AIDS.

Betinho's story made people realize that the transmission of HIV could happen through the blood supply. The timing of the highly publicized campaign was excellent, because the country was preparing a new constitution. The new Brazilian constitution guaranteed every citizen the right to health care and also included measures prohibiting the sale of blood. The Unified Health System (SUS, or *Sistema Único de Saúde*) was established in 1988 and was structured to provide free comprehensive health care to the entire Brazilian population, whether or not an individual had another form of health insurance. The constitutional guarantees to health care and the creation of the Unified Health System came about as a result of mobilizations of health professionals, academics, and new political parties. The creation of the SUS was a fundamental step for the subsequent implementation of the policy of free and universal access to AIDS drugs in Brazil. And activism and societal input to the new constitution was essential to both developments.

Betinho had universal appeal: he brought together Catholic leaders and gay activists, international donor organizations and hemophiliacs, anthropologists and doctors. These partnerships led to invaluable contributions to the debate on sexual diversity and sexual and reproductive rights and their intersections with the HIV/AIDS epidemic. Betinho was concerned not only with the disease but also the social dimensions, with trying to catalyze community awareness and action. He wanted to bring together very diverse groups to confront the epidemic. This was reflective of Betinho's deep investment in Brazilian politics and society. He was never advocating for only himself or his own cause; rather, he was always looking for ways to make Brazilian life more decent and just. This also had the benefit of giving him a broader social legitimacy in advocating in relation to HIV and in seeking out AIDS-related contributions.

Despite the new constitution, by the early 1990s, not only was the number of AIDS cases being underreported but hospital care for AIDS patients was lackluster in Rio and other cities. There were not enough beds to accommodate the number of people who needed hospitalization. At this time, the only treatment available was zidovudine (AZT), and that represented an improvement in terms of the number of deaths from opportunistic infections. These had been very high *before* AZT, but ultimately there were still many, many people who were very sick and in need of hospital care.

Betinho steered ABIA to call attention to the failure of the health authorities to mount an effective response. A favorite saying of Betinho's at that time was, "We cannot accept the theory that if the foot is too big for the shoe, we should cut the foot to size. The shoe is what needs to be changed." He strove to do just that by seeking to implement more inclusive public health policies. Betinho publicly challenged, in the media and at events, the individuals responsible for Brazil's federal AIDS program and the AIDS program in the state of Rio de Janeiro.

In 1991, Betinho and I sat together in a meeting with the coordinator of the AIDS program for the state of Rio de Janeiro. At that time I was working on AIDS-related issues through a nongovernmental organization (NGO) in Rio de Janeiro called the Institute of Religious Studies. One of the institute's projects was a program called Religious Support against AIDS, which aimed to work with different religious groups in Brazil in order to promote solidarity with people living with HIV/AIDS (PLWHA).

The coordinator seemed to us to be a very sincere man, soft-spoken and kind. However, programs for both AZT distribution and prevention were much weaker than we thought they could be, and one of the results was that very few Rio hospitals were equipped to actually receive and care for AIDS patients. As a large state, Rio was important to us in terms of strengthening HIV surveillance—monitoring the number of infections as well as the care and treatment of those who had acquired the virus. The city was the second largest in terms of AIDS cases in Brazil, a fact Betinho pointed out, and a good policy in Rio could potentially serve as an example for the rest of the country.

I sat next to Betinho as he outlined these circumstances, emphasizing his words with the rise and fall of his hands. As he spoke, his luminous green eyes bore down on the coordinator. His cane leaned against the armrest of his chair and, despite his gaunt appearance, his speech was full of vigor. He was not rude or aggressive; that was not Betinho's style. Instead, he demanded that the AIDS coordinator *do* something about the problems, making it clear through his voice where he thought responsibility lay. When the man finally cut Betinho off and responded as we had anticipated, with defensiveness, Betinho leaned back in his chair and listened. The man launched into a detailed speech about all of the obstacles that he faced, referring to budget constraints, the difficulty of implementing training in hospitals, and finally his own inability to tackle the problem alone. He threw his arms up in the air, in mock helplessness, and Betinho, along with the rest of us in the room, watched him go on and on. When the man finally paused and took a deep breath, Betinho leaned his frail body forward again and trained his powerful gaze on him.

"*This*," he said, "is why *you* are here. You are the person in charge of this program. You need to do something. The NGOs can help you, and we can collaborate, but this is *your problem*."

As he spoke, I found myself saying *yes, yes,* along with him in my head. Betinho refused to let the man excuse away his inaction. I looked at a few of the other activists who were in the room; from the expressions on their faces, it looked as if they were having similar thoughts. This encounter was typical for Betinho: he was expressing many of our frustrations in his eloquent and powerful way, and as always he was trying to systematize discussion surrounding the problem. He saw his role as one of creating awareness and increased pressure, so that action would be taken at the highest levels possible.

Looking back on this meeting, I can see Betinho's drive to increase the availability of care for HIV-positive citizens as a precursor to the meeting that would take place, almost 2 years later, with Paul Wolfenson, President of the World Bank. In 1992, Wolfenson and his staff expressed interest in meeting with members of Brazil's NGOs. The meeting was informal, and there were no more than 15 of us waiting in a small conference room at the top of one of the luxury hotels that punctuate the Rio de Janeiro skyline. Groups with different matters of focus were represented—as I looked around I saw people whose organizations worked for the improvement of health, literacy, environment, and other issues affecting Brazilian society.

Like myself, there were a few others who worked on matters surrounding HIV and AIDS. One of them, sitting next to me, straight up in his chair, eagerly awaiting Wolfenson's arrival, was Betinho. His wild gray hair seemed ready to fly from the top of his head, and his bushy eyebrows were raised in anticipation as he looked around the room.

When Wolfenson walked in a few moments later, he circled the room, shaking hands and making introductions. He was a jovial-looking man, with thick, wavy, salt-and-pepper hair and a round face. He was followed by two staff members and a translator. As Betinho reached across me to shake the president's hand, I could feel his energy gathering and growing.

Although I would not begin working for him until a year later, I knew well the reasons why Betinho viewed this meeting with such importance. Major development institutions such as the World Bank were known to grant funding in poorer countries for AIDS prevention work, but they refused to recognize the value of funding AIDS medications for the public. At that time the World Bank believed that, given limited resources, funds should be directed to prevention in order to limit the number of new infections. The primary arguments against allocating funding to "developing countries," including Brazil, for the purchase of medications were the costs and implied financial trade-offs as well as concerns about poor patient adherence to the treatment, which, they argued, could potentially result in the development of new strains of drug-resistant HIV.

The result was that in Brazil and other places those medications initially were available only to those who could afford them. Although the government's Unified

Health System was already passing out medications to patients, the quantities of drugs available were directly related to the limited amount of money Brazil had to spend on them. As Betinho had written in an article that appeared in the *Boletim Abia*, "to live or to die, in great measure, depends on the treatment that already exists. Those who have access survive. Those who do not die. In life, your bank account is charged, but death makes us all equal." At the time of the meeting with Wolfenson, Betinho had already begun to advocate militantly for increased access to AIDS medication, which was then primarily AZT, so that the drug would be available to all who needed it. He knew well that this kind of change could happen if minds could be changed at the national level of government in Brazil and at the international level in the funding priorities of the World Bank.

Betinho's frustration with the World Bank went far beyond the bank's policies on AIDS. He was upset by the drastic cuts in social services caused by the austerity measures (known as "structural adjustment") that were being imposed on Brazil and many other nations as conditions of loans, credits, or debt relief. Like many in the room, Betinho argued for a deep transformation of the bank's policies and practices so that the development process would become more democratic and accountable.

As Wolfenson began the meeting, he spoke of wanting to see change in the agenda of the World Bank. He was interested, he told us, in learning as much as he could from key NGOs, like the ones represented in the room, to help the bank distribute funds more successfully. As he was talking, I reached into my bag, where I had a copy of Betinho's book *The Cure of AIDS*, a bilingual publication (in Portuguese and English), with articles written on HIV and AIDS. I passed it to Betinho, hoping he would take my hint and present the book to Wolfenson.

He did. When there was a pause in the conversation, Betinho brought the book out and scrawled an inscription across the title page. With the other NGO members looking on in approval, he announced that the book was a gift, a resource for Wolfenson. Betinho gave the book directly to him, and the president flipped it open immediately. Upon seeing that the dedication was in Portuguese, he handed it to the translator, who read it over silently, then cleared his throat. "To Mr. Wolfenson," he began. "For the cure of AIDS and the cure of the World Bank."

All of us present at the meeting chuckled at this, but few of us were surprised. Betinho was like that; he never gave up the opportunity to "convert" a nonbeliever, even with such a reluctant and powerful entity such as the World Bank. And his risky move had been worth it: the World Bank's representative in Brazil paid Betinho a visit that very evening, and they talked the entire night through, not just about HIV and AIDS medications, but about poverty, hunger, land—all of the issues Betinho cared so much about.

Another way that ABIA was able to catalyze action was through the judicial process. Under Betinho's leadership, the organization began in the late 1980s and early 1990s to help HIV-positive citizens hold the Brazilian government to its constitutional promise of providing health care by suing either the state or the city in

which they lived. This worked to some extent: in 1988, medicines to treat opportunistic infections began to be distributed through the health system, and in 1991,
AZT began to be offered. However, not all who needed the medicines were able to
get them, and lawyers and doctors were brought together to work on the cases of
individual patients.

Through ABIA, Betinho financially supported the creation of a separate organization, called Pela VIDDA (For the Valorization, Integration, and Dignity of People with AIDS), serving to assist with the legal issues. Another important figure of
this time, Herbert Daniel, was working with ABIA and had an important role in
the creation of Pela VIDDA. As a militant of the gay movement in Brazil—and,
when he returned to the country from exile, a key figure in the creation of the
Green Party—Daniel gave voice to demands for protecting the civil rights of PLWHA.
Decrying what he defined as the "civil death" of PLWHA—the violation of the
rights of those with AIDS—he described the degree of prejudice and discrimination that those with AIDS had to face. The creation of Pela VIDDA gave more visibility to PLWHA and their needs. Daniel died in 1992, at age 45. That same year,
the book *AIDS in the World*, edited by Jonathan Mann, Daniel Tarantola, and Tho-
mas Netter, was published and was dedicated to Daniel in recognition of his role in
the promotion of rights for PLWHA. Pela VIDDA helped organize the lawyers and
doctors who would work together on patient cases. In many instances, by the time
the final decision was handed down in the courtroom, the patient had died. Many
lawsuits were brought against the health-care system, and the judges often ruled in
the patient's favor, citing the constitution. The lawsuits incorporated the language
of human rights and the strategic application of national laws—such as the Brazilian Constitution – to further place the health of people living with HIV and AIDS
on the political agenda and set an invaluable precedent for the Brazilian government's distribution of AIDS medications in 1996, when combination antiretroviral
therapy was announced.

While tirelessly pursuing government accountability for public health, Betinho
at the same time increasingly sought funding from the private sector in order to fill
the vacuum of systematic health care in the AIDS epidemic. Although he continued to push for government responsibility in the care and treatment of AIDS and
HIV patients, he recognized that the social work around the issue could and should
be done in part by private funding. By the early 1990s, there were many large corporations in Brazil, including Xerox, the Companhia Vale do Rio Doce (one of the
world's largest mining groups), and Petrobrás, the national oil company. Under
Betinho's direction, ABIA began to campaign aggressively toward them and other
members of the national business community. Betinho's reputation, in combination with his charisma, helped open doors for meetings with senior management at
these companies, and his persuasive skills established many new partnerships.

Betinho's desired response from big business was twofold: he wanted the private sector to assume social responsibility through financial contributions to ABIA
and other AIDS organizations but also to implement prevention programs in the

workplace and to offer comprehensive treatment for HIV-positive employees. These efforts culminated in the establishment of the "Solidarity Is Big Business" program, which led these major companies as well as others in Brazil to implement health-care programs for employees and prioritize corporate funding to AIDS- and HIV-related programs. ABIA established relationships of solidarity with these companies and could then rely on the partner company's political and financial support. In turn, the companies were ensured that their names would be well publicized in connection with preventing HIV and AIDS. The companies were happy with the positive exposure they received, and soon even more were successfully recruited. The program had the added effect of further publicizing the health crisis caused by AIDS and thus put even more pressure on the government to provide health care for affected citizens.

In 1996 came the announcement of antiretroviral (ARV) therapy. It was a combination of two or more medicines and largely replaced monotherapy, which was primarily AZT. Although AZT had been distributed by the government for 5 years at that point, the new ARVs ushered in new hope for a significant decrease in the number of deaths of people living with HIV and AIDS as well as reductions in hospitalization and treatment costs associated with opportunistic infections. Very quickly, ABIA and other organizations pushed for the distribution of ARVs free of charge. In November of 1996, President Fernando Henrique Cardoso signed a law establishing the free distribution of AIDS medicines, including ARVs to HIV-positive Brazilian citizens.

This did not mean that anyone needing the medications was immediately given them. Although many people did benefit quickly from the new medication combination, Betinho himself included, Brazil had to obtain mass quantities of these expensive drugs before the government could begin to distribute them. As the decade progressed, the number of Brazilians receiving ARV medications rapidly increased. In 1997, an estimated 35,900 people received the medications at no cost via the Unified Health System; only 4 years later, 105,000 people were receiving ARVs, and in 2007 approximately 200,000 people were receiving them. The amount of money the Brazilian government spent on the medications followed a similar upward trend: in 1996, approximately $34 million were spent on the drugs, and in 2001, $232 million were spent. From the perspective of the government, the program was worth the money, because the drugs did, in fact, prove to reduce HIV/AIDS-related mortality and reduce in-hospital admissions and treatment costs associated with opportunistic infections

The increase in spending on AIDS medications created concern about less funding for other needs of the Unified Health System. Citing the high costs charged by the international pharmaceutical companies, on several occasions Brazil has threatened to break the patents on certain ARVs if companies do not lower prices. Such a measure, called compulsory licensing, would be admissible under Brazilian patent law; it would prove to be an important negotiating tool in the country's efforts to lower drug prices over the following decade. The Brazilian Constitution's Article 68, for example, requires that foreign-owned products be manufactured in Brazil for 3 years before receiving a patent. If a foreign company fails to comply, a Brazilian company can then be allowed to begin production of the drug in order to fulfill a need.

From the beginning, however, Brazil favored methods of lowering the costs of the ARVs mainly by producing them domestically; Brazil's national production of ARVs occurred primarily in state-run laboratories but also in privately held ones. By 1999, some 47% of the country's ARV medications came from domestic firms and 53% from international pharmaceutical companies. By 2001, Brazil was producing 7 of the 13 ARVs that were needed. The remainder were still being bought on the international market and, citing the high costs charged by the international pharmaceutical companies, Brazil's government began to threaten to break patents via compulsory licensing if the prices were not reduced. Although Brazil had signed in 1996 the World Trade Organization's (WTO) TRIPS (Trade-Related Aspects of Intellectual Property Rights) Agreement, a treaty that established standards for intellectual property (including pharmaceutical patents) for exchange between WTO members. The Brazilian patent law allowed the country, under the circumstances mentioned above, to issue a compulsory license for medicines for domestic use. This provided the grounds on which to defy the international pharmaceutical companies. In February 2001, the Brazilian government announced that it was considering invoking compulsory licensing for the drugs nelfinavir (produced by Roche) and efavirenz (produced by Merck) if these companies did not lower their prices. Merck agreed to lower the cost of efavirenz by 60%, but negotiations with Roche proved futile, and in August of the same year the Brazilian government announced its intentions to break Roche's patent and produce nelfinavir domestically. A few weeks later, Roche agreed to cut costs significantly.

Brazil's willingness to threaten and use compulsory licensing of drugs has evoked both challenges and support. Also in 2001, after the Roche and Merck negotiations, the WTO received and accepted a request from the United States for a panel to begin questioning Brazil's use of compulsory licensing, essentially challenging the country's patent laws on behalf of American-based pharmaceutical companies. Later that same year, the UN Human Rights Commission approved a Brazilian-proposed resolution that established as a basic human right access to medical drugs during pandemics. Soon after, the United States withdrew the WTO panel against Brazil, and in November 2001, the WTO released the Doha Declaration, which allowed compulsory licensing in cases of national public health emergencies.

In 2004, the Brazilian National AIDS Program announced that it had successfully negotiated even greater reductions in the prices of nelfinavir and efavirenz as well as the drug lopinavir. Up to that point, the three drugs had, in combination, been consuming 63% of the budget for acquiring ARVs. The new prices are estimated to have saved Brazil almost $100 million that year. By 2005, when the number of available ARV medications had reached 15, Brazil was producing 8 of the drugs domestically. Had Brazil been required to supply patented imports, the cost of ARVs to Brazilian citizens would have been 32% higher. In May of 2007, Brazil signed a compulsory license that allows the country to make or import a generic version of the drug efavirenz.

These statistics highlight the relative success of the Brazilian distribution program thus far. Although very specific international circumstances had put Brazil in the position of producing and distributing ARVs to its people, the history of activism in Brazil must not be discounted, as it has played an equally important role. The current success of Brazil's distribution program for ARVs can be traced directly back to the 1980s, when popular pressure combined with progressive political forces to create a national health-care system based on the principles of universal access and comprehensiveness. These principles, in turn, shaped the development of the health-care system, and with continued activist pressure, the advocacy of the Brazilian government on behalf of its people in the international bargaining sphere.

Betinho was one of the many Brazilians who benefited from the new drugs. However, he spent less than a year taking ARVs; in 1997 he contracted hepatitis and had to stop taking the AIDS medications owing to their adverse effects. He grew frailer than he already had been and became increasingly ill. In a letter that he asked to be delivered to his wife, Maria Nakano, upon his death, he referred to her as his "cocktail" and wrote that "without her, I would have long ago been up in the São João Batista cemetery, suffering the coldness of eternity." In August of that year he died at home in his bed, surrounded by Maria, his family, and his friends. At his request, he was cremated, and his ashes were scattered in the mountainous region of Itatiaia, Rio de Janeiro.

His death came before the international controversy between pharmaceutical interests and the Brazilian government really began, but I know if he were here today, Betinho would feel pride at the role of leadership Brazil has taken in the international discussion surrounding AIDS treatments and human rights. The one prediction that Betinho made incorrectly about AIDS was in regards to its duration—he had predicted that ABIA, as an institution, would not be necessary after a few years, because by that time, either a cure for AIDS would have been found or the public sector's response to the disease would be so effective that organizations such as ABIA would no longer be needed. But ABIA is still needed, and although the Brazilian response to HIV/AIDS has been successful, the country's policy must continue to be analyzed in terms of sustainability and to ensure that past success does not turn into future complacency. Although Betinho would be proud, he would also still be adamantly pushing for more; he would seek out ways in which the Brazilian health-care system could be improved, and he would be fighting fervently for human rights on a global level. He is not here to witness AIDS in the new millennium, and I know that he would be furious to learn that the medical coverage of entire continents, such as Africa, is being left to chance. Betinho would argue that it is necessary to remain vigilant in regard to human rights, particularly for the rights of those who are most vulnerable.

Betinho loved to illustrate his points with fables and stories. When he shared his favorite tales, his face became animated with expression. On of his favorites was this:

> There was a fire in the forest, and while all the animals ran in fear, a little hummingbird went from the river to the fire carrying drops of water in her beak. The lion, seeing this, asked the hummingbird, "Oh, Hummingbird, do you think you will succeed in putting out the fire all by yourself?" And the hummingbird replied, "I do not know if I will succeed or not, but I am doing my part."

Betinho dreamed of human possibility. His philosophy was like a reconstruction of the Brazilian singer Milton Nascimento's line "blind faith with a sharpened knife." In the case of Betinho, it would be faith with a sharpened wit. Above all else, Betinho emanated the rare, profound, and unshakable faith that the world could be changed, the economy could be fixed, those responsible for public health could learn and become more competent, and the cure for AIDS would one day be discovered. As anyone who worked with Betinho knows, he was in a hurry. It was not the hurry of someone who was simply impatient; it was the hurry of someone who denied complacency and knew that prompt action is a requirement when one is working to transform structures of inequality and oppression. Richard Parker, who worked with Betinho, has vivid memories of him, many not related to AIDS. They are linked to things like the campaign for ethics in politics, the broad civil society coalition that Betinho helped to build in order to work for the impeachment of the corrupt government of the Brazilian President Fernando Collor. As Richard Parker remembers, what stands out most minds is the march through the main street on the plain where the government buildings in Brazil stand, when literally hundreds of the most important figures in Brazilian civil society marched to deliver a letter to Congress demanding Collor's impeachment. There was Betinho at the front, with the head of the OAB (the Brazilian order of lawyers) and other similar civil society groups. He was a very frail man—he weighed just 45 kilos (100 pounds) and would get winded easily. But there he was on that march, at the front, in the hot sun, making his way forward awkwardly– there was always some fear among us that he could stumble and fall because his movements were difficult and seemed painful. He was the first person to take the steps up the ramp leading into the Congress building that day, carrying the letter in his hand. It is this vision of Betinho, his combination of frailty and force of will, that reminds me so much of the determined hummingbird of his story. Nobody could watch Betinho in action without feeling a huge sense of respect for all that he embodied.

Over the course of several years, Betinho went from a persona non grata to an icon of the Brazilian National AIDS Program. After his death for some years, his image greeted visitors to the program's website. Betinho found out, in his unique way, how to leave his legacy by building a more just nation and world. These contributions had several central themes: solidarity, social justice, partnership, democracy, and ethics. Betinho invited all Brazilians to discuss these themes, thinking about our responsibility to make the world a better place for everyone and living and taking action to make this happen.

ACKNOWLEDGMENTS

I would like to thank the people who sent their comment, which have enriched this article: John Garrison, Global Civil Society Team, World Bank, Washington, DC.; Dulce Pandolfi, Director of the Brazilian Institute of Social and Economic Analysis (IBASE) and Researcher at the Historical Research and Documentation Center at the Getúlio Vargas Foundation, Rio de Janeiro; Richard Parker, Chair of the Department of Sociomedical Sciences in the Mailman School of Public Health at Columbia University, New York, and President of the Brazilian Interdisciplinary AIDS Association (ABIA); and Veriano Terto Jr., Executive Director, ABIA.

CITATIONS AND REFERENCES

FOREWORD

1. We reviewed this data in Walton, D.A., Farmer, P.E., Dillingham, R. (2005) Social and cultural factors in tropical medicine: Reframing our understanding of disease (pp. 26–35). In: R.L. Guerrant, D.H. Walker, P.F. Weller (Eds.), *Tropical Infectious Diseases: Principles, Pathogens, and Practice* (2nd ed). New York: Elsevier.
2. See: Farmer, P.E., Becerra, M. (2001) Biosocial research and the TDR agenda. *TDR News* 66:5–7; Farmer, P.E. (2001) *Infections and Inequalities: The Modern Plagues* (2nd ed). Berkeley: University of California Press; Farmer, P. (2000) Social medicine and the challenge of biosocial research (pp. 55–73). In: Innovative Structures in Basic Research: Ringberg-Symposium 4–7 October 2000. Munich, Germany: Generalverwaltung der Max-Planck-Gesellschaft, Referat Press und Öffentlichkeitsarbeit.
3. These are discussed in: Farmer, P.E., Robin, S., Ramilus, S.L., Kim, J.Y. (1991) Tuberculosis, poverty, and "compliance": Lessons from rural Haiti. Seminars in Respiratory Infections, 6(4):254–260.
4. Walton, D.A., Farmer, P.E., Lambert, W., Léandre, F., Koenig, S.P., Mukherjee, J.S. (2004) Integrated HIV prevention and care strengthens primary health care: lessons from rural Haiti. *Journal of Public Health Policy*, 25(2):137–158.
5. These battles are discussed in the 2006 Preface to: Farmer, P.E. (2006) *AIDS and Accusation: Haiti and the Geography of Blame* (2nd ed). Berkeley: University of California Press.

PART 1: HEALTH AND DEVELOPMENT

1. Institute of Medicine. (1988). *The Future of Public Health.* Washington, D.C.: National Academy Press.
2. Institute of Medicine. (2003). *The Future of the Public's Health in the 21st Century.* Washington, D.C.: National Academy Press.
3. Barnes, Louis B., C. Roland Christensen, and Abby J. Hansen. (1994). *Teaching and the Case Method.* Boston: Harvard Business School Press.
4. Lynn, Laurence E., Jr. (1999). *Teaching and Learning with Cases.* New York: Chatam.
5. Boehrer, John, and Marty Linsky. (1990). Teaching with cases: learning to question. In Marilla D. Svinicki, (Ed.)., *The Changing Face of College Teaching.* San Francisco, CA: Jossey-Bass.
6. Funded by the Ford Foundation's "Crossing Borders" initiative.
7. Packard, Randall, and Peter J. Brown. (1997). Rethinking Health, Development, and Malaria: Historicizing a Cultural Model in International Health. *Medical Anthropology, 17,* 181–194.
8. Bud, Robert. (2007). Antibiotics: the epitome of a wonder drug. Retrieved June 11, 2007, from BMJ 2007: http://www.bmj.com/cgi/content/full/334/suppl_1/s6#REF1
9. Birn, Anne-Emanuelle. (1996). Public health or public menace? The Rockefeller Foundation and public health in Mexico, 1920–1950.VOLUNTAS, 7(1), 35–56.
10. World Health Organization. (n.d.) *Smallpox.* Retrieved June 11, 2007, from World Health Organization Media Center Web site: http://www.who.int/mediacentre/factsheets/smallpox/en/
11. Henderson D. A. (1982). A successful eradication campaign: discussion. *Reviews of Infectious Diseases, 4,* 923–924.
12. Gladwell, M. (2002). Fred Soper and the global malaria eradication programme. *J Public Health Policy, 23*(4),479–97.
13. Gish, Oscar. (1979). The political economy of primary care and "health by the people": an historical exploration. *Social Science and Medicine, 13C,* 203–211.
14. Navarro, V. (1984). A critique of the ideological and political position of the Brandt Report and the Alma Ata Declaration. *International Journal of Health Services, 14*(2), 159–172.
15. PAHO. (2005). *Renewing Primary Health Care in the Americas.* New York: Pan American Health Organization.
16. The Alma Ata Declaration defined primary health care as "essential health care made universally accessible to individuals and families in the community by means acceptable to them, through their full participation and at a cost that the community can afford" (WHO/UNICEF. 1978 Report of the International Conference on Primary Health Care, Alma Ata. ICPHC/ALA/ 1978.10. (Quote from page 2.)
17. Social medicine seeks to understand the interrelationship between health, disease and social condition.

18. Navarro, V. (1984). A critique of the ideological and political position of the Brandt Report and the Alma Ata Declaration. *International Journal of Health Services, 14*(2), 159–172.
19. Morgan, Lynn. (1987) dependency theory in the political economy of health: an anthropological critique. *Medical Anthropology Quarterly, 1*(2), 131–154.
20. Otis, Laura. (1999) *Membranes: Metaphors of Invasion in Nineteenth-Century Literature, Science, and Politics*. Baltimore: Johns Hopkins University Press.
21. Brown, Peter. (1987). Microparasites and macroparasites. *Cultural Anthropology, 2*(1), 155–171.
22. Birn, Anne-Emanuelle. (2005, August 6–12). Gates's grandest challenge: transcending technology as public health ideology. *Lancet, 366*(9484), 514–519.
23. Easterly, William Russell. (2006). *The White Man's Burden: Why the West's Efforts to Aid the Rest Have Done So Much Ill and So Little Good*. New York: Penguin Press.
24. Asthana, Sheena. (1993). Primary health care and selective primary health care. In D. Phillips and Y. Verhasselt (Eds.), *Health and Development*. London: Routledge.
25. Ugalde, A. (1985). Ideological dimensions of community participation in Latin American health programs. *Social Science and Medicine, 21*(1), 41–53.
26. Heggenhougen, H. K. (1984). Will primary health care efforts be allowed to succeed? *Social Science and Medicine.* 19(3), 217–224.
27. Asthana, Sheena. (1993). Primary health care and selective primary health Care. In D. Phillips and Y. Verhasselt, (Eds.), *Health and Development*. London: Routledge.
28. Walsh, J. A., and K. S. Warren. (1979). Selective primary health care: an interim strategy for disease control in developing countries. *New England Journal of Medicine, 301*, 967–974.
29. Brown, Theodore, Marcos Cueto, and Elizabeth Fee. (January 2006). The World Health Organization and the Transition From "international" to "global" public health. *American Journal of Public Health, 96*(1), 62–72.

CHAPTER 8: APPLYING GLOBAL LESSONS TO SYRACUSE, N.Y.

1. Passages of the chapter come from my book: Lane, S. D. **(2008)**. *Why are our babies dying? Pregnancy, birth and death in America*. Boulder, CO: Paradigm Publishers. These passages are used with the permission of the publisher.
2. Board on Health Sciences Policy, Institute of Medicine (2003). *Unequal treatment: confronting racial and ethnic disparities in health care*. Washington, DC: National Academies Press.
3. Lane, S.D., & Rubinstein, R.A. (1996). "International health: problems and programs in anthropological perspective." In T. Johnson & C. Sargent (Eds.), *Medical anthropology: contemporary theory and method* (2nd ed., pp. 396–423). Westport, CT: Praeger.

4. I calculated the maternal deaths during the twentieth century using vital records data on births and the estimates of maternal deaths in (1) Achievements in public health, 1900–1999, healthier mothers and babies, *MMWR*, 1999;48(38): 849–858, and (2) Maternal mortality—United States, 1982–1996, *MMWR*, 1998; 47(34):705–707. The source for military deaths during the twentieth century was First measured century, PBS: http://www.pbs.org/fmc/book/11government8.htm. Based on these sources, my estimates of the two causes of death during the twentieth century are as follows: maternal deaths = 978,885; military deaths = 440,000.

5. "There are also records of a debate whether a woman who had died in giving birth should be buried on the church graveyard if she had died unchurched. Popular custom occasionally had another woman undergoing the ceremony for the woman who had died, but such practice was not favored by the church. It was eventually decided that an unchurched woman could be buried, but in a number of cases they were buried in a special part of the graveyard and superstitious belief had it that women between 15 and 45 were not supposed to be going to that particular part of the graveyard," [Franz, p. 241]. Franz A. (1909). Die kirchlichen Benediktionen im Mittelalter. Freiburg, Germany: Herder. See also Coster W. (1990). Purity, profanity and puritanism. The churching of women, 1500–1700 (pp. 377–387). In: W. J. Sheils & D. Wood (Eds.), Women in the church. Oxford, UK: Blackwell.

6. Royal, C. D. M., & Dunston, G. M. Changing the paradigm from "race" to human genome variation. Nature Publishing Group, http://www.nature.com/ng/journal/v36/n11s/pdf/ng1454.pdf.

7. Lane, S. D., Cibula, D., Milano, L. P., Shaw, M., B. Bourgeois, B., Schweitzer, F., et al. (2001). Racial and ethnic disparities in infant mortality: risk in social context. Journal of Public Health Management and Practice, 7(3), 30–46.

8. Carter, E. J. Jr. (2008) *ESF projects aim to revitalize american cities.* Available at http://fla.esf.edu/people/faculty/carter/revitalize.htm.

9. Fumkin, H. (2005), Guest editorial: Health, equity, and the built environment. *Environmental Health Perspectives 113*(50), A290–A291; Bashir, S. (2002). Home is where the harm is: Inadequate housing as a public health crisis. *American Journal of Public Health*, 92(5), 733–738; Kreiger, J., & Higgins, D. (2002). Housing and health: time again for public health action. *American Journal of Public Health 92*(5), 758–768; Cohen, D., Spear, S., Scribner, R. et al. (2000). Broken windows and the risk of gonorrhea." *American Journal of Public Health,* 90(2), 230–236.

10. New York State Department of Health (2004). *Eliminating childhood lead poisoning in New York State by 2010.* Albany, NY: NYS Department of Health. All analyses by the author.

11. Mauer, M. (1999). *Race to incarcerate.* New York: The New Press.

12. Lane, S. D., Rubinstein, R. A., Keefe, R., Freedman, M., Levandowski, B., Cibula D., et al. (2004). Marriage promotion and missing men: African American women in a demographic double bind. *Medical Anthropology Quarterly,* 18(4), 405–428.

13. Lane, S. D., Keefe, R., Rubinstein, R. A., Webster, N., Rosenthal, A., Cibula, D., et al. (2004). Structural violence and racial disparity in heterosexual HIV Infection. *Journal of Health Care for the Poor and Underserved, 15*(3), 319–335.

14. O'Brien, J., Arnold, J., & Sieh, M. (1996). Inmate described bleeding in note as part of their review of Lucinda Batts' death. County officials are looking at what happened to her note to a nurse. Syracuse, NY: *Post-Standard*, March 20, sec. A, p. 1. Scanlon S. (1996). Inmate's death linked to rupture of fallopian tube. *Post-Standard*, March 16, sec. A, p. 1.

15. Arnold, J. (1996). Inmate in coma after she collapses. Justice center officials say the inmate had been checked on regularly after she complained of pain. Syracuse, NY: *Post-Standard*, March 14, sec. C, p. 1.

16. O'Brien, J. (1996). State faults care of inmate. A report cites a doctor and three nurses at the Justice Center jail for ignoring signs that Lucinda Batts was seriously ill before she collapsed and died. Syracuse, NY: *Post-Standard*, November 2, sec. A, p. 1.

17. Levandowski, B., Teran, S., Schweitzer, F., Buchanan, D., Paul, B., & Lane, S.D. (2003). Obstetrical care coordination for incarcerated women. National Centers of Excellence in Women's Health: Second National Forum, Understanding health differences and disparities in women: Closing the gap. Virginia, May 13–14.

18. Arialdi, M., Miniño, M., Arias, E., Kochanek, K. D., Murphy S. L., Betty L. et al. (2002). Deaths: final data for 2000. *National Vital Statistics Reports* (Vol. 50, No. 15).Washington, DC: Division of Vital Statistics, September 16.

19. Mathews, T. J., Menacker, F., & MacDorman M. F. (2004). Infant mortality statistics from the 2002 period linked birth/infant death data set. *National Vital Statistics Reports* (Vol. 53, No. 10). Washington, DC: Division of Vital Statistics, November 24.

20. This analysis is based on the format developed by Sue Stableford of the Maine AHEC Health Literacy Center, who was a consultant for Syracuse Healthy Start. It is summarized in her training module: *Write it easy-to-read, level 2: a training manual*, (n.d.).

PART III: THE CALCULUS OF HEALTH

1. Logie, D. and J. Woodroffe. (1993, July 3). Structural adjustment: the wrong prescription for Africa? *British Medical Journal, 41*(4).

2. Riddy, Valéry. (2003). Fees-for-services, cost recovery, and equity in a district of Burkina Faso operating the Bamako Initiative. *Bulletin of the World Health Organization, 81*(7), 532–538.

3. Pederson, Duncan. (1990). Notes for a critical review of the Bamako initiative. Retrieved June 29, 2007 from http://idrinfo.idrc.ca/archive/corpdocs/086746/86746.pdf.

4. Akin, J., N. Birdsall, and D. Ferranti. (1987). *Financing Health Services in Developing Countries: An Agenda for Reform*. Washington, DC: World Bank.

5. Whitehead, Margaret, Goran Dahlgren, and Timothy Evans. (2001). Equity and health sector reforms: can low-income countries escape the medical poverty trap? *Lancet, 358*, 833–836.

6. Yates, Rob. (2006). *International Experiences in Removing User Fees for Health Services—Implications for Mozambique*. London: DFID.
7. Walsh, J.A., Warren, K.S. Selective Primary Health Care: An Interim Strategy for Disease Control in Developing Countries. *New England Journal of Medicine* 1979; 301(18), 967–74.
8. World Bank. (1993). *Investing in Health*. World Development Report, p. 6.
9. World Bank. (1993). *Investing in Health*. World Development Report, p. 61.
10. World Bank. (1993). *Investing in Health*. World Development Report, p. 93.
11. Briscoe, John. (1984). Water supply and health in developing countries: selective primary health care revisited. *American Journal of Public Health*, 74(9), 1009–1013.
12. Bond, Patrick. (2004). The political roots of South Arica's cholera epidemic. In: Meredith Fort, Mary Anne Mercer, and Oscar Gish (Eds.), *Sickness and Wealth: The Corporate Assault on Global Health*. Cambridge, MA: Southend Press.
13. Homedes, Núria, and Antonio Ugalde. (2005). Why neoliberal health reforms have failed in Latin America. *Health Policy, 71*, 83–96.
14. Giovanni Andrea Cornia, Richard Jolly, and Frances Stewart (Eds.) (1987). *Adjustment with a Human Face: Protecting the Vulnerable and Promoting Growth*, Vols 1 and 2. Oxford, UK: Clarendon Press.
15. Prahalad, C. K. (2004). *The Fortune at the Bottom of the Pyramid: Eradicating Poverty through Profits*. Cambridge: Wharton School Publishing.
16. Brentlinger, P., K. Sherr, and S. Gloyd Mercer. (2003). Letter to the editor, *Lancet Infectious Diseases, 3*, 467.
17. Agha, Sohail, Ronan Van Rossem, Guy Stallworthy, and Thankian Kusanthan. (2007). The impact of a hybrid social marketing intervention on inequities in access, ownership and use of insecticide-treated nets. *Malaria Journal, 6*(13).
18. Sachs, J. (2005). *The End of Poverty: Economic Possibilities for Our Time*. New York: Penguin.
19. AfricaAction. (2006, July 6). *Africa Out of the Limelight: the Debt Crisis One Year after the Gleneagles G8*. Retrieved March 30, 2007 from the Global Policy Forum's Web site: www.globalpolicy.org/socecon/develop/debt/2006/0706gleneaglesafr.htm
20. Birn, Anne-Emanuelle. (2006, August 16). The downside of billions. *The Toronto Star*.
21. Sanchez, Marcela. (2007, May 11). IMF, World Bank face irrelevance: Latin America finds its own means of development. *Washington Post*. Retrieved July 4, 2007 from http://www.washingtonpost.com/wpdyn/content/article/2007/05/10/AR2007051001718.html
22. BBC News. (2007). Ecuador expels World Bank envoy. Retrieved July 4, 2007 from http://news.bbc.co.uk/1/hi/world/americas/6598027.stm
23. Holston, J. (2007). *Insurgent Citizenship: Disjunctions of Democracy and Modernity in Brazil*. Princeton: Princeton University Press.
24. PAHO. (2007). Renewing primary health care in the Americas: a position paper of the Pan American Health Organization/World Health Organization. Retrieved May 8, 2007 from http://www.paho.org/English/AD/THS/primary-HealthCare.pdf.

CHAPTER 12: CELEBRATION OF A LIFE

Berkman, A., Garcia, J., Muñoz-Laboy, M., Paiva, V., Parker, R. (2005). A critical analysis of the Brazilian response to HIV/AIDS: lessons learned for controlling and mitigating the epidemic in developing countries. *Am J Public Health*, 95:1162–1172.

Brazil. (1988). *Constituição da República Federativa do Brasil de 1988.* Available at: https://www.planalto.gov.br/ccivil_03/Constituicao/Constituiçao.htm (accessed February 12, 2008).

Brazil. (1996). Law 9.313. *Dispõe sobre a distribuição gratuita de medicamentos aos portadores do HIV e doentes de AIDS.* Available at: http://www.aids.gov.br/assistencia/lei9313.htm (accessed February 12, 2008).

Brazil. National Institute of Industrial Property. (1996). *Lei da Propriedade Industrial, 9.279, 14 de Maio de 1996* [Industrial Property Law, 9,279, May 14, 1996]. Available at: http://www.wipo.int/clea/docs_new/pdf/en/br/br003en.pdf (accessed December 17, 2006).

Cohen, J. (2007). Brazil, Thailand override big pharma patents. *Science*, 316, 816. Available at: http://www.cptech.org/ip/health/aids/2g/science05112007.pdf (accessed February 12, 2008).

Daniel, H. (1989). *Vida Antes da Morte [Life before Death].* Rio de Janeiro, Brazil: Tipografia Jaboti.

Galvão, J. (2002). Access to antiretroviral drugs in Brazil. *Lancet*, 360:1862–1865.

Galvão, J. (2005). Brazil and access to HIV/AIDS drugs: a question of human rights and public health. *American Journal of Public Health*, 95 (7): 1110–1116.

Grangeiro, A., Teixeira, L., Bastos, F. I., & Teixeira, P. (2006). Sustainability of Brazilian policy for access to antiretroviral drugs. *Revista de Saúde Pública*, 40(Supl), 1–9.

Levi, G.C., Vitória, M.A. (2002). Fighting against AIDS: the Brazilian experience. *AIDS*, 16:2373–2383.

Mann, J., Tarantola, D., Netter, T. (1992). *AIDS in the world.* Cambridge, Mass.: Harvard University Press.

Okie, S. (2006). Fighting HIV—Lessons from Brazil. *The New England Journal of Medicine*, 354, 1977–1981.

Pandolfi, D., Heymann, L. (Orgs). (2005). *Um abraço, Betinho.* Rio de Janeiro, Brazil: Garamond.

Parker, R., Terto Jr V(Orgs). (2001). *A ABIA na Virada do Milênio.* Rio de Janeiro, Brazil: Associação Brasileira Interdisciplinar de AIDS. Available at: http://www.abiaids.org.br/_img/media/Livro%20Solidariedade.pdf (accessed February 12, 2008).

Scheffer, M., Salazar, A.L., Grou, K.B. (2005). *O Remédio via Justiça: um estudo sobre o acesso a novos medicamentos e exames em HIV/AIDS no Brasil por meio de ações judiciais.* Ministério da Saúde, Secretaria de Vigilância em Saúde, Programa Nacional de DST/AIDS. Brasília, Brazil. Available at: http://www.aids.gov.br/final/biblioteca/medicamentos_justica/medic-justica01.pdf (accessed February 12, 2008).

Skidmore, T. (1988). *The Politics of Military Rule in Brazil, 1964–85.* New York, NY: Oxford University Press.

Souza, H. (1997). O amor em tempos de Aids. *Boletim ABIA Especial*, p. 3. Available at: http://www.abiaids.org.br/_img/media/boletim%20abia.pdf (accessed February 12, 2008).

Souza, H. (1992). O dia da cura. *Jornal do Brasil*, Rio de Janeiro, January 30. Available at: http://www.aids.gov.br/betinho/dia_cura.htm (accessed February 12, 2008).

Souza, H. (1994). *A cura da AIDS* [The cure of AIDS]. Rio de Janeiro, Brazil: Relume Dumará.

United Nations High Commissioner for Human Rights. (2001). Access to medication in the context of pandemics such as HIV/AIDS. Commission on Human Rights Resolution 2001/33 (57th Session). Geneva, Switzerland: United Nations High Commissioner for Human Rights. Available at: http://www.unhchr.ch/Huridocda/Huridoca.nsf/(Symbol)/E.CN.4.RES.2001.33.En?Opendocument (accessed February 12, 2008).

World Bank. (1997). *Confronting AIDS: public priorities in a global epidemic*. Washington, DC: World Bank.

World Trade Organization. (2001). Declaration on the TRIPS Agreement and Public Health. Geneva, Switzerland: World Health Organization. WT/MIN (01)/Dec/2. Available at: http://www.wto.org/english/thewto_e/minist_e/min01_e/mindecl_trips_e.pdf (accessed February 12, 2008).

INDEX

CPSIA information can be obtained at www.ICGtesting.com
Printed in the USA
BVOW001441130713

325729BV00005B/30/P